FOR
REFERENCE ONLY

This book is due for return on or before the last date shown below.

D1348938

Human Papillomavirus

Alberto Rosenblatt
Homero Gustavo de Campos Guidi

Human Papillomavirus

A Practical Guide for Urologists

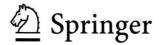 Springer

Alberto Rosenblatt, MD
Hospital Israelita Albert Einstein
Av. Albert Einstein 627/701
São Paulo-SP
Brazil
albrose1@gmail.com

Homero Gustavo de Campos Guidi, MD, PhD
Rua Teodoro Sampaio 744
São Paulo-SP
14th Floor
Brazil
hguidi@attglobal.net

ISBN: 978-3-540-70973-2   e-ISBN: 978-3-540-70974-9

DOI: 10.1007/978-3-540-70974-9

Library of Congress Control Number: 2008944023

Cover design: eStudioCalamar, Figueres/Berlin

Printed on acid-free paper

springer.com

This book is dedicated to our beloved parents
Agostinha and Mayer Rosenblatt
Isaura Guidi and Domingos Guidi
and to Sophie and Fernanda
for their constant support in every step of our lives.

Foreword

The award of the Nobel Prize in Medicine to Professor Harald zur Hausen in 2008 represented one of the most auspicious recognitions in the field of cancer prevention. Zur Hausen's pioneer work unleashed an entire domain of research on the molecular biology of human papillomavirus (HPV) and on its interaction with the human host. His work permitted the characterization of HPV infection as the cause of the vast majority of cervical cancers and of a large proportion of anogenital and upper aerodigestive tract malignancies. Understanding the unequivocal role of HPV infection in carcinogenesis led to two new fronts in cervical cancer prevention, namely, (i) the development of diagnostic assays for HPV DNA, which are now being incorporated into cervical cancer screening programs worldwide, and (ii) the regulatory approval of the first prophylactic HPV vaccines to prevent HPV infections with the genotypes of HPV that cause most cases of cervical cancer.

The burden of morbidity and mortality from cancers associated with HPV infection is greatest in developing cancers. Cervical cancer is the second most common cancer in women worldwide and the most common in many developing countries in Latin America, equatorial Africa, and in Southeast Asia. These countries now have a renewed hope in controlling a disease that has been very difficult to prevent via traditional Pap cytology screening, an undertaking that has worked well only in high-resource countries. One of the new vaccines also prevents the HPV types that cause the majority of genital warts and low-grade lesions of the lower genital tract. Such HPV types are also responsible for laryngeal papillomatosis. Collectively, these diseases, albeit classified as benign, are responsible for much suffering and loss of quality of life throughout the world. In all, the spectrum of malignant and benign diseases that can be prevented by the new prophylactic HPV vaccines affects women, men, and children everywhere, and leads to major healthcare expenditures related to diagnosis, management, and treatment.

In this book, Drs. Alberto Rosenblatt and Homero Gustavo de Campos Guidi have devoted considerable care in providing a comprehensive overview of the pathogenesis, diagnosis, treatment, and prevention of diseases causally associated with HPV infections. In many chapters, the authors also summarize the literature about diseases in which HPV seems to be an incidental finding and whose specific role has not yet been elucidated. As experienced, practicing urologists, Drs. Rosenblatt and Guidi provided a richly illustrated guide that clinicians will find very useful as an easy to navigate, yet authoritative reference to the diagnosis and treatment of HPV-associated diseases. Although the emphasis is on the urologist's approach to disease management, this book will also be appreciated by gynecologists, dermatologists, pediatricians, and infectious disease specialists. The authors also enlisted the contribution of two renowned colleagues, Drs. Luisa Villa and Simon Horenblas, for two chapters on laboratory detection methods and penile neoplasia, respectively.

Clinical and sub-clinical HPV infections are the most common sexually transmitted diseases. Although there is justifiable enthusiasm in the public health community with the novel prophylactic vaccines and sensitive screening tools, many challenges lie ahead. The science on preventive and therapeutic approaches to curb the burden of HPV diseases has grown exponentially in recent years. Clinicians need a practical guide to allow them to sift through the new methods that have passed the scrutiny of evidence-based medicine and can thus be used in the care of their patients. The authors, Drs. Rosenblatt and Guidi, and Springer, the publisher, are to be commended for *Human Papillomavirus – A Practical Guide for Urologists*, a contribution that fills this need with high scholarly value.

Montreal, Canada   Eduardo L. Franco

We are what we repeatedly do. Excellence, then, is not an act, but a habit.

Aristotle

Human papillomavirus infection is a globally widespread disease that affects young people and adults without sexual distinction. The sexually transmitted virus is responsible for the development of benign anogenital lesions as well as several premalignant and malignant anogenital and nongenital disorders.

Although obstetricians/gynecologists, urologists, and dermatologists are the medical specialists most often involved in the management of HPV-related diseases, practitioners in general ought to have a comprehensive understanding of the challenges caused by this infective agent.

The interested reader will find in the chapters of this practical guide all the current information concerning HPV and associated anogenital diseases, with particular emphasis on the management of the infected male.

Premalignant and malignant penile neoplasias as well as current management of anal and cervical intraepithelial disease are also reviewed in this book, providing the readers with an authoritative wealth of updated data. The addition of practically oriented tables and numerous colored figures provides quick access to the objective information, which is supported with over 800 references.

It is expected that the burden of HPV infection and associated diseases will certainly be reduced with the advent of current prophylactic vaccines. However, HPV infection is a recurrent disorder and this book will enable practitioners in general to understand and manage the male's most common genital-related disorders.

São Paulo, Brazil

Alberto Rosenblatt
Homero Gustavo de Campos Guidi

Acknowledgments

The authors acknowledge with deep appreciation Prof. Simon Horenblas and Dr. Luisa Lina Villa for their valuable contribution to this book. Prof. Horenblas's vast expertise in penile cancer and Dr. Villa's acclaimed investigative work with human papillomavirus provide us with two key chapters where updates on penile neoplasia and the current laboratory investigation of human papilloma virus are presented.

We express our gratitude to Dr. Carlos Walter Sobrado Jr., Dr. Sidney Roberto Nadal, Dr. Maricy Tacla, Dr. Marcia Jacomelli, Dr. Reinaldo J. Gusmão, Dr. Toshiro Tomishige, Dr. Monica Stiepcich, Dr. Rubens Pianna de Andrade, Dr. Libby Edwards, Prof. Robert A. Schwartz, Prof. Gerd Gross, and Prof. Gino Fornaciari for their generous contribution providing the innumerous and valuable figures that illustrate the chapters of the book.

We also specially thank Prof. Filomena Marino Carvalho for her significant insights regarding the nomenclature of genital squamous intraepithelial lesions as well as the illustrative cytology and histopathology slides, and Dr. Nadir Oyakawa, a pioneer in the field of HPV-related diseases in women and who prematurely left us at the height of her scientific career.

We thank the publishers who kindly gave us copyright permissions for the use of figures in this book.

Finally, we are deeply grateful to all the staff at Springer involved in the creation of this book, in particular, Ute Heilmann (Editorial Director, Clinical Medicine), Annette Hinze (Editor, Clinical Medicine), Wilma McHugh (Project Coordinator), and Dörthe Mennecke-Bühler (Assistant Editor, Clinical Medicine) for their professionalism, friendship, and guidance along the path to publication. We also thank Nandini Loganathan and the staff at SPi for their excellent job with the production of this book.

Contents

Human Papillomavirus History and Epidemiology

Alberto Rosenblatt and Homero Gustavo de Campos Guidi

1

Contents

1.1 Introduction

Human papillomavirus (HPV) infection is a significant source of morbidity and mortality among the young population and, together with HIV, is considered the most costly sexually transmitted disease (STD) in terms of estimated direct medical expenses (Chesson et al., 2004).

According to a recent Centers for Disease Control and Prevention (CDC) analysis (Forhan et al., 2008), one in four American women between the ages of 14 and 19 (approximately 3.2 million young girls) is infected with at least one of the most common STDs (i.e., HPV, *Chlamydia trachomatis*, trichomoniasis, and herpes simplex virus type 2). While genital chlamydia is the most commonly reported condition in the United States (Satterwhite, 2008), HPV is by far the most

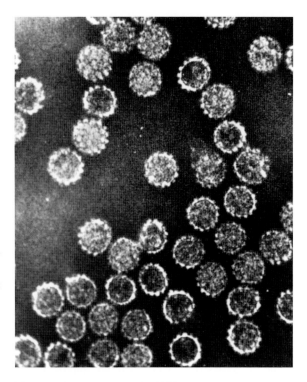

Fig. 1.1. Electron micrograph of HPVs

A. Rosenblatt (✉)
Albert Einstein Jewish Hospital, Sao Paulo, Brasil
e-mail: albrose1@gmail.com

A. Rosenblatt, H. G. de Campos Guidi, *Human Papillomavirus*,
DOI: 10.1007/978-3-540-70974-9-1, © Springer-Verlag Berlin Heidelberg 2009

1

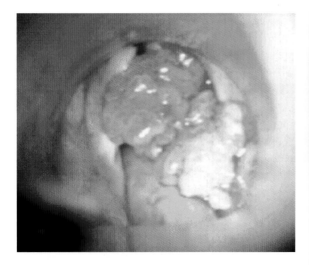

Fig. 1.2. Nasal cavity papillomas. (Source: Photograph courtesy of Reinaldo J. Gusmão, MD, PhD , São Paulo, Brazil)

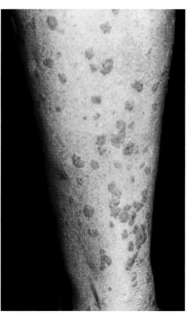

Fig. 1.4. Epidermodysplasia verruciformis. (Source: Barrasso and Gross (1997). Reproduced with permission from Prof. Gross G)

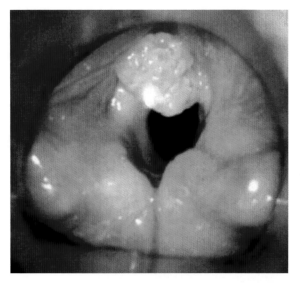

Fig. 1.3. HPV-related laryngeal papilloma. (Source: Photograph courtesy of Reinaldo J. Gusmão, MD, PhD , São Paulo, Brazil)

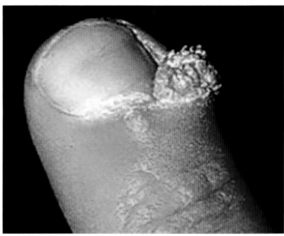

Fig. 1.5. Periungual wart. (Source: Photograph courtesy of Libby Edwards, MD, PhD, North Carolina, USA)

prevalent (18.3% in the CDC study compared to 3.9% for chlamydia).

HPV is considered more transmissible than other viral STDs (Burchell et al., 2006a), and Barnabas et al. (2006) estimated the per-partner male-to-female transmission probability of high-risk (oncogenic) type HPV 16 to be 60%.

HPV is a nonenveloped DNA virus with carcinogenic properties (Fig. 1.1). There are approximately 200 different HPV types, of which nearly 100 have been fully sequenced (de Villiers et al., 2004).

According to their molecular biological data and epidemiological association with anogenital cancers, mucosal HPV types are categorized into high-risk and low-risk types (zur Hausen, 1986, 2000).

High-risk HPV types (16, 18, 31, 33, 35, 39, 45, 51, 52, 56, 58, 59, 68, 73, and 82) have been implicated in the pathogenesis of genital and nongenital carcinomas (including their high-grade precursor lesions).

Low-risk HPV types (6, 11, 42, 43, 44, 54, 61, 70, 72, 81, and CP6108 (candHPV89)) cause benign anogenital lesions (warts) and low-grade squamous intraepithelial lesions of the cervix. Low-risk types 6 and 11 are also responsible for the development of papillomas in the oral/nasal cavity (Fig. 1.2) or the larynx (Fig. 1.3) that afflict individuals worldwide.

Therefore, although classified as low-risk types, HPV 6 and 11 have also been categorized as possibly carcinogenic (Cogliano et al., 2005; IARC Working Group on the Evaluation of Carcinogenic Risks to Humans, 2007).

HPV types 26, 53, and 66 are considered high-risk mucosal lesions, although they can also be found in benign lesions.

Cutaneous HPV genotypes are responsible for the development of the rare hereditary dermatological disease epidermodysplasia verruciformis (EV) (Fig. 1.4), and HPV 5 and 8 are the types most frequently detected. Moreover, plantar (HPV 1) and common warts (HPV 2, 4, 26, 27, 29) (Fig. 1.5) are also caused by cutaneous genotypes.

This chapter reviews historical aspects of the HPV infection from the ancient Hellenic-Roman era to the present. In addition, current epidemiologic data related to the HPV infection are discussed, with a focus on the burden on men. The most recent population prevalence, the dynamics of transmissibility (including nonsexual routes in children and adults), and novel prevention strategies are also detailed.

The biology and life cycle of HPV are discussed in Chaps. 9 and 11. Prophylactic HPV vaccines are reviewed in detail in Chap. 11.

1.2 Historical Perspective

The concept of sexual contact as a factor in causing disease was recognized as early as the ancient Hellenic and Roman times. HPV-related genital lesions (also known as genital warts, veneral warts, and condyloma acuminata) have been described in ancient writings as "morbid outgrowths" or "genital excrescences." Genital warts were referred to as "thymus" by Hippocrates (Adams, 1886) and as "ficus" (figs) by Roman physicians (Routh et al., 1997), because of the similarity with the plant *Thymus capitatus* (Fig. 1.6) and *Ficus sycomorus* (Fig. 1.7), respectively.

The word condyloma is derived from the Greek "round tumor," suggesting that anal warts might resemble a knob, while the term "acuminata" comes from

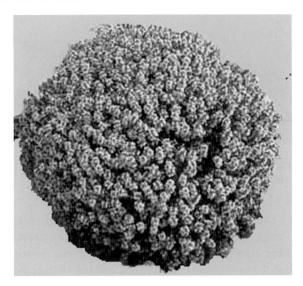

Fig. 1.6. *Thymus capitatus*

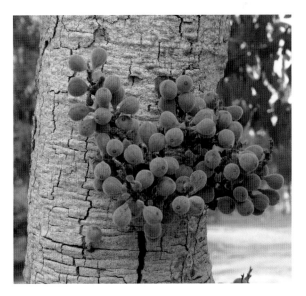

Fig. 1.7. *Ficus sycomorus*

the Latin word for "pointed." Perianal warts were usually associated with homosexual activity and, in the late first and early second centuries, the roman poet Decimus Junius Juvenalis (also known as Juvenal) wrote about this correlation in his *Satires* (Bafverstedt, 1967).

Ancient Greek and Roman physicians used to treat condylomata with alum and surgical excision (McDonagh, 1920; Buret, 1891), burning (Kelsey, 1882), and Hippocrates recommended using the herb *Parthenium parviflorum* for lesions located in the glans (Adams, 1886).

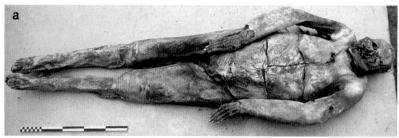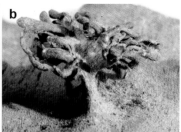

Fig. 1.8. (**a**) Italian Renaissance mummy. (**b**) Wart-like lesion in the right inguinal region. (Source: Fornaciari (2003). Reproduced with permission from Elsevier)

During the syphilis epidemics that emerged in Europe in 1492, STDs (including genital condyloma) were considered manifestations of a veneral poison and thus associated with syphilis, and even influenced the terminology of specific lesions of this disease (i.e., condyloma lata) (Wikstrom, 1995). However, by the end of the eighteenth century, genital warts and gonorrhea began to be recognized as distinct diseases unrelated to syphilis (Bell, 1793), with further confirmation occurring only in the next century (Ricord, 1838).

One of the first instances of documented evidence of a historical HPV infection was found in an Italian Renaissance mummy recovered from the Basilica of S. Domenico Maggiore in Naples, Italy. Maria d'Aragona, Marquise of Vasto (1503–1568), exhibited a wart-like lesion in the right inguinal region (Fig. 1.8a, b). Histological examination of the lesion suggested condyloma acuminatum and additional molecular studies performed revealed the presence of oncogenic type HPV 18 (Fornaciari, 2006). The same mummy exhibited a cutaneous ulcerated lesion in the left arm containing a large number of treponemal filaments, which clearly demonstrates the spread of multiple sexually transmitted infections (STIs) over time.

The infectious nature of the condyloma acuminata was first established in 1919 (Wiley et al., 2002; Kingery, 1923), and Strauss et al. (1949) detected viral particles in human warts by electron microscopy in 1949.

HPV DNA physical properties were described by Crawford and Crawford in 1963 (Crawford and Crawford, 1963), and the isolation of low-risk HPV 6 and 11 from genital warts occurred in 1980 (Gissmann and zur Hausen, 1980).

An association between HPV and the development of cervical cancer was initially proposed by zur Hausen in 1976 (zur Hausen 1976), and further studies later confirmed the role of high-risk HPV types in human

carcinogenesis (Schwarz et al., 1985; Durst et al., 1987; zur Hausen, 1991).

1.3   Epidemiology

HPV is the world's most common STD (Trottier and Franco, 2006), and the global prevalence is estimated at 291 million women (Burchell et al., 2006b). In the United States, an estimated 6.2 million persons are newly infected with the virus every year (Weinstock et al., 2004), and epidemiologic studies predict that approximately 100 million women worldwide will be infected with the oncogenic types HPV 16 or HPV 18 at least once in their lifetime.

Although recent data showed a reduction in sexual intercourse acts and an increase in condom use among U.S. high school students during 1991–2007, HIV- and STD-related risky behaviors are still prevalent in this group of young individuals (Centers for Disease Control and Prevention, 2008).

HPV affects more than two-thirds of North Americans aged 15–49 years, and molecular evidence of current or prior HPV infection is present in 20 million individuals (Koutsky, 1997; Koutsky et al., 1988).

However, Dunne et al. (2007) recently reported that the HPV infection prevalence in American women aged 14–59 years is 26.8%, which corresponds to almost 25 million individuals using the 2000 Census data. The same study showed that HPV prevalence was highest in sexually active women aged 20–24 years (49.3%) with a gradual decline up to age 59.

Epidemiologic evidence confirming the sexual transmission of the disease appeared in 1954, when a cohort of women exhibited vulvar warts after 4–6

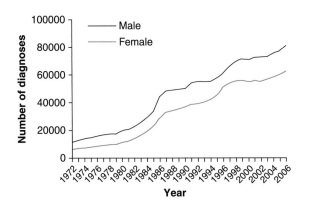

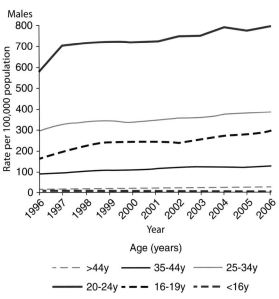

Fig. 1.9. Diagnoses of genital warts seen in genitourinary clinics in England, Wales, and Scotland: 1971–2006. (Source: Health Protection Agency (2007). Reproduced with permission)

Fig. 1.10. UK rates of male diagnoses of genital warts and age-group: 1996–2006. (Source: Health Protection Agency (2007). Reproduced with permission)

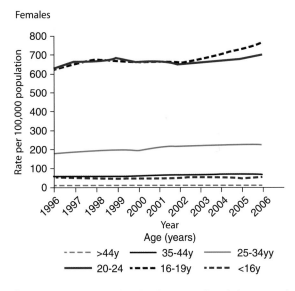

Fig. 1.11. UK rates of female diagnoses of genital warts and age-group: 1996–2006. (Source: Health Protection Agency (2007). Reproduced with permission)

weeks of their spouse's return from the Korean War. Medical records of the male partners demonstrated recently acquired penile warts in all of the involved soldiers (Barrett et al., 1954).

In the United Kingdom, HPV incidence in men increased almost 400% from 1971 to 1994 (Simms and Fairley, 1997). In 2006, 83,745 new cases of anogenital warts were diagnosed in genitourinary clinics throughout the United Kingdom (Fig. 1.9), with a predominance of male infections (Health Protection Agency, 2007). Moreover, diagnoses of HPV-related warts in male subjects increased by 34%, with the highest rates seen in the 20–24-year age-group (CDR, 2006) (Fig. 1.10).

However, rates of genital warts and numbers of diagnoses in women in the United Kingdom were particularly high in the under-20-year age-group (<16 years: 55/100,000 and 16–19 years: 767/100,000) (Fig. 1.11).

Koshiol et al. (2004) reported an increase in the rates of genital warts from 117.8 cases per 100,000 person-years at risk in 1998 to 205 cases per 100,000 person-years at risk in 2001.

In a retrospective analysis assessing the U.S. prevalence of genital warts in 18- to 59-year-old individuals, Dinh et al. (2008) found that 5.6% have had genital warts in the past. Genital warts are more prevalent among 20- to 39-year-old subjects (Fleischer et al., 2001), with a reported higher prevalence of the disease in female (7.2%) than in male subjects (4%) (Dinh et al., 2008).

The economic burden of HPV-related diseases has also been analyzed. The treatment of an incident (new) case of genital warts involved costs of U.S. $436

Genital warts have been estimated to be as common as breast and prostate cancers, with an approximate annual rate of 100 per 100,000 (Franco, 1996).

(Insinga et al., 2003), and the U.S. annual medical cost associated with the disease reached U.S. $200 million in 2004 (Insinga et al., 2005). Cervical cancer costs ranged between U.S. $300 million and $400 million, according to the same report.

Corresponding studies performed in Europe have estimated the mean direct cost per patient with new genital warts at €378 and for resistant genital warts at €1,142 (Hillemanns et al., 2008).

1.4 HPV in Women

HPV infection is highly contagious with a per-partner transmission probability of genital warts estimated at 60% (Oriel, 1971). Coinfection with multiple HPV types and sequential infection with phylogenetically related types and novel types are a common occurrence (Thomas et al., 2000).

In a recent cross-sectional study assessing the incidence of genital warts in Germany, Hillemanns et al. (2008) found new and recurrent cases in 113.7 and 34.7 per 100,000, respectively, for women aged 14–65 years. The highest incidence for new and recurrent cases was observed in women aged 14–25 years (171.0 per 100,000) and in those aged 26–45 years (53.1 per 100,000), respectively.

The prevalence of HPV infection is increased in younger women and usually decreases through the fourth and fifth decades of life (de Villiers et al., 1987; Meisels, 1992; Herrero et al., 2000; Garcia-Pineres et al., 2006). However, in a cross-sectional study evaluating sexually active women in four continents, Franceschi et al. (2006) observed that HPV infection was high across all age-groups in low-resource settings in Asia and Africa.

Cervical intraepithelial neoplasia (low-grade squamous intraepithelial lesion (LSIL) or high-grade SIL (HSIL)) develops in 4% of infected women (Mougin et al., 2001), and high-risk HPV presence and persistence is a required condition for HSIL development and progression to cervical cancer (Liaw et al., 1999; Ylitalo et al., 2000; Schlecht et al., 2001; Kjaer et al., 2002) (see also Chap. 8).

A recent large population-based study performed in Denmark has found an HPV prevalence of 26.4%, with a peak of 50.2% in young women aged 20–24 years. The

prevalence of oncogenic HPV types has increased from 19.2% in women with normal cytology to 100% in those presenting with cervical intraepithelial neoplasia grade 3 (CIN 3)/cervical cancer. In addition, HPV 16 has been the most common type found (Kjaer et al., 2008).

The biological mechanisms likely involved for the increased susceptibility of young female subjects to HPV infection are cervical immaturity, inadequate production of protective cervical mucus, and increased cervical ectopy (Kahn et al., 2002).

Postmenopausal women in selected groups have an increased prevalence of low-risk and unclassified HPV types (Herrero et al., 2000), which is likely related to the negative effect in host immune response that is associated with the persistent HPV infection (Garcia-Pineres et al., 2006).

Reactivation of previously undetectable infections acquired earlier in life as a result of diminished immunity caused by hormonal influences, and/or novel HPV infections acquired with different sexual partners is another explanation for the increased prevalence of HPV in postmenopausal women (Bosch et al., 2008).

Recent multicountry data show that men and women aged 40–80 years regard sex as an important part of life and continue to engage in sexual activity (Nicolosi et al., 2004; Moreira et al., 2006). Moreover, studies also demonstrate that older men are still involved in risky sex, and the use of drugs for erectile dysfunction likely contributes to the high-risk sexual behavior. In a recent cross-sectional analysis, Cooperman et al. (2007) reported that less than 20% of HIV-negative individuals aged 49–80 used condoms with their sexual partners.

1.4.1 Risk Factors

The sexual behavior of men (the so-called male factor) can influence the risk of HPV infection and related diseases in their female sexual partners (Brinton et al., 1989).

The risk of infection is related to the reported lifetime number of male partners (Dillner et al., 1996;

Carter et al., 1996), although in a recent cross-sectional study that evaluated a large group of Danish females, Nielsen et al. (2008) found that an increased number of recent sexual partners was associated with a higher risk of infection with oncogenic HPV types in younger women.

Age is another determining factor for HPV infection, and several studies show that the risk of acquiring incident infection is increased in young women (Jamison et al., 1995; Rousseau et al., 2000; Giuliano et al, 2002; Sellors et al., 2003; Trottier and Franco, 2006).

Other reported risk factors associated with the disease are failure to use condoms, having intercourse with uncircumcised men, and a history of herpes simplex virus or chlamydia infections (Castellsague et al., 2002; Moscicki et al., 2001).

HPV infection can be acquired even without vaginal penetration, since any genital skin contact is sufficient for virus transmission (Moscicki, 2005). Dunne et al. (2007) recently detected HPV DNA in 5.2% of females who reported they had never experienced sexual intercourse.

The risk of female subjects acquiring HPV with a first heterosexual experience has been assessed as 28.5% and 50% at 1 and 3 years after the monogamous episode, respectively (Winer et al., 2008).

Data from several studies indicate that HPV 16 is usually the most common type acquired (Giuliano et al., 2002; Richardson et al., 2003), although HPV 18, 39, 84, 51, 58, 31, and 52 have also been regularly detected (Allen and Siegfried, 2000; Munoz et al., 2003; Munoz et al., 2004).

In the prevalence study performed by Dunne et al. (2007), high-risk HPV 16 and low-risk HPV 6 was detected in 1.5% and 1.3% of women, respectively, and the detection of the HPV types included in the quadrivalent prophylactic vaccine (HPV 6, 11, 16, and 18) was 3.4%. However, none of the females studied was simultaneously infected with all four HPV vaccine types.

Furthermore, it is estimated that HPV 16 and/or HPV 18 is present in 32% of women presenting normal cytology (de Sanjose et al., 2007), and both types are detected in 95–100% of cervical carcinomas.

However, despite the high infection rates, approximately 90% of HPV infections are usually cleared (eliminated) within 24 months of the initial contact (Ho et al., 1998; Giuliano et al., 2002; Richardson et al., 2003; Brown et al., 2005; Rodriguez et al., 2007).

A longitudinal study performed in a cohort of former university students that were examined 4–12 years after their initial HPV diagnosis has shown that nearly 1 in 5 women (16.3%) exhibited one or more of the same previously detected HPV types. The long-term HPV persistence was only 5%, but correlated positively with an abnormal Pap test result, presence of genital warts, and detection of the same HPV type during the course of the infection (Sycuro et al., 2008).

1.5 HPV in Men

The majority of HPV infections in men are symptomless and unapparent, and detection is only possible when molecular diagnostic techniques are used (see also Chap. 2).

Prevalence rates in men (Table 1.1) appear to be similar to those in women when HPV DNA detection techniques are used (Baken et al., 1995; Hernandez et al., 2006; Dunne et al., 2006; Giuliano et al., 2008b), with (prevalence) rates as high as 73% being reported (Bleeker et al., 2005a).

A recent meta-analysis has shown that HPV seroprevalence of specific anti-HPV antibodies is lower in men than in women (Dunne et al., 2006).

Stone et al. (2002) analyzed the seroprevalence of oncogenic HPV 16 infection in the United States and found it significantly higher in women (17.9%) than in men (7.9%). Moreover, Hariri et al. (2008) analyzed the U.S. seroprevalence of low-risk HPV 11 infection and reported that women have higher prevalence rates than men (5.7% vs 3.6%, respectively).

Age has not been significantly associated with HPV prevalence, incidence, and duration of infection in men (Giuliano et al., 2008a, b). However, Giuliano et al. (2008a) observed a bimodal distribution with age for oncogenic infections, with decreased prevalence of high-risk HPV types found in younger and older male subjects. The prevalence peak occurred at ages 30–34 years for oncogenic HPV types, while the prevalence of nononcogenic infections peaked among men aged 45–70 years. Furthermore, Stone et al. (2002) showed that the overall prevalence peak occurred among men aged 30–39 years.

Duration of HPV infection in men seems to be shorter than in women, suggesting that a more expeditious viral

Table 1.1 Estimates of the prevalence of HPV infection by study (Source: Adapted from Partridge and Koutsky, 2006. Reproduced with permission from Elsevier)

References	No.	Age (years)	HPV prevalence (%)			
			DNA	Warts	High-risk HPV types	Low-risk HPV types
Baken et al. (1995)	48	>17	63		~18	~12
Van Doornum et al. (1994)	85	U/NR	28.2	U/NR	U/NR	U/NR
Hippelainen et al. (1993)	432	U/NR	23.6	5.6	U/NR	U/NR
Bosch et al. (1996)	354	45.4[a]	4.9	2.1[b]	9.0	
Wikstrom et al. (2000)	235	18–54	20.4	U/NR	U/NR	U/NR
Lazcano-Ponce et al. (2001)	120	14–55	42.7		19.8	17.7
Franceschi et al. (2002)	533	19–82	16.0	U/NR	U/NR	0.5
Svare et al. (2002)	216	>18	44.9	25[b]	U/NR	U/NR
Baldwin et al. (2003)	436	18–70	28.2		12.0	14.8
Weaver et al. (2004)	318	18–25	35.0	U/NR	U/NR	U/NR
Shin et al. (2004)	381	U/NR	8.7	U/NR	4.2	2.6
Bleeker et al. (2005a)	181	22–67	72.9	U/NR	58.6	27.1
Nicolau et al. (2005)	50	19–53	70.0	U/NR	U/NR	U/NR
Kjaer et al. (2005)	337	19–22	33.8	U/NR	U/NR	U/NR
Lajous et al. (2005)	1030	16–40	44.6	5.8	34.8	23.9
Rombaldi et al. (2006)	99	18–56	54.5	9.3	HPV 16 (3.5)	HPV 6 (56.1)
Hernandez et al. (2006)	136	18–63	42.8–41.3	U/NR	U/NR	U/NR
Nielson et al. (2007)	463	18–40	65.4 (at any site)	U/NR	10.6	22.0
Giuliano et al. (2008b)	290	18–44	52.8	U/NR	31.7	30.0
Giuliano et al. (2008a)	1,160	18–70	65.2	None	12.0	20.7

U/NR unknown/not reported
[a]Mean age
[b]Percentage of men who reported previous history of genital warts

clearance occurs in the male partner (Hippelainen et al., 1993), with most infections resolving after 1 year (Van Doornum et al., 1994; Lajous et al., 2005; Giuliano et al., 2008b). However, in a prospective follow-up study among Danish soldiers, Kjaer et al. (2005) found that infection with multiple HPV types strongly correlated with viral persistence and the presence of oncogenic HPV types increased the persistence risk.

Monogamous intercourse with a male partner for more than 8 months has been associated with a lower risk of HPV infection acquisition among women (Winer et al., 2003), which could be related to the shorter duration of HPV infection in men.

Conversely, HPV incidence rates in men are reported to be higher when compared with age-matched women. In a recent study that evaluated incidence and risk factors of genital HPV among heterosexually active male university students 18–20 years of age, Partridge et al. (2007) found that the cumulative incidence of new HPV infection was 62.4% at 2 years, with low-risk HPV 84 and high-risk HPV 16 the most frequent types detected.

Prevalence rates in immunosupressed patients (Halpert et al., 1986) and HIV-positive men who have sex with men (MSM) are even higher, with reported rates of HPV DNA detected in 64.7% of the anal specimens of Dutch homosexual men (van der Snoek et al., 2003).

Several studies have investigated the prevalence of type-specific HPV infection and the virus anatomic distribution in men. High-risk HPV 16 has been the most prevalent type detected (Bosch et al., 1996; Wikstrom et al., 2000; Lazcano-Ponce et al., 2001; Franceschi et al., 2002; Baldwin et al., 2003; Weaver et al., 2004; Nielson et al., 2007; Giuliano et al., 2008b); however, a predominance of low-risk types (36.3% low-risk vs. 29.2% high-risk types) was found in a recent anogenital and semen sampling analysis of 463 men aged 18–40 years (Nielson et al., 2007), as well as in another prospective study of male sexual partners of women with CIN (Rombaldi et al., 2006).

Giuliano et al. (2008a) also reported an increased prevalence of nononcogenic types (20.7% nononcogenic types only vs. 12.0% oncogenic types only) among 1,160 men from Brazil, Mexico, and the United States, with HPV 6 being detected in 6.6% of cases.

In addition, there has been a predominance of low-risk HPV types in studies that evaluated genital wart HPV typing (Yun and Joblin, 1993; Boxman et al., 1999; Hadjivassiliou et al., 2007).

Data from several investigators show that the penis shaft harbors most of the HPV DNA detected (Nielson et al., 2007, Giuliano et al., 2007; Nicolau et al., 2005). However, a recent analysis performed by Smith et al. (2007) in African male subjects reported a high HPV DNA prevalence in the glans/coronal sulcus (39%). Furthermore, the study concluded that urethral sampling in men added no sensitivity for HPV detection.

Intriguing results from a recent study have shown that the glans penis and scrotum were the most frequent targets of infection from women (Hernandez et al., 2008b). However, data from several reports have demonstrated a low incidence of scrotal lesions (Nicolau et al., 2005; Giuliano et al., 2007; Weaver et al., 2004; Flores et al., 2008). Therefore, one may speculate that although the scrotal region is not usually subjected to microabrasive trauma during intercourse, contamination can still occur through anogenital skin contact and vaginal secretions.

The prevalence of HPV DNA in the male partners of HPV-infected women has also been analyzed.

Reported data from studies performed in Spain and Colombia have demonstrated a higher HPV DNA prevalence in the male partner of women with cervical cancer than in women not presenting the disease (Castellsague et al., 1997). Nicolau et al. (2005) reported a high prevalence of HPV DNA (70%) in male partners of HPV-infected women, and the internal surface of the prepuce was the most affected site.

Hernandez et al. (2008b) recently evaluated HPV transmission in 25 heterosexual, monogamous couples. In this prospective study, male-to-female transmission (i.e., from the penis to the cervix) was substantially lower than transmission from the female to the male partner.

Studies evaluating HPV type prevalence in sex partners have shown that concordance is high and it is associated with increased viral load (Bleeker et al., 2005a) and with recent sexual intercourse (Baken et al., 1995).

In addition, Giovannelli et al. (2007) showed that a combination of penile and urethral brushing was the most adequate approach in men to evaluate HPV type concordance in sexual couples.

In a recent multicountry analysis of HPV prevalence and type distribution among heterosexual males, Giuliano et al. (2008a) reported that HPV types varied widely across the countries studied. Among high-risk types, HPV 16 was the most common type detected in Brazil and the United States, whereas HPV 59 was commonly detected in Mexico. Among the nononcogenic types, HPV 62 was most commonly detected in Brazil, whereas in Mexico and the United States HPV 84 was the most common. Prevalence rates of the HPV types that are prevented by the current prophylactic HPV vaccines were 6.5% for HPV 16, 1.7% for HPV 18, 6.6% for HPV 6, and 1.5% for HPV 11. Furthermore, according to the study, the prevalence of HPV infection and quadrivalent vaccine-related HPV types (6, 11, 16, and 18) was highest in Brazil.

1.5.1 Risk Factors

Significant risk factors associated with HPV infection in men are related to sexual behavior, particularly lifetime sexual behavior and recent number of sexual partners (Hippelainen et al., 1993; Franceschi et al., 2002; Svare et al., 2002; Vaccarella et al., 2006; Nielson et al., 2007). Condom use and cigarette smoking (ten or more cigarettes per day) have also been identified as modifiable risk factors.

Studies that have analyzed HPV infection in circumcised individuals show conflicting results (Castellsague et al., 2002; Baldwin et al., 2004; Shin et al., 2004; Weaver et al., 2004; Vaccarella et al., 2006), although Hernandez et al. (2008a) recently demonstrated a lower HPV prevalence in the glans/corona of circumcised men. In addition, the same study reported that infection with high-risk and multiple HPV types was more prevalent in uncircumcised men, suggesting a protective effect of circumcision against prevalent HPV infection (see also Sect. 3.9 in Chap. 3).

1.6   HPV Transmission Modes

Genital HPV transmission occurs through direct skin contact between sexual partners, and several studies have shown that transmission is likely even without vaginal and/or anal penetration (Tay et al., 1990; Winer et al., 2003; Frega et al., 2003).

The recent report of HPV transmission between the female anus and the scrotum with nonpenetrative sexual contact (Hernandez et al., 2008b) and the data confirming that the perianal area is a frequent site of HPV contamination support this observation. In addition, the occurrence of male self-transmission involving the scrotum and other proximate genital sites (i.e., penis) could suggest the scrotum as a viable infection reservoir (Hernandez et al., 2008b). However, additional studies are needed to confirm this finding (see also Sect. 3.2 in Chap. 3; Sects. 7.3 and 7.4 in Chap. 7).

Yet, Puranen et al. (1996) showed that transmission through moist seats and floors is unlikely in locations with adequate sanitary conditions.

Genital HPV types have been detected in the fingers and fingernail tips of individuals with genital warts, and a finger-genital route has been suggested (Sonnex et al., 1999). In addition, Hernandez et al. (2008b) reported that viral transmission from the woman's hands to the male partner's genitals occurred in four cases of a prospective transmission study that evaluated heterosexual, monogamous couples. The investigators concluded that HPV self-inoculation is a likely event in both genders, particularly in men.

Studies suggest that oral HPV infection is sexually acquired (D'Souza et al., 2007; Schwartz et al., 1998), although auto- and hetero-inoculation can also occur.

The increased risk of HPV-related tonsillar squamous cell carcinoma in patients presenting with HPV-associated anogenital cancers suggests that genital–oral transmission is likely (Frisch and Biggar, 1999; Hemminki et al., 2000).

In addition, a recent case-control study has found that a high (i.e., 26 or more) lifetime number of vaginal-sex partners and six or more lifetime oral-sex partners were associated with oropharyngeal cancer (D'Souza et al., 2007).

However, in a prospective Finnish study, Rintala et al. (2006) failed to show an association between sexual habits and oral HPV infection. In addition, the role of saliva as a vector transmitter is yet unknown.

> HPV infection and HPV-related diseases occur even in women in monogamous relationships and Pap test screening should be regularly performed in these individuals (Marrazzo, 2000, 2001).

1.6.1   HPV Transmission in Children

Perinatal HPV transmission has been shown to occur in the external genital mucosa, oral cavity, nasal mucosa, and particularly in the larynx of prepubertal children (Fig. 1.12), although there is no evidence to support transmission to the cervix (see also Sect. 11.6 in Chap. 11).

HPV DNA has been detected in 37–73% of nasopharyngeal aspirates or buccal swabs of newborn babies

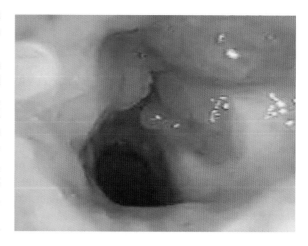

Fig. 1.12. HPV-related laryngeal papilloma. (Source: Photograph courtesy of Marcia Jacomelli, MD, PhD, São Paulo, Brazil)

(Sedlacek et al., 1989; Fredericks et al., 1993; Pakarian et al., 1994; Puranen et al., 1997).

In a recent study evaluating a possible hematogenous (i.e., transplacental) transmission route of HPV, Rombaldi et al. (2008) showed HPV-associated placental infection in 23.3% of the patients and transplacental transmission of the virus in 12.2%. These results suggest that transplacental transmission of HPV can occur, and the potential consequences of fetal exposure to the virus should be further investigated.

Vertical transmission (from an infected mother to the child) is increased when maternal genital HPV DNA is present or high viral loads are detected at the time of delivery (Alberico et al., 1996; Kaye et al., 1994).

Studies analyzing concordance of HPV types detected in newborn babies and their mothers have shown concordance results of 57–69% (Syrjanen and Puranen, 2000). This finding suggests that postpartum HPV contamination of infants may occur from a variety of sources, including breast milk (Sarkola et al., 2008), from siblings or caretakers via skin contact (Obalek et al., 1990; Handley et al., 1997), or even through exposure to contaminated fomites (Syrjanen and Puranen, 2000).

A prospective analysis evaluating HPV infection in infants showed that oral HPV infection had been acquired by 42% and it had cleared and persisted in 11 and 10% of the children enrolled in the study, respectively. In contrast, genital HPV had persisted in only 1.5% of the infants during their first 26 months of life (Rintala et al., 2005), suggesting that genital infection persistence in early age is an infrequent event (Moscicki, 1996).

However, Cason et al. (1995) detected high rates (73%) of perinatal transmission of oncogenic HPV 16 and HPV 18 in contaminated infants 24 h after delivery, with persistent HPV 16 DNA and HPV 18 DNA detected in 83.3 and 20% of cases at 6 months of age, respectively.

HPV seropositivity to low-risk HPV 6 and high-risk HPV 16 types is noticeably more prevalent in children and adolescents than in adults, suggesting that infection with these types is common (Muller et al., 1995; Cason et al., 1995).

HPV-related lesions (genital warts) in boys are usually located in the perianal area, although the penis can also be affected (Copulsky et al., 1975; Kumar et al., 1990; Oriel, 1992). HPV lesions in young girls occur in the vulvar (Fig. 1.13), vaginal, urethral, and perianal areas (Fig. 1.14).

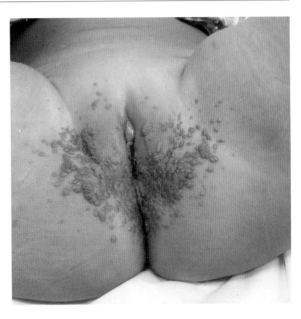

Fig. 1.13. Vulvar and perianal condyloma in a 16-month-old girl. (Source: Photograph courtesy of Nadir Oyakawa, MD, PhD, São Paulo, Brazil)

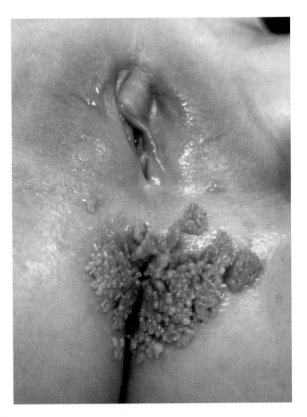

Fig. 1.14. Anal and perianal condyloma in a 2-year-old girl. (Source: Photograph courtesy of Nadir Oyakawa, MD, PhD, São Paulo, Brazil)

HPV 6 and HPV 11 are detected in the majority of anogenital lesions in children (Gibson et al., 1990; Obalek et al., 1993). However, anogenital HPV in children can also be associated with nonmucosal HPV types, and cutaneous HPV 2 has been the usual type detected (Obalek et al., 1990; Obalek et al., 1993; Handley et al., 1997).

In addition to this finding, several studies have confirmed the low prevalence of sexual abuse as the cause of anogenital warts in children (Sinclair et al., 2005; Jones et al., 2007). The investigators suggest that auto- or hetero-inoculation from cutaneous warts may be the usual nonsexual transmission route of anogenital warts in prepubertal children (Handley et al., 1997; Jones et al., 2007).

1.6.2   Considerations Regarding Unusual Transmission Routes

1.6.2.1   Transmission from CO_2 Plume

Experimental studies have confirmed the presence of clinically active HPV particles within the plume of smoke emanated from laser equipment and electrocautery (Ferenczy et al., 1990). The inadvertent inhalation of noxious viral particles while performing laser surgery

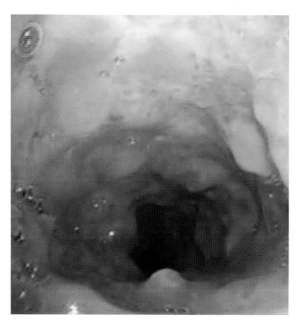

Fig. 1.15. HPV-related tracheal papilloma. (Source: Photograph courtesy of Marcia Jacomelli, MD, PhD, São Paulo, Brazil)

for HPV places the surgeon, as well as other members of the operating team and room staff, at risk of developing respiratory tract papillomatosis (Hallmo and Naess, 1991) (Fig. 1.15). Therefore, appropriate preventive measures should be adopted to avoid this occupational health hazard (see Chaps. 3 and 10).

1.7   Prevention

1.7.1   Condoms

Studies suggest that condom use offers limited or no protection against HPV infection, because the virus can still be transmitted through contact with areas of unprotected genital skin. However, there is some evidence that condom use may be associated with regression of CIN lesions (Hogewoning et al., 2003), as well as with a reduced risk of developing genital warts, CIN 2 or 3, and invasive cervical carcinoma (Manhart and Koutsky, 2002; Winer et al., 2006). Furthermore, Bleeker et al. (2003) demonstrated that condom use was associated with regression of HPV-related penile lesions in men (see also Chap. 3).

> Condom use should be strongly recommended (particularly among young individuals), because it offers effective protection against several other sexually transmitted infections (STIs), including HIV (Holmes et al., 2004).

1.7.2   Vaccines

Prophylactic HPV vaccines are highly immunogenic and have shown safety and efficacy in preventing HPV infection and related diseases in young women. Recently licensed Gardasil (Merck & Co., Whitehouse Station, NJ, USA) and Cervarix (GlaxoSmithKline, Rixensart, Belgium) target a subset of oncogenic HPV genotypes regarded as the most common disease-causing HPV types. In addition, Gardasil prevents against infection with low-risk HPV types largely associated with genital warts.

However, protection is not afforded against all cancer-associated HPV types, and current vaccines are not effective for individuals already infected with the HPV types contained in the vaccine formulation.

Currently, indications for vaccine administration favor young female subjects, and clinical trials evaluating vaccine efficacy in different target groups (older women and male subjects) are underway. Furthermore, the majority of cervical cancer deaths worldwide occur in developing countries, where current vaccine characteristics (e.g., need for refrigeration, three separate doses administered by injection, and particularly the high cost of the vaccine) might not facilitate a comprehensive global implementation.

Therefore, the production of multivalent second-generation vaccines that would be administered as a single dose orally or via a nasal spray rather than by injection are long awaited. And preferably, vaccines targeting diseases that are highly prevalent in low-resource countries should have low production costs and no need for a cold chain.

1.7.3 Antiviral Microbicides

The development of antiviral compounds that might be used as topical microbicides to block HPV transmission by sexual contact is a promising cost-effective strategy.

Carrageenan (Carraguard), a sulfated polysaccharide extracted from red algae, has been described as an effective HPV genital infection inhibitor (Buck et al., 2006; Roberts et al., 2007). Carrageenan works by preventing HPV attachment to cells and it resembles heparan sulfate, an HPV cell-attachment factor. In addition, carrageenan blocks HPV infection through a second, postattachment heparan sulfate-independent effect (Buck et al., 2006). Carragard has failed to protect against HIV in a recent phase-III study, but HPVs demonstrate enhanced susceptibility to the product. Further clinical studies are needed to assess the potential of carrageenan as a topical microbicide against HPV.

Defensins are proteins associated with innate antiviral immunity (Selsted and Ouellette, 2005; Klotman and Chang, 2006).

Studies suggest that human α-defensins (human α-defensins 1–3 [known as human neutrophil peptides (HNPs) 1–3] and particularly, human α-defensin 5 [HD-5]), may contribute to host defenses against infection with sexually transmitted HPV types. These observations raise the possibility that α-defensins could

be used as an ingredient of next-generation, broad-spectrum topical microbicide candidates being developed (Buck et al., 2006).

In contrast, several studies have shown that non-oxynol-9 (COL-1492) vaginal gel, an over-the-counter spermicide, provides no protection against HPV and other STDs, and could even potentiate HPV infection and persistence (Van Damme et al., 2002; Marais et al., 2006; Roberts et al., 2007).

References

Adams F (1886) The genuine works of Hippocrates: Translated from the Greek with a preliminary discourse and annotations, vol 2. William Wood, New York

Alberico S, Pinzano R, Comar M, Toffoletti F, Maso G, Ricci G, Guaschino S (1996) [Maternal-fetal transmission of human papillomavirus]. Minerva Ginecol 48: 199–204

Allen AL, Siegfried EC (2000) What's new in human papillomavirus infection. Curr Opin Pediatr 12: 365–369

Bafverstedt B (1967) Condylomata acuminata-past and present. Acta Derm Venereol 47: 376–381

Baken LA, Koutsky LA, Kuypers J, Kosorok MR, Lee SK, Kiviat NB, Holmes KK (1995) Genital human papillomavirus infection among male and female sex partners: Prevalence and type-specific concordance. J Infect Dis 171: 429–432

Baldwin SB, Wallace DR, Papenfuss MR, Abrahamsen M, Vaught LC, Giuliano AR (2004) Condom use and other factors affecting penile human papillomavirus detection in men attending a sexually transmitted disease clinic. Sex Transm Dis 31: 601–607

Baldwin SB, Wallace DR, Papenfuss MR, Abrahamsen M, Vaught LC, Kornegay JR, Hallum JA, Redmond SA, Giuliano AR (2003) Human papillomavirus infection in men attending a sexually transmitted disease clinic. J Infect Dis 187: 1064–1070

Barnabas RV, Laukkanen P, Koskela P, Kontula O, Lehtinen M, Garnett GP (2006) Epidemiology of HPV 16 and cervical cancer in Finland and the potential impact of vaccination: Mathematical modelling analyses. PLoS Med 3: e138

Barrasso R, Gross GE (1997) External genitalia: Diagnosis. In: Gross GE, Barrasso R (eds) Human papillomavirus infection, a clinical atlas. Ullstein Mosby, Berlin, pp 296–331

Barrett TJ, Silbar JD, Mc GJ (1954) Genital warts-a venereal disease. J Am Med Assoc 154: 333–334

Bell B (1793) Treatise on gonorrhoea virulenta and lues venerea, vol 1. Watson Mudie, Edinburgh

Bleeker MC, Hogewoning CJ, Berkhof J, Voorhorst FJ, Hesselink AT, van Diemen PM, van den Brule AJ, Snijders PJ, Meijer CJ (2005a) Concordance of specific human papillomavirus types in sex partners is more prevalent than would be expected by chance and is associated with increased viral loads. Clin Infect Dis 41: 612–620

Bleeker MC, Hogewoning CJ, Voorhorst FJ, van den Brule AJ, Snijders PJ, Starink TM, Berkhof J, Meijer CJ (2003) Condom use promotes regression of human papillomavirus-associated penile lesions in male sexual partners of women with cervical intraepithelial neoplasia. Int J Cancer 107: 804–810

Bosch FX, Burchell AN, Schiffman M, Giuliano AR, de Sanjose S, Bruni L, Tortolero-Luna G, Kjaer SK, Munoz N (2008) Epidemiology and natural history of human papillomavirus infections and type-specific implications in cervical neoplasia. Vaccine 26(Suppl 10): K1–K16

Bosch FX, Castellsague X, Munoz N, de Sanjose S, Ghaffari AM, Gonzalez LC, Gili M, Izarzugaza I, Viladiu P, Navarro C, Vergara A, Ascunce N, Guerrero E, Shah KV (1996) Male sexual behavior and human papillomavirus DNA: key risk factors for cervical cancer in Spain. J Natl Cancer Inst 88: 1060–1067

Boxman IL, Hogewoning A, Mulder LH, Bouwes Bavinck JN, ter Schegget J (1999) Detection of human papillomavirus types 6 and 11 in pubic and perianal hair from patients with genital warts. J Clin Microbiol 37: 2270–2273

Brinton LA, Reeves WC, Brenes MM, Herrero R, Gaitan E, Tenorio F, de Britton RC, Garcia M, Rawls WE (1989) The male factor in the etiology of cervical cancer among sexually monogamous women. Int J Cancer 44: 199–203

Brown DR, Shew ML, Qadadri B, Neptune N, Vargas M, Tu W, Juliar BE, Breen TE, Fortenberry JD (2005) A longitudinal study of genital human papillomavirus infection in a cohort of closely followed adolescent women. J Infect Dis 191: 182–192

Buck CB, Day PM, Thompson CD, Lubkowski J, Lu W, Lowy DR, Schiller JT (2006) Human alpha-defensins block papillomavirus infection. Proc Natl Acad Sci U S A 103: 1516–1521

Burchell AN, Richardson H, Mahmud SM, Trottier H, Tellier PP, Hanley J, Coutlee F, Franco EL (2006a) Modeling the sexual transmissibility of human papillomavirus infection using stochastic computer simulation and empirical data from a cohort study of young women in Montreal, Canada. Am J Epidemiol 163: 534–543

Burchell AN, Winer RL, de Sanjose S, Franco EL (2006b) Chapter 6: Epidemiology and transmission dynamics of genital HPV infection. Vaccine 24(Suppl 3): S3/52–S3/61

Buret F (1891) Syphilis to-day and among the ancients, vol 1: Syphilis in ancient and prehistoric times. F.A. Davis, Philadelphia, pp 124–154

Carter JJ, Koutsky LA, Wipf GC, Christensen ND, Lee SK, Kuypers J, Kiviat N, Galloway DA (1996) The natural history of human papillomavirus type 16 capsid antibodies among a cohort of university women. J Infect Dis 174: 927–936

Cason J, Kaye JN, Jewers RJ, Kambo PK, Bible JM, Kell B, Shergill B, Pakarian F, Raju KS, Best JM (1995) Perinatal infection and persistence of human papillomavirus types 16 and 18 in infants. J Med Virol 47: 209–218

Castellsague X, Bosch FX, Munoz N, Meijer CJ, Shah KV, de Sanjose S, Eluf-Neto J, Ngelangel CA, Chichareon S, Smith JS, Herrero R, Moreno V, Franceschi S (2002) Male circumcision, penile human papillomavirus infection, and cervical cancer in female partners. N Engl J Med 346: 1105–1112

Castellsague X, Ghaffari A, Daniel RW, Bosch FX, Munoz N, Shah KV (1997) Prevalence of penile human papillomavirus DNA in husbands of women with and without cervical neoplasia: a study in Spain and Colombia. J Infect Dis 176: 353–361

Centers for Disease Control and Prevention (2008) Trends in HIV- and STD-related risk behaviors among high school students–United States, 1991-2007. MMWR Morb Mortal Wkly Rep 57: 817–822

Chesson HW, Blandford JM, Gift TL, Tao G, Irwin KL (2004) The estimated direct medical cost of sexually transmitted diseases among American youth, 2000. Perspect Sex Reprod Health 36: 11–19

Cogliano V, Baan R, Straif K, Grosse Y, Secretan B, El Ghissassi F (2005) Carcinogenicity of human papillomaviruses. Lancet Oncol 6: 204

Cooperman NA, Arnsten JH, Klein RS (2007) Current sexual activity and risky sexual behavior in older men with or at risk for HIV infection. AIDS Educ Prev 19: 321–333

Copulsky J, Whitehead ED, Orkin LA (1975) Condyloma acuminata in a three-year-old boy. Urology 05: 372–373

Crawford LV, Crawford EM (1963) A comparative study of polyoma and papilloma viruses. Virology 21: 258–263

D'Souza G, Kreimer AR, Viscidi R, Pawlita M, Fakhry C, Koch WM, Westra WH, Gillison ML (2007) Case-control study of human papillomavirus and oropharyngeal cancer. N Engl J Med 356: 1944–1956

de Sanjose S, Diaz M, Castellsague X, Clifford G, Bruni L, Munoz N, Bosch FX (2007) Worldwide prevalence and genotype distribution of cervical human papillomavirus DNA in women with normal cytology: A meta-analysis. Lancet Infect Dis 7: 453–459

de Villiers EM, Fauquet C, Broker TR, Bernard HU, zur Hausen H (2004) Classification of papillomaviruses. Virology 324: 17–27

de Villiers EM, Wagner D, Schneider A, Wesch H, Miklaw H, Wahrendorf J, Papendick U, zur Hausen H (1987) Human papillomavirus infections in women with and without abnormal cervical cytology. Lancet 2: 703–706

Dillner J, Kallings I, Brihmer C, Sikstrom B, Koskela P, Lehtinen M, Schiller JT, Sapp M, Mardh PA (1996) Seropositivities to human papillomavirus types 16, 18, or 33 capsids and to Chlamydia trachomatis are markers of sexual behavior. J Infect Dis 173: 1394–1398

Dinh TH, Sternberg M, Dunne EF, Markowitz LE (2008) Genital warts among 18- to 59-year-olds in the United States, National Health and Nutrition Examination Survey, 1999–2004. Sex Transm Dis 35: 357–360

Dunne EF, Nielson CM, Stone KM, Markowitz LE, Giuliano AR (2006) Prevalence of HPV infection among men: A systematic review of the literature. J Infect Dis 194: 1044–1057

Dunne EF, Unger ER, Sternberg M, McQuillan G, Swan DC, Patel SS, Markowitz LE (2007) Prevalence of HPV infection among females in the United States. JAMA 297: 813–819

Durst M, Croce CM, Gissmann L, Schwarz E, Huebner K (1987) Papillomavirus sequences integrate near cellular oncogenes in some cervical carcinomas. Proc Natl Acad Sci U S A 84: 1070–1074

Ferenczy A, Bergeron C, Richart RM (1990) Carbon dioxide laser energy disperses human papillomavirus deoxyribonucleic acid onto treatment fields. Am J Obstet Gynecol 163: 1271–1274

Fleischer AB, Jr., Parrish CA, Glenn R, Feldman SR (2001) Condylomata acuminata (genital warts): Patient demographics and treating physicians. Sex Transm Dis 28: 643–647

Flores R, Abalos AT, Nielson CM, Abrahamsen M, Harris RB, Giuliano AR (2008) Reliability of sample collection and laboratory testing for HPV detection in men. J Virol Methods 149: 136–143

Forhan SE, Gottlieb SL, Sternberg MR, Xu F, Datta SD, Berman S, Markowitz LE (2008) Prevalence of sexually transmitted infections and bacterial vaginosis among Female adolescents in the United States: Data from the National Health and Nutritional Examination Survey (NHANES) 2003–2004. In: National STD Prevention Conference, Chicago, IL

Fornaciari G (2006) [The Aragonese mummies of the Basilica of Saint Domenico Maggiore in Naples]. Med Secoli 18: 843–864

Fornaciari G, Zavaglia K, Giusti L, Vultaggio C, Ciranni R (2003) Human papillomavirus in a 16th century mummy. Lancet 362: 1160

Franceschi S, Castellsague X, Dal Maso L, Smith JS, Plummer M, Ngelangel C, Chichareon S, Eluf-Neto J, Shah KV, Snijders PJ, Meijer CJ, Bosch FX, Munoz N (2002) Prevalence and determinants of human papillomavirus genital infection in men. Br J Cancer 86: 705–711

Franceschi S, Herrero R, Clifford GM, Snijders PJ, Arslan A, Anh PT, Bosch FX, Ferreccio C, Hieu NT, Lazcano-Ponce E, Matos E, Molano M, Qiao YL, Rajkumar R, Ronco G, de Sanjose S, Shin HR, Sukvirach S, Thomas JO, Meijer CJ, Munoz N (2006) Variations in the age-specific curves of human papillomavirus prevalence in women worldwide. Int J Cancer 119: 2677–2684

Franco EL (1996) Epidemiology of anogential warts and cancer. In: Reid R, Lorincz A (eds) Human papillomaviruses I. W.B. Saunders, Philadelphia, pp 597–623

Fredericks BD, Balkin A, Daniel HW, Schonrock J, Ward B, Frazer IH (1993) Transmission of human papillomaviruses from mother to child. Aust N Z J Obstet Gynaecol 33: 30–32

Frega A, Cenci M, Stentella P, Cipriano L, De Ioris A, Alderisio M, Vecchione A (2003) Human papillomavirus in virgins and behaviour at risk. Cancer Lett 194: 21–24

Frisch M, Biggar RJ (1999) Aetiological parallel between tonsillar and anogenital squamous-cell carcinomas. Lancet 354: 1442–1443

Garcia-Pineres AJ, Hildesheim A, Herrero R, Trivett M, Williams M, Atmetlla I, Ramirez M, Villegas M, Schiffman M, Rodriguez AC, Burk RD, Hildesheim M, Freer E, Bonilla J, Bratti C, Berzofsky JA, Pinto LA (2006) Persistent human papillomavirus infection is associated with a generalized decrease in immune responsiveness in older women. Cancer Res 66: 11070–11076

Gibson PE, Gardner SD, Best SJ (1990) Human papillomavirus types in anogenital warts of children. J Med Virol 30: 142–145

Giovannelli L, Bellavia C, Capra G, Migliore MC, Caleca M, Giglio M, Perino A, Matranga D, Ammatuna P (2007) HPV group- and type-specific concordance in HPV infected sexual couples. J Med Virol 79: 1882–1888

Gissmann L, zur Hausen H (1980) Partial characterization of viral DNA from human genital warts (Condylomata acuminata). Int J Cancer 25: 605–609

Giuliano AR, Harris R, Sedjo RL, Baldwin S, Roe D, Papenfuss MR, Abrahamsen M, Inserra P, Olvera S, Hatch K (2002) Incidence, prevalence, and clearance of type-specific human papillomavirus infections: The Young Women's Health Study. J Infect Dis 186: 462–469

Giuliano AR, Lazcano-Ponce E, Villa LL, Flores R, Salmeron J, Lee JH, Papenfuss MR, Abrahamsen M, Jolles E, Nielson CM, Baggio ML, Silva R, Quiterio M (2008a) The human papillomavirus infection in men study: Human papillomavirus prevalence and type distribution among men residing in Brazil, Mexico, and the United States. Cancer Epidemiol Biomarkers Prev 17: 2036–2043

Giuliano AR, Lu B, Nielson CM, Flores R, Papenfuss MR, Lee JH, Abrahamsen M, Harris RB (2008b) Age-specific prevalence, incidence, and duration of human papillomavirus infections in a cohort of 290 US men. J Infect Dis 198: 827–835

Giuliano AR, Nielson CM, Flores R, Dunne EF, Abrahamsen M, Papenfuss MR, Markowitz LE, Smith D, Harris RB (2007) The optimal anatomic sites for sampling heterosexual men for human papillomavirus (HPV) detection: The HPV detection in men study. J Infect Dis 196: 1146–1152

Hadjivassiliou M, Stefanaki C, Nicolaidou E, Bethimoutis G, Anyfantakis V, Caroni C, Katsambas A (2007) Human papillomavirus assay in genital warts – correlation with symptoms. Int J STD AIDS 18: 329–334

Hallmo P, Naess O (1991) Laryngeal papillomatosis with human papillomavirus DNA contracted by a laser surgeon. Eur Arch Otorhinolaryngol 248: 425–427

Halpert R, Fruchter RG, Sedlis A, Butt K, Boyce JG, Sillman FH (1986) Human papillomavirus and lower genital neoplasia in renal transplant patients. Obstet Gynecol 68: 251–258

Handley J, Hanks E, Armstrong K, Bingham A, Dinsmore W, Swann A, Evans MF, McGee JO, O'Leary J (1997) Common association of HPV 2 with anogenital warts in prepubertal children. Pediatr Dermatol 14: 339–343

Hariri S, Dunne EF, Sternberg M, Unger ER, Meadows KS, Karem KL, Markowitz LE (2008) Seroepidemiology of human papillomavirus type 11 in the United States: Results from the third National Health and Nutrition Examination Survey, 1991–1994. Sex Transm Dis 35: 298–303

Health Protection Agency (2006) Trends in anogenital warts and anogenital herpes simplex virus infection in the United Kingdom: 1996 to 2005. CDR Wkly 16: 1–4

Health Protection Agency (2007) Trends in genital warts and genital herpes diagnoses in the United Kingdom. In: Health Protection Weekly Report, vol 1. Health Protection Agency, UK

Hemminki K, Dong C, Frisch M (2000) Tonsillar and other upper aerodigestive tract cancers among cervical cancer patients and their husbands. Eur J Cancer Prev 9: 433–437

Hernandez BY, McDuffie K, Goodman MT, Wilkens LR, Thompson P, Zhu X, Wong W, Ning L (2006) Comparison of physician- and self-collected genital specimens for detection of human papillomavirus in men. J Clin Microbiol 44: 513–517

Hernandez BY, Wilkens LR, Zhu X, McDuffie K, Thompson P, Shvetsov YB, Ning L, Goodman MT (2008a) Circumcision and human papillomavirus infection in men: A site-specific comparison. J Infect Dis 197: 787–794

Hernandez BY, Wilkens LR, Zhu X, Thompson P, McDuffie K, Shvetsov YB, Kamemoto LE, Killeen J, Ning L, Goodman MT (2008b) Transmission of human papillomavirus in heterosexual couples. Emerg Infect Dis 14: 888–894

Herrero R, Hildesheim A, Bratti C, Sherman ME, Hutchinson M, Morales J, Balmaceda I, Greenberg MD, Alfaro M, Burk RD, Wacholder S, Plummer M, Schiffman M (2000) Population-based study of human papillomavirus infection and cervical neoplasia in rural Costa Rica. J Natl Cancer Inst 92: 464–474

Hillemanns P, Breugelmans JG, Gieseking F, Benard S, Lamure E, Littlewood KJ, Petry KU (2008) Estimation of the incidence of genital warts and the cost of illness in Germany: A cross-sectional study. BMC Infect Dis 8: 76

Hippelainen M, Syrjanen S, Koskela H, Pulkkinen J, Saarikoski S, Syrjanen K (1993) Prevalence and risk factors of genital human papillomavirus (HPV) infections in healthy males: A study on Finnish conscripts. Sex Transm Dis 20: 321–328

Ho GY, Bierman R, Beardsley L, Chang CJ, Burk RD (1998) Natural history of cervicovaginal papillomavirus infection in young women. N Engl J Med 338: 423–428

Hogewoning CJ, Bleeker MC, van den Brule AJ, Voorhorst FJ, Snijders PJ, Berkhof J, Westenend PJ, Meijer CJ (2003) Condom use promotes regression of cervical intraepithelial neoplasia and clearance of human papillomavirus: A randomized clinical trial. Int J Cancer 107: 811–816

Holmes KK, Levine R, Weaver M (2004) Effectiveness of condoms in preventing sexually transmitted infections. Bull World Health Organ 82: 454–461

Insinga RP, Dasbach EJ, Myers ER (2003) The health and economic burden of genital warts in a set of private health plans in the United States. Clin Infect Dis 36: 1397–1403

Insinga RP, Dasbach EJ, Elbasha EH (2005) Assessing the annual economic burden of preventing and treating anogenital human papillomavirus-related disease in the US: Analytic framework and review of the literature. Pharmacoeconomics 23: 1107–1122

IARC Working Group on the Evaluation of Carcinogenic Risks to Humans (2007). Human papillomaviruses. IARC Monogr Eval Carcinog Risks Hum 90: 1–636

Jamison JH, Kaplan DW, Hamman R, Eagar R, Beach R, Douglas JM, Jr. (1995) Spectrum of genital human papillomavirus infection in a female adolescent population. Sex Transm Dis 22: 236–243

Jones V, Smith SJ, Omar HA (2007) Nonsexual transmission of anogenital warts in children: A retrospective analysis. Scientific WorldJournal 7: 1896–1899

Kahn JA, Rosenthal SL, Succop PA, Ho GY, Burk RD (2002) The interval between menarche and age of first sexual intercourse as a risk factor for subsequent HPV infection in adolescent and young adult women. J Pediatr 141: 718–723

Kaye JN, Cason J, Pakarian FB, Jewers RJ, Kell B, Bible J, Raju KS, Best JM (1994) Viral load as a determinant for transmission of human papillomavirus type 16 from mother to child. J Med Virol 44: 415–421

Kelsey CB (1882) Diseases of the rectum and anus. William Wood, New York

Kingery LB (1923) The etiology of common warts: Their production in second generation. JAMA 76: 440

Kjaer SK, Breugelmans G, Munk C, Junge J, Watson M, Iftner T (2008) Population-based prevalence, type- and age-specific distribution of HPV in women before introduction of an HPV-vaccination program in Denmark. Int J Cancer 123: 1864–1870

Kjaer SK, Munk C, Winther JF, Jorgensen HO, Meijer CJ, van den Brule AJ (2005) Acquisition and persistence of human papillomavirus infection in younger men: A prospective follow-up study among Danish soldiers. Cancer Epidemiol Biomarkers Prev 14: 1528–1533

Kjaer SK, van den Brule AJ, Paull G, Svare EI, Sherman ME, Thomsen BL, Suntum M, Bock JE, Poll PA, Meijer CJ (2002) Type specific persistence of high risk human papillomavirus (HPV) as indicator of high grade cervical squamous intraepithelial lesions in young women: Population based prospective follow up study. BMJ 325: 572

Klotman ME, Chang TL (2006) Defensins in innate antiviral immunity. Nat Rev Immunol 6: 447–456

Koshiol JE, Laurent SA, Pimenta JM (2004) Rate and predictors of new genital warts claims and genital warts-related healthcare utilization among privately insured patients in the United States. Sex Transm Dis 31: 748–752

Koutsky L (1997) Epidemiology of genital human papillomavirus infection. Am J Med 102: 3–8

Koutsky LA, Galloway DA, Holmes KK (1988) Epidemiology of genital human papillomavirus infection. Epidemiol Rev 10: 122–163

Kumar B, Gupta R, Sharma SC (1990) Penile condylomata acuminata in a male child: A case report. Genitourin Med 66: 226–227

Lajous M, Mueller N, Cruz-Valdez A, Aguilar LV, Franceschi S, Hernandez-Avila M, Lazcano-Ponce E (2005) Determinants of prevalence, acquisition, and persistence of human papillomavirus in healthy Mexican military men. Cancer Epidemiol Biomarkers Prev 14: 1710–1716

Lazcano-Ponce E, Herrero R, Munoz N, Hernandez-Avila M, Salmeron J, Leyva A, Meijer CJ, Walboomers JM (2001) High prevalence of human papillomavirus infection in Mexican males: Comparative study of penile-urethral swabs and urine samples. Sex Transm Dis 28: 277–280

Liaw KL, Glass AG, Manos MM, Greer CE, Scott DR, Sherman M, Burk RD, Kurman RJ, Wacholder S, Rush BB, Cadell DM, Lawler P, Tabor D, Schiffman M (1999) Detection of human papillomavirus DNA in cytologically normal women and subsequent cervical squamous intraepithelial lesions. J Natl Cancer Inst 91: 954–960

Manhart LE, Koutsky LA (2002) Do condoms prevent genital HPV infection, external genital warts, or cervical neoplasia? A meta-analysis. Sex Transm Dis 29: 725–735

Marais D, Carrara H, Kay P, Ramjee G, Allan B, Williamson AL (2006) The impact of the use of COL-1492, a nonoxynol-9 vaginal gel, on the presence of cervical human papillomavirus in female sex workers. Virus Res 121: 220–222

Marrazzo JM (2000) Genital human papillomavirus infection in women who have sex with women: A concern for patients and providers. AIDS Patient Care STDS 14: 447–451

Marrazzo JM, Koutsky LA, Kiviat NB, Kuypers JM, Stine K (2001) Papanicolaou test screening and prevalence of genital human papillomavirus among women who have sex with women. Am J Public Health 91: 947–952

McDonagh JER (1920) Venereal diseases. Mosby, St. Louis

Meisels A (1992) Cytologic diagnosis of human papillomavirus. Influence of age and pregnancy stage. Acta Cytol 36: 480–482

Moreira ED, Jr., Kim SC, Glasser D, Gingell C (2006) Sexual activity, prevalence of sexual problems, and associated help-seeking patterns in men and women aged 40–80 years in Korea: Data from the Global Study of Sexual Attitudes and Behaviors (GSSAB). J Sex Med 3: 201–211

Moscicki AB (1996) Genital HPV infections in children and adolescents. Obstet Gynecol Clin North Am 23: 675–697

Moscicki AB (2005) Impact of HPV infection in adolescent populations. J Adolesc Health 37: S3–S9

Moscicki AB, Hills N, Shiboski S, Powell K, Jay N, Hanson E, Miller S, Clayton L, Farhat S, Broering J, Darragh T, Palefsky J (2001) Risks for incident human papillomavirus infection and low-grade squamous intraepithelial lesion development in young females. JAMA 285: 2995–3002

Mougin C, Dalstein V, Pretet JL, Gay C, Schaal JP, Riethmuller D (2001) [Epidemiology of cervical papillomavirus infections. Recent knowledge]. Presse Med 30: 1017–1023

Muller M, Viscidi RP, Ulken V, Bavinck JN, Hill PM, Fisher SG, Reid R, Munoz N, Schneider A, Shah KV, et al. (1995) Antibodies to the E4, E6, and E7 proteins of human papillomavirus (HPV) type 16 in patients with HPV-associated diseases and in the normal population. J Invest Dermatol 104: 138–141

Munoz N, Bosch FX, de Sanjose S, Herrero R, Castellsague X, Shah KV, Snijders PJ, Meijer CJ (2003) Epidemiologic classification of human papillomavirus types associated with cervical cancer. N Engl J Med 348: 518–527

Munoz N, Mendez F, Posso H, Molano M, van den Brule AJ, Ronderos M, Meijer C, Munoz A (2004) Incidence, duration, and determinants of cervical human papillomavirus infection in a cohort of Colombian women with normal cytological results. J Infect Dis 190: 2077–2087

Nicolau SM, Camargo CG, Stavale JN, Castelo A, Dores GB, Lorincz A, de Lima GR (2005) Human papillomavirus DNA detection in male sexual partners of women with genital human papillomavirus infection. Urology 65: 251–255

Nicolosi A, Laumann EO, Glasser DB, Moreira ED, Jr., Paik A, Gingell C (2004) Sexual behavior and sexual dysfunctions after age 40: The global study of sexual attitudes and behaviors. Urology 64: 991–997

Nielsen A, Kjaer SK, Munk C, Iftner T (2008) Type-specific HPV infection and multiple HPV types: prevalence and risk factor profile in nearly 12,000 younger and older Danish women. Sex Transm Dis 35: 276–282

Nielson CM, Flores R, Harris RB, Abrahamsen M, Papenfuss MR, Dunne EF, Markowitz LE, Giuliano AR (2007) Human papillomavirus prevalence and type distribution in male anogenital sites and semen. Cancer Epidemiol Biomarkers Prev 16: 1107–1114

Obalek S, Jablonska S, Favre M, Walczak L, Orth G (1990) Condylomata acuminata in children: frequent association with human papillomaviruses responsible for cutaneous warts. J Am Acad Dermatol 23: 205–213

Obalek S, Misiewicz J, Jablonska S, Favre M, Orth G (1993) Childhood condyloma acuminatum: Association with genital and cutaneous human papillomaviruses. Pediatr Dermatol 10: 101–106

Oriel JD (1971) Natural history of genital warts. Br J Vener Dis 47: 1–13

Oriel JD (1992) Sexually transmitted diseases in children: Human papillomavirus infection. Genitourin Med 68: 80–83

Pakarian F, Kaye J, Cason J, Kell B, Jewers R, Derias NW, Raju KS, Best JM (1994) Cancer associated human papillomaviruses: Perinatal transmission and persistence. Br J Obstet Gynaecol 101: 514–517

Partridge JM, Hughes JP, Feng Q, Winer RL, Weaver BA, Xi LF, Stern ME, Lee SK, O'Reilly SF, Hawes SE, Kiviat NB, Koutsky LA (2007) Genital human papillomavirus infection in men: Incidence and risk factors in a cohort of university students. J Infect Dis 196: 1128–1136

Partridge JM, Koutsky LA (2006) Genital human papillomavirus infection in men. Lancet Infect Dis 6: 21–31

Puranen M, Syrjanen K, Syrjanen S (1996) Transmission of genital human papillomavirus infections is unlikely through the floor and seats of humid dwellings in countries of high-level hygiene. Scand J Infect Dis 28: 243–246

Puranen MH, Yliskoski MH, Saarikoski SV, Syrjanen KJ, Syrjanen SM (1997) Exposure of an infant to cervical human papillomavirus infection of the mother is common. Am J Obstet Gynecol 176: 1039–1045

Richardson H, Kelsall G, Tellier P, Voyer H, Abrahamowicz M, Ferenczy A, Coutlee F, Franco EL (2003) The natural history of type-specific human papillomavirus infections in female university students. Cancer Epidemiol Biomarkers Prev 12: 485–490

Ricord P (1838) Traité pratique des maladies vénériennes. J. Rouvier and E. le Bouvier, Paris

Rintala M, Grenman S, Puranen M, Syrjanen S (2006) Natural history of oral papillomavirus infections in spouses: A prospective Finnish HPV Family Study. J Clin Virol 35: 89–94

Rintala MA, Grenman SE, Jarvenkyla ME, Syrjanen KJ, Syrjanen SM (2005) High-risk types of human papillomavirus (HPV) DNA in oral and genital mucosa of infants during their first 3 years of life: Experience from the Finnish HPV Family Study. Clin Infect Dis 41: 1728–1733

Roberts JN, Buck CB, Thompson CD, Kines R, Bernardo M, Choyke PL, Lowy DR, Schiller JT (2007) Genital transmission of HPV in a mouse model is potentiated by nonoxynol-9 and inhibited by carrageenan. Nat Med 13: 857–861

Rodriguez AC, Burk R, Herrero R, Hildesheim A, Bratti C, Sherman ME, Solomon D, Guillen D, Alfaro M, Viscidi R, Morales J, Hutchinson M, Wacholder S, Schiffman M (2007) The natural history of human papillomavirus infection and cervical intraepithelial neoplasia among young women in the Guanacaste cohort shortly after initiation of sexual life. Sex Transm Dis 34: 494–502

Rombaldi RL, Serafini EP, Mandelli J, Zimmermann E, Losquiavo KP (2008) Transplacental transmission of human papillomavirus. Virol J 5: 106

Rombaldi RL, Serafini EP, Villa LL, Vanni AC, Barea F, Frassini R, Xavier M, Paesi S (2006) Infection with human papillomaviruses of sexual partners of women having cervical intraepithelial neoplasia. Braz J Med Biol Res 39: 177–187

Rousseau MC, Franco EL, Villa LL, Sobrinho JP, Termini L, Prado JM, Rohan TE (2000) A cumulative case-control study of risk factor profiles for oncogenic and non-oncogenic cervical human papillomavirus infections. Cancer Epidemiol Biomarkers Prev 9: 469–476

Routh HB, Bhowmik KR, Parish LC (1997) Myths, fables and even truths about warts and human papillomavirus. Clin Dermatol 15: 305–307

Sarkola M, Rintala M, Grenman S, Syrjanen S (2008) Human papillomavirus DNA detected in breast milk. Pediatr Infect Dis J 27: 557–558

Satterwhite CL (2008) Up, up, and away? Trends in chlamydial infections in the U.S. In: National STD Prevention Conference, Chicago, IL

Schlecht NF, Kulaga S, Robitaille J, Ferreira S, Santos M, Miyamura RA, Duarte-Franco E, Rohan TE, Ferenczy A, Villa LL, Franco EL (2001) Persistent human papillomavirus infection as a predictor of cervical intraepithelial neoplasia. JAMA 286: 3106–3114

Schwartz SM, Daling JR, Doody DR, Wipf GC, Carter JJ, Madeleine MM, Mao EJ, Fitzgibbons ED, Huang S, Beckmann AM, McDougall JK, Galloway DA (1998) Oral cancer risk in relation to sexual history and evidence of human papillomavirus infection. J Natl Cancer Inst 90: 1626–1636

Schwarz E, Freese UK, Gissmann L, Mayer W, Roggenbuck B, Stremlau A, zur Hausen H (1985) Structure and transcription of human papillomavirus sequences in cervical carcinoma cells. Nature 314: 111–114

Sedlacek TV, Lindheim S, Eder C, Hasty L, Woodland M, Ludomirsky A, Rando RF (1989) Mechanism for human papillomavirus transmission at birth. Am J Obstet Gynecol 161: 55–59

Sellors JW, Karwalajtys TL, Kaczorowski J, Mahony JB, Lytwyn A, Chong S, Sparrow J, Lorincz A (2003) Incidence, clearance and predictors of human papillomavirus infection in women. CMAJ 168: 421–425

Selsted ME, Ouellette AJ (2005) Mammalian defensins in the antimicrobial immune response. Nat Immunol 6: 551–557

Shin HR, Franceschi S, Vaccarella S, Roh JW, Ju YH, Oh JK, Kong HJ, Rha SH, Jung SI, Kim JI, Jung KY, van Doorn LJ, Quint W (2004) Prevalence and determinants of genital infection with papillomavirus, in female and male university students in Busan, South Korea. J Infect Dis 190: 468–476

Simms I, Fairley CK (1997) Epidemiology of genital warts in England and Wales: 1971 to 1994. Genitourin Med 73: 365–367

Sinclair KA, Woods CR, Kirse DJ, Sinal SH (2005) Anogenital and respiratory tract human papillomavirus infections among children: Age, gender, and potential transmission through sexual abuse. Pediatrics 116: 815–825

Smith JS, Moses S, Hudgens MG, Agot K, Franceschi S, Maclean IW, Ndinya-Achola JO, Parker CB, Pugh N, Meijer CJ, Snijders PJ, Bailey RC (2007) Human papillomavirus detection by penile site in young men from Kenya. Sex Transm Dis 34: 928–934

Sonnex C, Strauss S, Gray JJ (1999) Detection of human papillomavirus DNA on the fingers of patients with genital warts. Sex Transm Infect 75: 317–319

Stone KM, Karem KL, Sternberg MR, McQuillan GM, Poon AD, Unger ER, Reeves WC (2002) Seroprevalence of human papillomavirus type 16 infection in the United States. J Infect Dis 186: 1396–1402

Strauss MJ, Shaw EW, et al. (1949) Crystalline virus-like particles from skin papillomas characterized by intranuclear inclusion bodies. Proc Soc Exp Biol Med 72: 46–50

Svare EI, Kjaer SK, Worm AM, Osterlind A, Meijer CJ, van den Brule AJ (2002) Risk factors for genital HPV DNA in men resemble those found in women: a study of male attendees at a Danish STD clinic. Sex Transm Infect 78: 215–218

Sycuro LK, Xi LF, Hughes JP, Feng Q, Winer RL, Lee SK, O'Reilly S, Kiviat NB, Koutsky LA (2008) Persistence of genital human papillomavirus infection in a long-term follow-up study of female university students. J Infect Dis 198: 971–978

Syrjanen S, Puranen M (2000) Human papillomavirus infections in children: The potential role of maternal transmission. Crit Rev Oral Biol Med 11: 259–274

Tay SK, Ho TH, Lim-Tan SK (1990) Is genital human papillomavirus infection always sexually transmitted? Aust N Z J Obstet Gynaecol 30: 240–242

Thomas KK, Hughes JP, Kuypers JM, Kiviat NB, Lee SK, Adam DE, Koutsky LA (2000) Concurrent and sequential acquisition of different genital human papillomavirus types. J Infect Dis 182: 1097–1102

Trottier H, Franco EL (2006) The epidemiology of genital human papillomavirus infection. Vaccine 24(Suppl 1): S1–S15

Vaccarella S, Lazcano-Ponce E, Castro-Garduno JA, Cruz-Valdez A, Diaz V, Schiavon R, Hernandez P, Kornegay JR, Hernandez-Avila M, Franceschi S (2006) Prevalence and determinants of human papillomavirus infection in men attending vasectomy clinics in Mexico. Int J Cancer 119: 1934–1939

Van Damme L, Ramjee G, Alary M, Vuylsteke B, Chandeying V, Rees H, Sirivongrangson P, Mukenge-Tshibaka L, Ettiegne-Traore V, Uaheowitchai C, Karim SS, Masse B, Perriens J, Laga M (2002) Effectiveness of COL-1492, a nonoxynol-9 vaginal gel, on HIV-1 transmission in female sex workers: A randomised controlled trial. Lancet 360: 971–977

van der Snoek EM, Niesters HG, Mulder PG, van Doornum GJ, Osterhaus AD, van der Meijden WI (2003) Human papillomavirus infection in men who have sex with men participating in a Dutch gay-cohort study. Sex Transm Dis 30: 639–644

Van Doornum GJ, Prins M, Juffermans LH, Hooykaas C, van den Hoek JA, Coutinho RA, Quint WG (1994) Regional distribution and incidence of human papillomavirus infections among heterosexual men and women with multiple sexual partners: A prospective study. Genitourin Med 70: 240–246

Weaver BA, Feng Q, Holmes KK, Kiviat N, Lee SK, Meyer C, Stern M, Koutsky LA (2004) Evaluation of genital sites and sampling techniques for detection of human papillomavirus DNA in men. J Infect Dis 189: 677–685

Weinstock H, Berman S, Cates W, Jr. (2004) Sexually transmitted diseases among American youth: Incidence and prevalence estimates, 2000. Perspect Sex Reprod Health 36: 6–10

Wikstrom A (1995) Clinical and serological manifestations of genital human papillomavirus infection. Acta Derm Venereol Suppl (Stockh) 193: 1–85

Wikstrom A, Popescu C, Forslund O (2000) Asymptomatic penile HPV infection: A prospective study. Int J STD AIDS 11: 80–84

Wiley DJ, Douglas J, Beutner K, Cox T, Fife K, Moscicki AB, Fukumoto L (2002) External genital warts: Diagnosis, treatment, and prevention. Clin Infect Dis 35: S210–S224

Winer RL, Feng Q, Hughes JP, O'Reilly S, Kiviat NB, Koutsky LA (2008) Risk of female human papillomavirus acquisition associated with first male sex partner. J Infect Dis 197: 279–282

Winer RL, Hughes JP, Feng Q, O'Reilly S, Kiviat NB, Holmes KK, Koutsky LA (2006) Condom use and the risk of genital human papillomavirus infection in young women. N Engl J Med 354: 2645–2654

Winer RL, Lee SK, Hughes JP, Adam DE, Kiviat NB, Koutsky LA (2003) Genital human papillomavirus infection: Incidence and risk factors in a cohort of female university students. Am J Epidemiol 157: 218–226

Ylitalo N, Josefsson A, Melbye M, Sorensen P, Frisch M, Andersen PK, Sparen P, Gustafsson M, Magnusson P, Ponten

J, Gyllensten U, Adami HO (2000) A prospective study showing long-term infection with human papillomavirus 16 before the development of cervical carcinoma in situ. Cancer Res 60: 6027–6032

Yun K, Joblin L (1993) Presence of human papillomavirus DNA in condylomata acuminata in children and adolescents. Pathology 25: 1–3

zur Hausen H (1976) Condylomata acuminata and human genital cancer. Cancer Res 36: 794

zur Hausen H (1986) Genital papillomavirus infections. In: Rigby PW, Wilkie NM (eds) Viruses and cancer. Cambridge University Press Cambridge, pp 83–90

zur Hausen H (1991) Human papillomaviruses in the pathogenesis of anogenital cancer. Virology 184: 9–13

zur Hausen H (2000) Papillomaviruses causing cancer: Evasion from host-cell control in early events in carcinogenesis. J Natl Cancer Inst 92: 690–698

Laboratory Methods for Detection of Human Papillomavirus Infection

2

Luisa Lina Villa

Contents

2.1 Introduction

The diagnosis of human papillomavirus (HPV) infection can be inferred from morphological, serological, and clinical findings. In productive infections, such as warts, virus particles of about 50 nm diameter can be detected by electron microscopy and by immune detection of the virus capsid proteins (L1, L2). Immunological detection of HPV in human cells or tissues has been hindered by three main factors: (a) the late, capsid proteins are only expressed in productive infections; (b) the early proteins are often expressed in low amounts in infected tissues; and (c) the lack of high-quality, sensitive, and specific antibodies against the viral proteins. Antibodies generated against bovine papillomavirus (BPV) late proteins have been widely used because of the observed cross-reaction with HPV late proteins; however, they have low sensitivity and fail to discriminate between HPV types, which is essential for disease risk determination. Detection of HPV early proteins is even more complicated due to the low expression levels generally observed in cells or tissues derived from HPV-positive lesions. Antibodies against E6 or E7 are available but their use is mostly restricted to in vitro assays including the direct visualization in cells or tissues (immunohistochemistry) or in protein extracts (Western blots and immune precipitation assays), not always with consistent results.

HPV cannot be propagated in tissue culture and hence in most cases its accurate identification relies on molecular biology techniques. With a double-stranded DNA genome of about 8,000 base pairs (bp) in length and a well-known physical structure and gene organization, tests of choice for detecting HPV from clinical specimens are based on nucleic acid probe technology. Direct detection of HPV genomes and its transcripts can be achieved with hybridization procedures that include Southern and Northern blots, dot blots, in situ hybridization (ISH), Hybrid Capture (HC; formerly DIGENE Co., now QIAGEN, MA, USA), and DNA sequencing (reviewed in Iftner and Villa, 2003). A variety of signal-detection procedures are available that can further increase the sensitivity of these assays. The only procedure potentially capable of recognizing all HPV types and variants present in the biological specimen is DNA sequencing of the viral genome, either after cloning into plasmids or by direct sequencing of a polymerase chain

L.L. Villa
Ludwig Institute for Cancer Research,
São Paulo, Brazil
e-mail: llvilla@ludwig.org.br

A. Rosenblatt, H. G. de Campos Guidi, *Human Papillomavirus*,
DOI: 10.1007/978-3-540-70974-9-2, © Springer-Verlag Berlin Heidelberg 2009

reaction (PCR) fragment. This method, however, is presently labor-intensive and requires expensive equipment. Moreover, direct sequencing of specimens containing multiple HPVs awaits further developments.

For HPV genome analysis, hybridization in solid phase, such as Southern blot for DNA and Northern blot for RNA molecules, is an excellent procedure that can generate information with quality, but is time-consuming and requires large amounts of highly purified nucleic acids. Moreover, it requires well preserved, ideally full-size molecules, and therefore cannot be done with any biological specimen, particularly those derived from fixed tissues in which DNA degradation is often observed. It is also technically cumbersome and time-consuming, not being amenable to large-scale population studies. ISH is a technique by which specific nucleotide sequences are identified in cells or tissue sections with conserved morphology, thereby allowing the precise spatial localization of the target genomes in the biological specimen. One great advantage of ISH is that it can be applied to routinely fixed and processed tissues, which overcomes the relatively low analytical sensitivity of this method. This can be increased by combining PCR to ISH, a procedure known as in situ PCR (Nuovo et al., 1992). ISH has been used to detect messenger RNA (mRNA) as a marker of gene expression, where levels of viral proteins are low (Stoler et al., 1997). The major limitations of the method are the potential for error in HPV typing because of probe cross-hybridization. However, recent improvements have made it possible for this method to be widely used for HPV DNA and RNA detection in tissues, with high sensitivities and specificities. Viral DNA and RNA can also be detected by a series of assays based on PCR. In this case, the viral genomes are selectively amplified by a series of polymerization steps, which result in an exponential and reproducible increase in the HPV nucleotide sequences present in the biological specimen (Iftner and Villa, 2003). A summary of the characteristics and usefulness of different HPV detection assays is presented in Table 2.1.

Studies conducted during the last two decades have clearly demonstrated the role of HPV infections and risk of cervical neoplasia in women (Bosch et al., 2008). In men, however, this knowledge is just starting to accumulate. An accurate definition of infection and identification of HPV-associated diseases in the male genital tract is critical (Dunne et al., 2006; Partridge and Koutsky, 2006). Moreover, the natural history of HPV-related diseases and transmission of HPV between individuals cannot be fully understood without the establishment of proper measures of the prevalence and incidence of HPV infections in male subjects. The dynamics of HPV infection in special populations, including immune-deficient individuals, can also be improved with precise measures of HPV exposure including both HPV DNA and serology. This chapter discusses the different technologies available for detecting HPV infections. Moreover, the differences in anatomical sites and types of specimen collection in men are highlighted.

2.2   HPV DNA Methods

Presently, the two methodologies most widely used for genital type detection that have equivalent sensitivities and specificities are Hybrid Capture version 2 (HC2) and PCR with generic primers. Both assays are suitable for high-throughput testing, with automated execution and reading, which is a necessary step to be considered for use in large epidemiological studies and in clinical settings.

HC2 is based on hybridization in solution of long synthetic RNA probes complementary to the genomic sequence of 13 high-risk (16, 18, 31, 33, 35, 39, 45, 51, 52, 56, 58, 59, and 68) and five low-risk (6, 11, 42, 43, 44) HPV types, which are used to prepare high (B) and low (A) probe cocktails that are used in two separate reactions. DNA present in the biological specimen is then hybridized in solution with each of the probe cocktails allowing the formation of specific HPV DNA-RNA hybrids. These hybrids are then captured by antibodies bound to the wells of a microtiter plate that specifically recognize RNA-DNA hybrids. The immobilized hybrids are detected by a series of reactions that generate a luminescent product that can be measured in a luminometer. The intensity of emitted light, expressed as relative light units, is proportional to the amount of target DNA present in the specimen, providing a semiquantitative measure of the viral load. HC2 is currently available in a 96-well microplate format, is easy to perform in clinical settings, and is suitable for automation (Lorincz and Anthony, 2001). Furthermore, HC2 does not require special facilities to

Table 2.1 Characteristics of HPV test technologies

	Test	Analytical	Clinical	Comments
		Sensitivity/specificity	Sensitivity/specificity for CIN3/cervical cancer	
Based on cell morphology	Pap smear/tissues	Not applicable	Low/high	Limited because of their low-sensitivities
	Colposcopy	Not applicable	Moderate/low	
	Visual inspection	Not applicable	Low/low	Highly dependent on sampling and tissue preservation
Detection of HPV proteins	Immunocito/histochemistry[a]	Low/high	Low/low	
		Low/high	Low/low	Cannot type HPV
	Electron microscopy[a]	Low/high	Low/moderate	
	Western blots[a]			
Detection of HPV genomes				
Direct methods	Southern blot[a,b]	Moderate/high	Moderate/high	
	ISH[a,b]	Moderate/moderate	Moderate/moderate	
	Dot blot	Low/high	Low/high	
Signal amplification	HC[c,d,e]	High/high	High/high	
Target amplification	PCR[c,d,e]	High/high	Very high-high/high-moderate	
	Real-time PCR[d,e]	Very high/high	Very high[f]	
Detection of anti-HPV antibodies				
	ELISA peptides	Low/low	Low/low	
	VLP	Moderate/high	Low/low	
	Fused E6/E7	High/moderate	Low-moderate/high	

[a]Technically cumbersome and/or time-consuming
[b]Requires DNA and tissue preservation
[c]Less dependent on sampling; can be done in crude samples
[d]Suitable for high-throughput testing and automation
[e]Provides viral load information
[f]No data available

avoid cross-contamination, because it does not rely on target amplification to achieve high sensitivity, as do PCR protocols. Often only the high-risk cocktail is used, and this reduces the time and cost of the test. The U.S. Food and Drug Administration recommended cutoff value for test-positive results is 1.0 relative light unit (equivalent to 1 pg HPV DNA per 1 ml of sampling buffer).

A newly developed HC assay uses RNA probes as in HC2, but has been developed to be used in low-resource settings (*careHPV*, QIAGEN NV). It is designed to be a rapid test, able to detect 14 HPV types in about 2.5 h,

and can be performed outside a specialized laboratory by staff with minimal training. The ability of the *careHPV* test to detect premalignant lesions was found to be 90% in a large study conducted in the rural area of China (Qiao et al., 2008).

The sensitivity and specificity of *PCR-based methods* can vary, depending mainly on the primer set, the size of the PCR product, the reaction conditions and performance of the DNA polymerase used in the reaction, the spectrum of HPV types amplified and the ability to detect multiple types, and the availability of a type-specific assay. PCR can theoretically produce one billion copies from a single double-stranded DNA molecule after 30 cycles of amplification. Therefore, care must be taken to avoid false-positive results derived from cross-contaminated specimens or reagents. Several procedures are available to avoid this potential problem in using PCR protocols for HPV DNA detection.

The most widely used PCR protocols employ consensus primers that are directed to a highly conserved region of the L1 gene, since they are potentially capable of detecting all mucosal HPV types. Among these are the single pair of consensus primers GP5/6 and its extended version GP5+/6+ (de Roda Husman et al., 1995; Jacobs et al., 1995) as well as the MY09/11 degenerate primers and its modified version, PGMY09/11 (Gravitt et al., 2000). Full distinction of more than 40 types can be achieved by hybridization with type-specific probes that can be performed in different formats, and restriction fragment length polymorphism analysis by gel electrophoresis (Bernard et al., 1994), dot blot hybridization, line strip assays, and microtiter plates that are amenable to automation. Recent developments include the Amplicor HPV test kit (Roche Diagnostics, CA, USA) designed to amplify with non-degenerate primers a short fragment (170 bp) of the L1 gene of 13 high-risk genotypes. A PCR-based linear array HPV product, which exploits the pGMY09/11 amplification system and is capable of identifying 37 HPV genotypes, including all high- and low-risk genotypes in the human anogenital region, is also commercially available (Linear Array HPV Genotyping Test, Roche Diagnostics).

Another pair of consensus primers is available that amplifies a smaller fragment (65 bp compared to 150 bp for the GP primers and 450 bp for MY09/11) of the L1 gene. This short PCR fragment (SPF)-PCR is designed to discriminate between a broad spectrum of HPVs in a reverse line blot hybridization (LiPA) (Kleter et al., 1999). Tests that rely on shorter fragments of the viral genome are considered to be more sensitive and amenable for less-preserved specimens. The SPF and GP5+/6+ systems are widely used in epidemiological studies and have being adapted to formats amenable for high-throughput testing. A fast and reliable HPV typing method has been developed using nonradioactive reverse line blotting (RLB) of GP5+/6+ PCR-amplified HPV genotypes. In this way 40 HPV-positive clinical samples can be simultaneously typed for 37 HPV types (14 HR and 23 LR types) (van den Brule et al., 2002).

Recently, PCR protocols based on a 5'-exonuclease assay and real-time detection of the accumulation of fluorescence were developed and named real-time PCR. Compared to other assays, such as HC, this is considered to be an accurate method of estimating viral load, while controlling for variation in the cellular content of the sample by quantification of a nuclear gene. Several studies have shown that the risk of developing cervical neoplasia is associated with higher copy numbers of different HPV types (Gravitt et al., 2003; Moberg et al., 2004; Schlecht et al., 2003). However, there are inherent differences in the assays to determine viral load that could obscure the interpretation and clinical relevance of the results obtained. Further studies to evaluate the clinical relevance of viral load are warranted.

Testing for the presence of more than one HPV type in the biological specimen is preferentially done by PCR-based methods, since HC2 does not discriminate between HPV types. In general, it seems that PCR systems using multiple primers such as PGMY09/11 and SPF-PCR are more robust for detecting multiple infections than systems using single consensus primers such as GP5+/6+. This may especially be true in cases of mixed infections where one type is present in large amounts, but all types present could be identified by very sensitive reverse line blot assays or linear arrays, as described above.

2.3   HPV RNA Methods

HPV RNA is being considered as an important target for the molecular diagnosis of HPV infections. Testing for viral RNA aims to evaluate the HPV genome expression (and hence their activity in the infected cells), unlike HPV DNA assays that detect only the presence of viral genomes. The rationale is that the presence of transcripts of the HPV oncogenes E6 and E7 is a more accurate and specific marker of cells at risk or already transformed by high-risk HPVs. HPV 16 E6 and E7 transcripts can be detected with high sensitivity in clinical specimens by employing PCR-based methods including reverse transcriptase PCR (RT-PCR) (Sotlar et al., 1998), quantitative RT-PCR, and real-time PCR (Lamarcq et al., 2002). Recent studies have shown that testing for E6/E7 transcripts of HPV types 16, 18, 31, 33, and 45 with an RNA-based real-time nucleic acid sequence-based amplification assay (NASBA; PreTect HPV-Proofer; Norchip, Norway) was more specific in detecting individuals that developed high-grade cervical disease than HPV DNA detection by PCR with GP5+/6+ consensus primers (Molden et al., 2005). Moreover, detection of such oncogenic transcripts identified which HPV high-risk infections persisted without having to perform repeat testing (Cuschieri et al., 2004). Another important application for HPV RNA studies has been suggested by Klaes et al. (1999), who developed a method (*APOT*, amplification of papillomavirus oncogene transcripts) to differentiate between episomal and integrated HPV oncogene transcripts. The rationale behind this method is that in cervical cancers HPV genomes are often integrated into the host chromosomes, while in normal and premalignant tissues the viral DNA is usually kept as episomes. Using this assay, they were able to show a strong correlation between detection of integrated high-risk HPV transcripts and presence of high-grade cervical neoplasia. The main problem with these techniques is that RNA is a much more labile molecule than DNA, and therefore less available in most biological specimens depending on the time and type of storage conditions. Therefore, there is great interest in collection media capable of preserving both DNA and RNA molecules. These include collection media which contain methanol, shown to preserve both the cell morphology and integrity of DNA, RNA, and proteins (Cuschieri et al., 2005; Nonogaki et al., 2004).

2.4 Serological Assays

At present there is no agreed standard methodology for serological assays that measure antibody acquired in a present or past HPV infection, although virtually all reported studies employ enzyme immunoassays (Konya and Dillner, 2001). Before neutralizing antibody assays were made available (Pastrana et al., 2004), most serological assays were type-specific HPV VLP ELISA (Carter et al., 2001). More recently, an automated multiplex assay based on the use of Luminex beads was developed for the detection of different serotypes with the same sensitivity and specificity achieved in the single-type assays (Dias et al., 2005).

Standardized methodologies that measure total serum antibody, neutralizing antibody, and type-specific antibody concentrations will be necessary. Not all of these assays will be routine, but if and when employed they must be standard and consistent. These assays will require the establishment of an International Standard(s) with an arbitrarily assigned unit measure or international units (IU). These issues were recognized by the World Health Organization (WHO), who established collaborative studies to evaluate reference reagents for type-specific HPV serologic assays (http://whqlibdoc.who.int/hq/2004/WHO_IVB_04.22.pdf and Ferguson et al., 2006). Importantly, about half of the individuals exposed to HPV never develop measurable titers of antibodies, although this scenario will change drastically as HPV prophylactic vaccination is implemented in different areas around the world. This information is and will be predominantly known in women, which underscores the need to better understand the natural course of HPV infection and corresponding immune responses to HPV in men (Svare et al., 1997).

It is very important to stress that the analytical sensitivities and specificities of HPV tests vary largely, depending on the assay characteristics, the type and quality of the biological specimen, and the type and quality of the reagents employed, including the use of different DNA polymerases that affect test performance. Moreover, caution should be used to interpret such comparisons, because the assays differ in their ability to detect different HPV types either as single or multiple infections. In general, there are good to excellent agreement rates between tests performed with HC2 and generic-PCR employing MY09/11 and GP5+/6+ systems. This emphasizes the availability of several robust HPV tests. Nevertheless, standardized methods and validated protocols, reagents, and reference samples should be available to assure the best test performance in different settings.

Although the analytical sensitivities of some HPV detection assays can be very high, and therefore valuable for addressing the burden of HPV infections epidemiologically, their corresponding clinical significance is not so evident (Snijders et al., 2003). This is because several HPV infections do not persist and therefore do not lead to clinically relevant disease. Anogenital HPV infections are very common in young, sexually active populations, including both women and men. However, in the latter, the natural history of persistence and disease development is largely unknown.

2

2.5 Detecting HPV Infection in Men

Results from different studies of HPV infections in men are not always consistent and vary considerably according to the anatomical site sampled, the type of collection, and the HPV DNA test used to ascertain HPV presence and type (Baldwin et al., 2003; Dunne et al., 2006; Giuliano et al., 2008b, c; Nielson et al., 2007). Among a series of clinical and histopathological techniques, PCR has emerged as the most sensitive method to define HPV infection in men. Indeed, this is the methodology being used in large cohort studies of the natural history of HPV infection and risk of neoplasia in men (Giuliano et al., 2008a; Svare et al., 2002) (see also Chaps. 1, 5, and 6).

Specimen Collection Site: Single and multiple anatomical sites of the male genitalia are often sampled. They include the penile shaft, coronal sulcus/glans (including the prepuce in uncircumcised men), scrotum, urethra, as well as urine and semen (Aguilar et al., 2006; Benevolo et al., 2008; Fife et al., 2003; Giuliano et al., 2008a; Nielson et al., 2007). It has been shown that specimens from the urethra and semen contribute little toward the analysis of HPV DNA prevalence and that specimens should be collected from the shaft, glans, and scrotum in a combined sample (Giuliano et al., 2007).

Collection Method: Another most important aspect when analyzing HPV infection in men is the variability attributable to the collection method. Several methods to obtain samples from the male genitalia have been described. They include the removal of exfoliated cells from the penis surface either by direct scraping with a swab or brush (dry or pre-wetted in saline) (see also Sect. 3.5 in Chap. 3) or by first abrading the skin with a nail file followed by removal of cells with a swab (Weaver et al., 2004). This in fact is the method that is being applied to collect cells from the penis of men included in a large clinical trial for the quadrivalent HPV L1 VLP prophylactic vaccine (Giuliano, 2007). Recently, a systematic study has shown that skin cells exfoliated with a swab can be used reliably for HPV testing (Flores et al., 2008). Moreover, HPV prevalence results obtained from self-collected samples in men show good agreement with clinician-collected samples, which may be considered a suitable alternative for studies on HPV transmission (Hernandez et al., 2006; Ogilvie et al., 2008).

In summary, several methods to detect HPV infections are available. The choice of a particular method is very much dependent on its analytical as well as its clinical sensitivities and specificities. In the male genitalia, HPV detection is further complicated by the low amount of DNA obtained from exfoliated skin cells, which highlights the importance of validating the collection and detection method of choice. There are sufficient and validated tools for performing studies of anogenital HPV infections in men, and results are rapidly accumulating. This experience should contribute to accelerate our knowledge about the natural history of HPV infection and risk of anogenital disease in men.

References

Aguilar LV, Lazcano-Ponce E, Vaccarella S (2006) Human papillomavirus in men: Comparison of different genital sites. Sex Transm Infect 82(1): 31–33

Baldwin SB, Wallace DR, Papenfuss MR, et al. (2003) Human papillomavirus infection in men attending a sexually transmitted disease clinic. J Infect Dis 187(7): 1064–1070

Benevolo M, Mottolese M, Marandino F, et al. (2008) HPV prevalence among healthy Italian male sexual partners of women with cervical HPV infection. J Med Virol 80(7): 1275–1281

Bernard H, Chan S, Manos MM, et al. (1994) Identification and assessment of known and novel human papillomavirus by polymerase chain reaction amplification, restriction fragment polymorphisms, nucleotide sequence, and phylogeny algorithms. J Infect Dis 170: 1077–1085

Bosch FX, Burchell AN, Schiffman M, et al. (2008) Epidemiology and natural history of human papillomavirus infections and type-specific implications in cervical neoplasia. Vaccine 26 (Suppl 10): K1–K16

Carter JJ, Madeleine MM, Shera K, et al. (2001) Human papillomavirus 16 and 18 L1 serology compared across anogenital cancer sites. Cancer Res 61(5): 1934–1940

Cuschieri KS, Beattie G, Hassan S, et al. (2005) Assessment of human papillomavirus mRNA detection over time in cervical specimens collected in liquid based cytology medium. J Virol Methods 124: 211–215

Cuschieri KS, Whitley MJ, Cubie H (2004) Human papillomavirus type specific DNA and RNA persistence – implications for cervical disease progression and monitoring. J Med Virol 73: 65–70

de Roda Husman AM, Snijders PJ, Stel HV, et al. (1995) Processing of long-stored archival cervical smears for human papillomavirus detection by the polymerase chain reaction. Br J Cancer 72: 412–417

Dias D, Van Doren J, Schlottmann S, et al. (2005) Optimization and validation of a multiplexed luminex assay to quantify antibodies to neutralizing epitopes on human papillomaviruses 6, 11, 16, and 18. Clin Diagn Lab Immunol 12(8): 959–969

Dunne EF, Nielson CM, Stone KM, et al. (2006) Prevalence of HPV infection among men: A systematic review of the literature. J Infect Dis 194(8): 1044–1057

Ferguson M, Heath A, Johnes S, et al., Collaborative Study Participants (2006) Results of the first WHO international collaborative study on the standardization of the detection of antibodies to human papillomaviruses. Int J Cancer 118(6): 1508–1514

Fife KH, Coplan PM, Jansen KU, et al. (2003) Poor sensitivity of polymerase chain reaction assays of genital skin swabs and urine to detect HPV 6 and 11 DNA in men. Sex Transm Dis 30(3): 246–248

Flores R, Abalos AT, Nielson CM, et al. (2008) Reliability of sample collection and laboratory testing for HPV detection in men. J Virol Methods 149(1): 136–143

Giuliano AR (2007) Human papillomavirus vaccination in males. Gynecol Oncol 107(2 Suppl 1): S24–S26

Giuliano AR, Lazcano-Ponce E, Villa LL, et al. (2008a) The human papillomavirus infection in men study: Human papillomavirus prevalence and type distribution among men residing in Brazil, Mexico, and the United States. Cancer Epidemiol Biomarkers Prev 17(8): 2036–2043

Giuliano AR, Lu B, Nielson CM, et al. (2008b) Age-specific prevalence, incidence, and duration of human papillomavirus infections in a cohort of 290 US men. J Infect Dis 198(6): 827–835

Giuliano AR, Nielson CM, Flores R, et al. (2007) The optimal anatomic sites for sampling heterosexual men for human papillomavirus (HPV) detection: The HPV detection in men study. J Infect Dis 196(8): 1146–1152

Giuliano AR, Tortolero-Luna G, Ferrer E, et al. (2008c) Epidemiology of human papillomavirus infection in men, cancers other than cervical and benign conditions. Vaccine 26(Suppl 10): K17–K28

Gravitt PE, Peyton C, Wheeler C, et al. (2003) Reproducibility of HPV 16 and HPV 18 viral load quantitation using TaqMan real-time PCR assays. J Virol Methods 112(1–2): 23–33

Gravitt PE, Peyton CL, Alessi TQ, et al. (2000) Improved amplification of genital human papillomaviruses. J Clin Microbiol 38: 357–361

Hernandez BY, McDuffie K, Goodman MT, et al. (2006) Comparison of physician- and self-collected genital specimens for detection of human papillomavirus in men. J Clin Microbiol 44(2): 513–517

Iftner T, Villa LL (2003) Chapter 12: Human papillomavirus technologies. J Natl Cancer Inst Monogr 31: 80–88

Jacobs MV, de Roda Husman AM, van den Brule AJ, et al. (1995) Group-specific differentiation between high- and low-risk human papillomavirus genotypes by general primer-mediated PCR and two cocktails of oligonucleotide probes. J Clin Microbiol 33: 901–905

Klaes R, Woerner SM, Ridder R, et al. (1999) Detection of high-risk cervical intraepithelial neoplasia and cervical cancer by amplification of transcripts derived from integrated papillomavirus oncogenes Cancer Res 59(24): 6312–6316

Kleter B, van Doorn LJ, Schrauwen L, et al. (1999) Development and clinical evaluation of a highly sensitive PCR-reverse hybridization line probe assay for detection and identification of anogenital human papillomavirus. J Clin Microbiol 37: 2508–2517

Konya J, Dillner J (2001) Immunity to oncogenic human papillomaviruses. Adv Cancer Res 82: 205–238

Lamarcq L, Deeds J, Ginzinger D, et al. (2002) Measurements of human papillomavirus transcripts by real time quantitative reverse transcription-polymerase chain reaction in samples collected for cervical cancer screening. J Mol Diagn 4(2): 97–102

Lorincz A, Anthony J, (2001) Advances in HPV detection by hybrid capture. Papillomavirus Rep 145: 154

Moberg M, Gustavsson I, Gyllensten U (2004) Type-specific associations of human papillomavirus load with of developing cervical carcinoma in situ. Intl J Cancer 112(5): 854–859

Molden T, Kraus I, Skomedal H, et al. (2005) Comparison of human papillomavirus messenger RNA and DNA detection: A cross-sectional study of 4,136 women >30 years of age with a 2-year follow-up of high-grade squamous intraepithelial lesion. Cancer Epidemiol Biomarkers Prev 14(2): 367–373

Nielson CM, Flores R, Harris RB, et al. (2007) Human papillomavirus prevalence and type distribution in male anogenital sites and semen. Cancer Epidemiol Biomarkers Prev 16(6): 1107–1114

Nonogaki S, Wakamatsu A, Longatto Filho A, et al. (2004) Hybrid capture II and polymerase chain reaction for identifying HPV infections in samples collected in a new collection medium. A comparison. Acta Cytol 48(4): 514–520

Nuovo GJ, Moritz J, Walsh LL, et al. (1992) Predictive value of human papillomavirus DNA detection by filter hybridization and polymerase chain reaction in women with negative results of colposcopic examination. Anatom Pathol 98(5): 489–492

Ogilvie G, Taylor D, Krajden M, et al. (2008) Self collection of genital human papillomavirus in heterosexual men. Sex Transm Infect Dec 9 [Epub ahead of print]

Partridge JM, Koutsky LA (2006) Genital human papillomavirus infection in men. Lancet Infect Dis 6(1): 21–31

Pastrana DV, Buck CB, Pang YY, et al. (2004) Reactivity of human sera in a sensitive, high-throughput pseudovirus-based papillomavirus neutralization assay for HPV16 and HPV18. Virology 321(2): 205–216

Qiao YL, Sellors JW, Eder PS, Bao YP, Lim JM, Zhao FH, Weigl B, Zhang WH, Peck RB, Li L, Chen F, Pan QJ, Lorincz AT (2008) A new HPV-DNA test for cervical cancer screening in developing regions: A cross sectional study of clinical accuracy in rural China. Lancet Oncology 9(10): 926–936

Schlecht N, Trevisan A, Duarte-Franco E, et al. (2003) Viral load as a predictor of the risk of cervical intraepithelial neoplasia. Int J Cancer 103: 519–524

Snijders PJ, van den Brule AJ, Meijer CJ (2003) The clinical relevance of human papillomavirus testing: relationship between analytical and clinical sensitivity. J Pathol 1(1): 1–6

Sotlar K, Selinka H-C, Menton M, et al. (1998) Detection of human papillomavirus type 16 E6/E7 oncogene transcripts in dysplastic and nondysplastic cervical scrapes by nested RT-PCR. Gynecol Oncol 69: 114–121

Stoler MH, Wolinsky SM, Whitbeck A, et al. (1997) Differentiation-linked human papillomavirus types 6 and 11 transcription in genital condylomata revealed by in situ hybridization with message-specific RNA probes. Virology 172: 331–340

Svare EI, Kjaer SK, Nonnenmacher B, et al. (1997) Seroreactivity to human papillomavirus type 16 virus-like particles is lower in high-risk men than in high-risk women. J Infect Dis 176(4): 876–883

Svare EI, Kjaer SK, Worm AM, et al. (2002) Risk factors for genital HPV DNA in men resemble those found in women: a study of male attendees at a Danish STD clinic. Sex Transm Infect 78(3): 215–218

Van den Brule AJ, Pol R, Fransen-Daalmeijer N, Schouls LM, et al. (2002) GP5+/6 PCR followed by reverse line blot analysis enables rapid and high-throughput identification of human papillomavirus genotypes. J Clin Microbiol 40(3): 779–787

Weaver BA, Feng Q, Holmes KK, et al. (2004) Evaluation of genital sites and sampling techniques for detection of human papillomavirus DNA in men. J Infect Dis 189(4): 677–685

Human Papillomavirus and External Genital Lesions

3

Alberto Rosenblatt and Homero Gustavo de Campos Guidi

Contents

3.1 Introduction

Genital lesions associated with human papillomavirus (HPV) infection affect children and adults of both genders and are a medical problem worldwide.

According to Fleischer et al. (2001), obstetricians/ gynecologists, urologists, and dermatologists are the specialists most involved with the disease and the ones that HPV-infected patients usually seek for counseling and treatment. Because of the increasing number of individuals that are being infected by the virus and the burden inflicted by the disease, it is imperative that every medical practitioner and particularly specialists in these fields acquire the necessary expertise in the management of HPV.

This chapter discusses the management of subclinical infection and clinical disease, including novel therapeutic options for HPV-related external genital lesions. In addition, it reviews current concepts regarding

A. Rosenblatt (✉)
Albert Einstein Jewish Hospital, Sao Paulo, Brasil
e-mail: albrose1@gmail.com

A. Rosenblatt, H. G. de Campos Guidi, *Human Papillomavirus*,
DOI: 10.1007/978-3-540-70974-9-3, © Springer-Verlag Berlin Heidelberg 2009

circumcision and HPV infection, as well as preventive measures against the disease (see also Chap. 11).

3.2 Overview

Although HPV infection in the male population has not received as much attention as in its female counterpart, Weaver et al. (2004) reported that both genders have similar infection rates.

Furthermore, young male and female adults are most likely to seek medical treatment for the disease, mainly because of the stigma attached to a sexually transmitted disease (STD) (Koshiol et al., 2004; Insinga et al., 2003).

HPVs are classified as the Papillomaviridae family and approximately 200 different HPV types have currently been identified. According to their tissue tropism, HPVs can be also subdivided into mucosatropic and cutaneotropic, with a predilection for squamous epithelial cells rather than columnar, cuboidal, or transitional epithelial cells (Gillison and Shah, 2003).

HPV infection occurs by direct inoculation of the virus into the epidermal layers, and skin trauma may play an important role, causing epithelial microdefects that facilitate virus invasion (Mansur, 2002).

Following invasion, the virus undergoes a variable period of latency with limited viral DNA replication occurring in the basal layers of the epithelium. Expression of HPV nonstructural proteins (E6 and E7) delays cell-cycle arrest and differentiation, causing epithelial cells to proliferate. The ensuing process will then result in the production of a clinically apparent lesion (Doorbar and Sterling, 2001).

As the virus migrates into differentiating keratinocytes, HPV DNA replication is amplified, with final virus assembly occurring in the superficial squames. Highly infectious virions are then shed into the environment and viremia is nonexistent, since only superficial epithelial cells are infected (Tseng et al., 1999) (Fig. 3.1) (see also Sect. 9.3 in Chap. 9 and Sect. 11.3 in Chap. 11).

According to Gonçalves and Donadi (2004), viral activity is likely to depend on the host immune status. In immunocompetent patients, most genital HPV infections are cleared spontaneously by the body's defenses through a cell-mediated immune mechanism (see also Chap. 9).

HPV infection is thought to be acquired predominantly through sexual contact in adolescents and adults, although transmission by nonsexual routes is possible

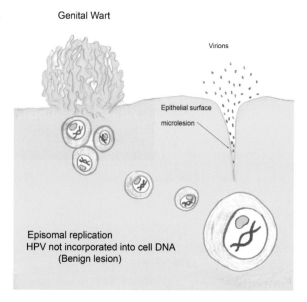

Fig. 3.1. Schematic representation of HPV-related benign lesion formation

and was described by Pao et al. (1993), Tay et al. (1990), and Sonnex et al. (1999) (see also Sect. 1.6 in Chap. 1).

HPV type-specific concordance between specimens obtained from heterosexually active couples occurs often and confirms the contagious nature of the disease (Baken et al., 1995; Bleeker et al., 2005a; Giovannelli et al., 2007; Hernandez et al., 2008b).

Moreover, Brown et al. (1999b) estimated the infectivity rate between sexual partners at 60%, although Van Doornum et al. (1994) reported that men have fewer persistent infections than women. Available data from a study of a large group of Finnish male subjects also suggest that spontaneous viral clearance may occur more rapidly in men (Hippelainen et al., 1993).

The prevalence of HPV infection ranges from 2.3 to 34.8% for high-risk types and from 2.3 to 23.9% for low-risk types (Weaver et al., 2004; Lazcano-Ponce et al., 2001; Kataoka et al., 1991; Wikstrom et al., 2000; Franceschi et al., 2002; Baldwin et al., 2003; Lajous et al., 2005). HPV 16 is the most prevalent high-risk type detected, although variability exists among different geographic areas. However, Partridge and Koutsky (2006) reported the possibility of reduced penile skin receptivity toward oncogenic HPV types.

Genital warts are common among sexually active young men, occurring in approximately 1% of the U.S. sexually active group aged 15–49 years.

The peak incidence of genital warts occurs in the 20–24-year age-group and the lifetime cumulative risk of developing genital warts is almost 10%, according to Franco (1996). Moreover, there has been a predominance of low-risk HPV types in several studies that evaluated genital wart HPV typing (Yun and Joblin, 1993; Boxman et al., 1999; Hadjivassiliou et al., 2007), with a U.S. seroprevalence of low-risk HPV 11 estimated at 4.7%. However, since the introduction of the quadrivalent HPV vaccine, genital warts have become a vaccine-preventable disease.

> **Current U.S. Centers for Disease Control (CDC) Recommendation to Patients with Genital Warts (Workowski and Berman, 2007)**
>
> - HPV infection and recurrence are common among sexually active individuals.
> - Incubation period can be long and variable.
> - Duration of infection and methods of prevention are not definitively known.

3.3 Clinical Manifestations

Following contamination, HPV infection may follow one of three paths:

(a) *Latent infection* – The virus remains in a quiescent state, without producing any gross or microscopic evidence of disease (asymptomatic)
(b) *Subclinical infection*
(c) *Clinical disease*

- Asymptomatic
- Symptomatic

Most HPV infections in men are symptomless and unapparent (Mao et al., 2003).

> **Expert Advice**
>
> Persistence (i.e., HPV DNA genes are being detected regularly) and latency (i.e., HPV DNA is detectable although not replicating) are usually synonymous with long-term infections, regardless of symptoms.

3.3.1 Subclinical Infection

3.3.1.1 Presentation

- Normal appearance of skin or mucosa
- Mild hyperemia
- Mucosal fissuring
- Superficial moist desquamation, unpleasant odor and white thick secretion when associated with fungal infection

3.3.1.2 Symptoms

- Mostly asymptomatic
- Pruritus
- Burning sensation and increased skin sensitivity (even to water)
- Dyspareunia

3.3.2 Clinical Disease

Condyloma Acuminatum (Anogenital Warts)

- Incidence – 2.4 cases per 1,000 per year
- Estimated annual incidence in individuals aged 20–24 years – 1.2%, according to Persson et al. (1996)

Condyloma acuminatum is the most common and classical clinical presentation of genital HPV infection (excluding subclinical or latent infection), and 70–100% of exophytic genital warts are usually associated with HPV 6 or HPV 11 infections, with a small risk of malignant transformation (Brown et al., 1999a; Coleman et al., 1994; Greer et al., 1995; Li et al., 1995).

3.3.2.1 Presentation

The classic acuminate condylomata (Fig. 3.2a, b) are pointed, cauliflower-like lesions with a fleshy, vascular appearance, usually found on moist surfaces, although they can also be found outside the genital area.

- The lesions range in size from a few millimeters to several centimeters (Fig. 3.3a, b), and individual warts may coalesce forming large exophytic masses.

Keratotic lesions have a thickened, rough surface and are usually found on dry surfaces, such as the penile shaft (Fig. 3.4).

- Lesions appear as single or multiple well-circumscribed verrucous or keratotic papules and plaques (Fig. 3.5a, b).

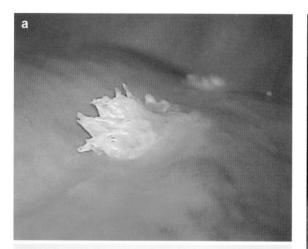

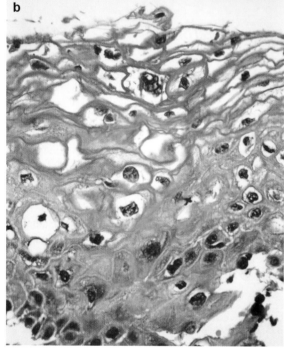

Fig. 3.2. (**a**) Condyloma acuminatum on the penis shaft. (**b**) Viral condyloma acuminatum (histology) (Source: Photograph courtesy of Filomena Marino Carvalho MD, PhD, São Paulo, Brazil)

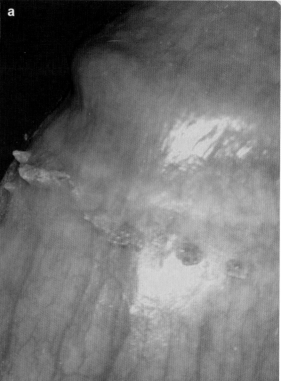

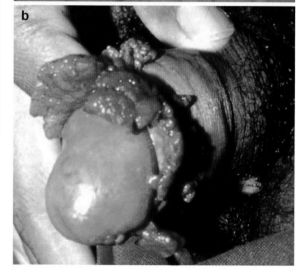

Fig. 3.3. (**a**) Small subcoronal warty lesions. (**b**) Condylomatous lesions around the coronal sulcus

Smooth papular warts are dome-shaped lesions, usually found in relatively dry locations such as the keratotic lesions (Fig. 3.6).

- They may appear in clusters and the color ranges from flesh-colored to pink to reddish-brown.
- When located in the glans penis and coronal sulcus, the nonpigmented papules and small warts are translucent and show a clear vascular punctuation on the top, allowing their distinction from pearly papules (Barrasso and Gross, 1997) (see below Sect. 3.4).

Expert Advice

Condyloma lesions are rare in the glans penis (except in the coronal sulcus) (Fig. 3.7), and occur frequently in immunosuppressed and HIV-infected individuals. In these patients, glans penis lesions are associated with high-risk HPV types (Fig. 3.8a, b) and more aggressive histological findings (Fig. 3.9).

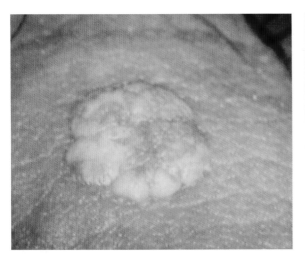

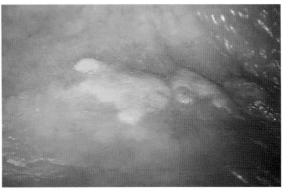

Fig. 3.6. Papular warts located on the penis shaft

Fig. 3.4. Single, well-circumscribed verrucous lesion on the shaft of the penis

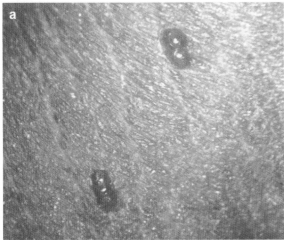

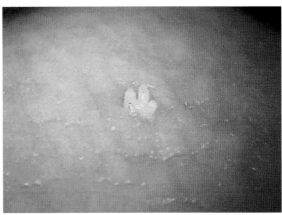

Fig. 3.7. Glove finger-type lesion located on the glans penis

3.3.2.2 Multifocality

HPV-related lesions in the male population can develop anywhere on the penis (Fig. 3.10), urethral meatus (Fig. 3.11), and urethra (see Chap. 4). They can also be found in the pubic area and the inguinal crease (Fig. 3.12), but the scrotum (Fig. 3.13a, b) and perineum are infrequent locations. The perianal area and particularly the intra-anal region is a common location among men who have sex with men (MSM), but non-sexual transmission routes (i.e., finger–genital) are also implicated. Exotic presentations (Fig. 3.14a–c) can also occur, particularly in immunosuppressed patients.

Data from several studies show that the penis shaft harbors most of the HPV DNA detected (Cook et al., 1993; Nielson et al., 2007; Giuliano et al., 2007; Nicolau et al., 2005). However, in a recent analysis

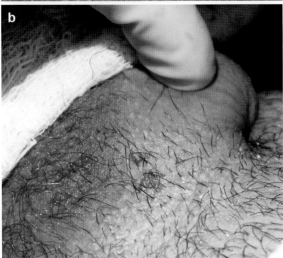

Fig. 3.5. (**a**) Well-circumscribed keratotic shaft papules. (**b**) HPV-related keratotic lesions at the base of the penis

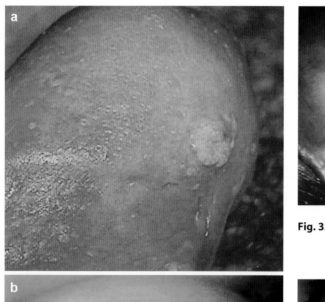

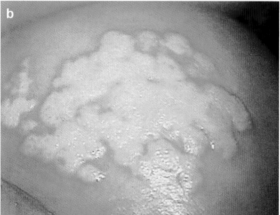

Fig. 3.8. (**a**) Glans papular lesion in HIV-positive patient; virology HPV 16. (**b**) Glans penis lesion in HIV-positive patient; virology HPV 18

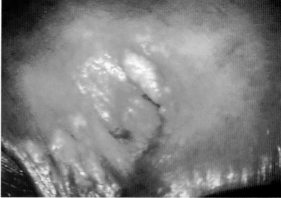

Fig. 3.10. HPV-related lesion in the frenulum recessus

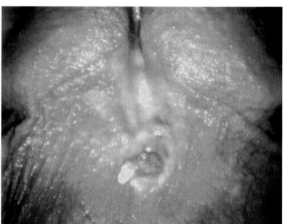

Fig. 3.11. Wart at the hypospadic meatus

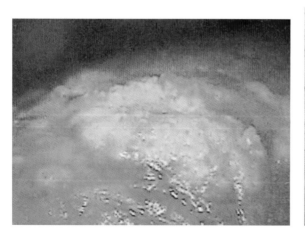

Fig. 3.9. Rapidly progressing glans penis lesion

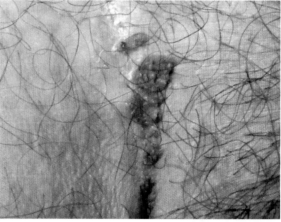

Fig. 3.12. Condyloma acuminatum in the inguinal crease

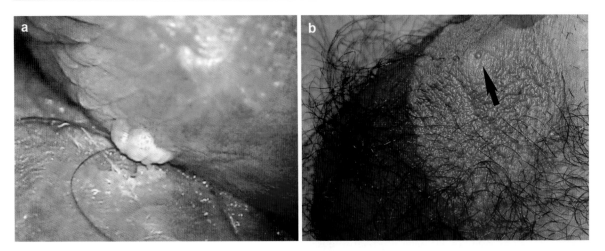

Fig. 3.13. (**a**) "Kissing" lesions (scrotal lesion developing through contact of the HPV-related penis lesion). (**b**) Small, HPV-related, scrotal pigmented papule (*arrow*)

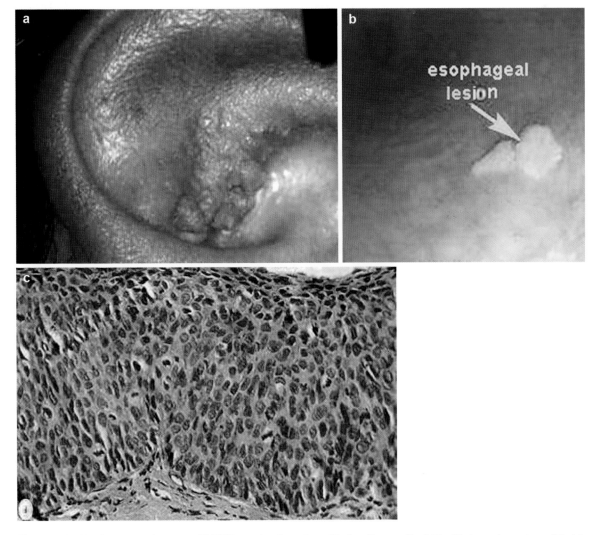

Fig. 3.14. (**a**) Exotic presentation – ear. (**b**) HPV-associated esophageal lesion (Source: Tomishige Photograph courtesy of Toshiro Tomishige MD, PhD, São Paulo, Brazil). (**c**) Esophageal lesion – severe dysplasia (HPV-positive) (Source: Photograph courtesy of Monica Stiepcich MD, PhD, São Paulo, Brazil)

performed on African men by Smith et al. (2007), a high HPV DNA prevalence was detected in the glans/coronal sulcus (39%).

The proximal penile area is a common location of HPV-related lesions among men who routinely use condoms, because the virus can still be transmitted through contact with areas of unprotected genital skin (Fig. 3.15). Besides, microabrasions caused by the friction of the rolled portion of the condom are common at the base of the penis.

In uncircumcised men

- Distal warts are more prevalent.
- The preputial cavity (glans penis, coronal sulcus, inner aspect of the foreskin and frenulum) is particularly affected (Buechner, 2002).

In circumcised men the shaft of the penis is often involved.

Among women, frequent locations are the posterior introitus, the labia majora and minora (Fig. 3.16), and the clitoris. Less common locations are the vagina, cervix, perineum, anus, and urethra.

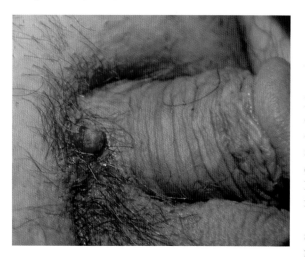

Fig. 3.15. Condyloma located at the base of the penis

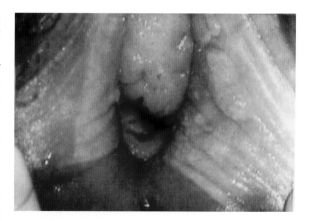

Fig. 3.16. HPV-related vulvar intraepithelial neoplasia 1 (VIN 1). (Source: Photograph courtesy of Nadir Oyakawa, MD, PhD, São Paulo, Brazil)

3.3.2.3 Symptoms

- Often asymptomatic
- Pruritus
- Mild burning
- Bleeding and pain (usually associated with large lesions or secondary infection)

3.3.3 HPV-Related Flat Penile Lesions

Flat condyloma is frequently associated with subclinical infection and this lesion is difficult to detect without special techniques. The clinical findings resemble a chronic inflammatory condition causing intermittent episodes of balanoposthitis, with or without visible flat lesions. However, flat condyloma can also be present in totally asymptomatic individuals.

Bleeker et al. (2005b) recently evaluated the male sexual partners of women with cervical intraepithelial neoplasia (CIN). These individuals presented a higher prevalence of HPV-related flat penile lesions, as well

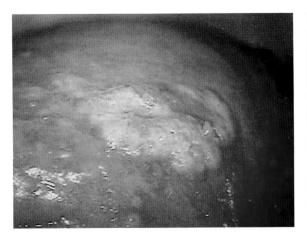

Fig. 3.17. Glans lesion; virology HPV 16

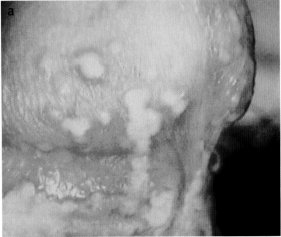

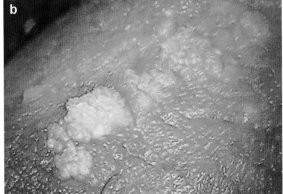

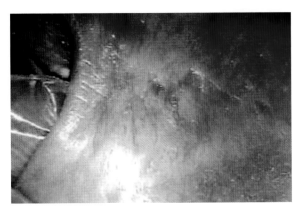

Fig. 3.18. Hyperemic mucosa and fissuring

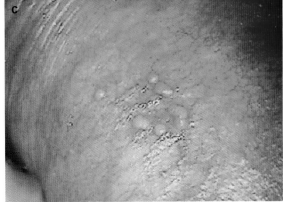

as a larger size of these lesions, when compared with a male population from a non-STD clinic.

Moreover, recent data (Bleeker et al., 2006) have shown that flat penile lesions are usually associated with increased viral copy numbers of particularly high-risk HPV types (Fig. 3.17), and the investigators have further suggested that these lesions contribute to the viral spread.

Fig. 3.19. (**a**) Flat condyloma (glans penis and inner aspect of the foreskin). (**b**) Condyloma and flat condyloma lesions. (**c**) Flat condyloma

3.3.3.1 Presentation

- Normal appearance of the mucosa
- Hyperemia and/or fissuring (Fig. 3.18)
- Visible slightly raised or macular lesions (Fig. 3.19 a–c)

3.3.3.2 Symptoms

- Asymptomatic
- Itching and burning
- Dyspareunia

3

3.4   Differential Diagnosis

3.4.1   Benign Penile Pearly Papules (Hirsutoid Papillomas) (Fig. 3.20)

- Asymptomatic.
- Usually appear at puberty and are present in 20% of young adult males without racial predilection.
- More commonly found in uncircumcised men.
- Flesh-colored or pink papules with rounded tips and discrete bases.
- They are located primarily around the coronal sulcus and presenting one or more rows around this structure ("hirsute corona" (Fig. 3.21a, b)), although also found on the distal penile shaft lateral to the frenulum, or on the posterior aspect of the glans penis.
- Histology shows angiofibroma.
- No treatment is required but reassurance given of benign condition.

3.4.2   Fibroepithelial Polyps (Fig. 3.22)

- Asymptomatic.
- Occasionally inflammatory symptoms secondary to local trauma.
- Soft, skin-colored, pedunculated lesions resembling warts.

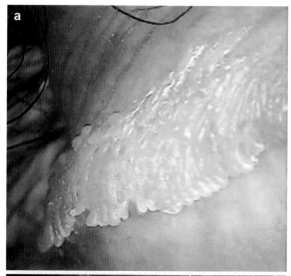

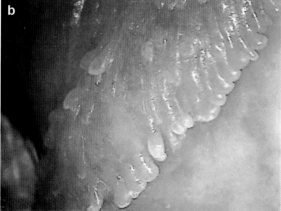

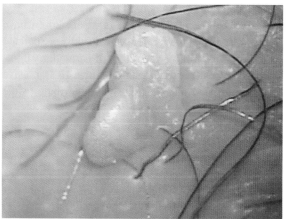

Fig. 3.21. (**a**) Large and exuberant pearly papules around coronal sulcus (**b**) detail of "hirsute corona"

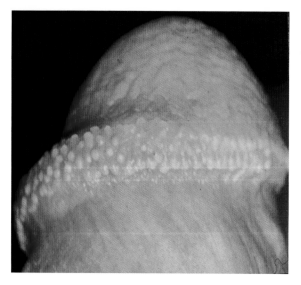

Fig. 3.20. Pearly papules

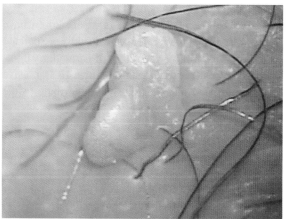

Fig. 3.22. Fibroepithelioma

- No treatment is required but reassurance given of benign condition.
- Excision is indicated if lesion is subjected to frequent trauma.

3.4.3 Prominent Sebaceous Glands (Ectopic Sebaceous Glands, Fordyce Spots) (Fig. 3.23)

- Asymptomatic
- Small, raised, flesh-colored-to-yellow papules with a smooth surface located on the shaft of the penis
- No treatment required

3.4.4 Sebaceous Glands (Fig. 3.24)

- Asymptomatic
- Large, normal sebaceous glands usually located on the proximal third of the penile shaft, especially on the ventral surface
- No treatment required

3.4.5 Seborrheic Keratoses (Fig. 3.25a, b)

- Asymptomatic.
- Usually appears in individuals older than 30 years of age.
- Brown macules, plaques, and papules that may be confused with warts or even melanoma when hyperpigmented (Pierson et al., 2003).
- Waxy, "stuck-on" appearance; sometimes lesions may drop off spontaneously and reappear.
- Usually no treatment required but excision or destruction with liquid nitrogen can be performed for cosmetic reasons.

3.4.6 Angiokeratoma (Fordyce Angiokeratoma) (Fig. 3.26a–c)

- Asymptomatic.
- Small, blue-to-red papules, usually located on the scrotum, shaft of penis, or lower abdomen; glans can occasionally be affected.

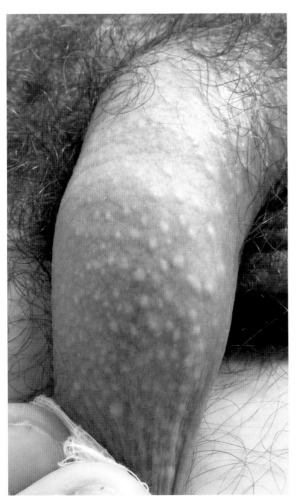

Fig. 3.23. Fordyce spots

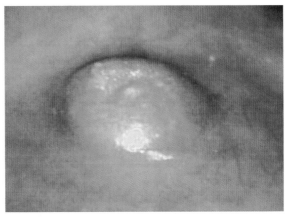

Fig. 3.24. Sebaceous glands of the penis shaft mimicking molluscum contagiosum

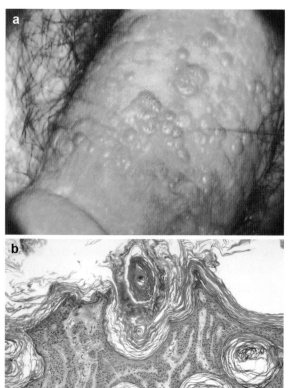

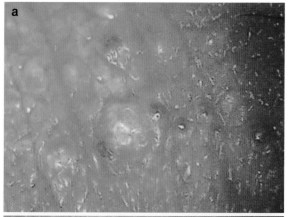

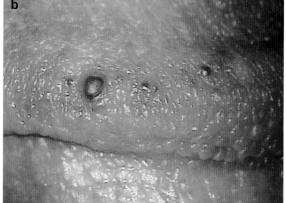

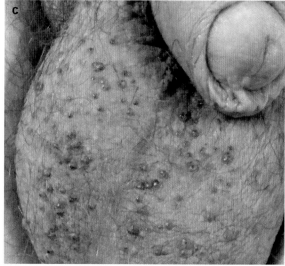

Fig. 3.25. (**a**) Seborrheic keratoses mimicking genital warts. (**b**) Seborrheic keratoses (histology) (Source: Photograph courtesy of Filomena Marino Carvalho MD, PhD, São Paulo, Brazil)

- Histology shows ectatic thin-walled vessels in the superficial dermis with overlying epidermal hyperplasia.
- No treatment required.

3.4.7   Verrucous Epidermal Nevi and Pigmented Nevi *(Fig. 3.27 a–d)*

- Verrucous epidermal nevi typically occur at birth or infancy, but in rare occasions lesions develop at puberty.
- Single or multiple warty papules of any size that coalesce to form well-defined keratotic plaques usually in a linear fashion.
- Extragenital location is usual but lesions have been described in the perianal area (Bandyopadhyay and Sen, 2003) and penis (Narang and Kanwar, 2006).

Fig. 3.26. (**a**) Angiokeratoma of the penis shaft. (**b**) Angiokeratoma of the glans. (**c**) Angiokeratoma of the scrotum

- Histology shows circumscribed hamartomatous lesions composed almost exclusively of keratinocytes.
- No treatment required.

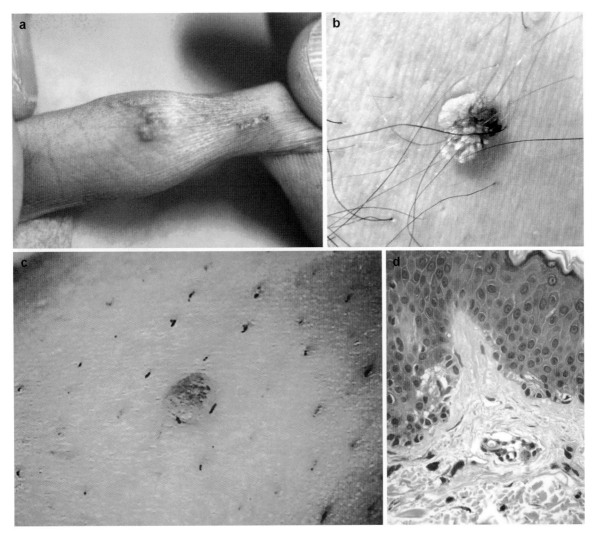

Fig. 3.27. (**a**) Verrucous epidermal nevus. (Source: Narang and Kanwar (2006). Reproduced with permission from Medknow Publications). (**b**) Verrucous nevus in the pubic area. (**c**) Pigmented nevus mimicking wart. (**d**) Nevus (histology) (Source: Photograph courtesy of Filomena Marino Carvalho MD, PhD, São Paulo, Brazil)

3.4.8 Molluscum Contagiosum (Fig. 3.28 a, b)

- Increasing prevalence in young adults.
- Can be initially confused with folliculitis and furunculosis.
- Asymptomatic or discrete pruritus.
- Firm, flesh-colored, dome-shaped papules with classic central umbilication in the majority of cases.
- Usually located in the pubic area, penile shaft, proximal and medial thighs.
- A waxy central core (rich in viral particles) is extracted when the lesion is incised.
- Tzanck smear is a useful diagnostic method.
- Spontaneous resolution is frequent.
- Treatment with lesion destruction is indicated to reduce transmission.

Expert Advice

Cryptococcosis in HIV/AIDS patients may produce lesions that mimic those of molluscum contagiosum. Therefore, biopsy is recommended in these patients.

3.4.9 Lichen Nitidus

- Inflammatory condition (granulomatous nodules).
- Penis is preferentially affected.

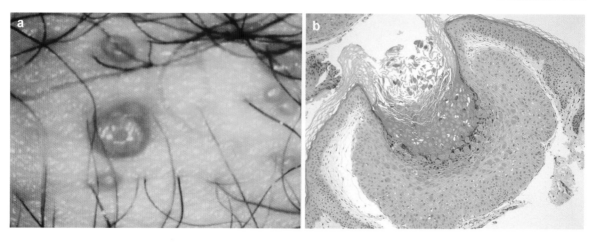

Fig. 3.28. (**a**) Molluscum contagiosum. (**b**) Molluscum contagiosum (histology) (Source: Photograph courtesy of Filomena Marino Carvalho MD, PhD, São Paulo, Brazil)

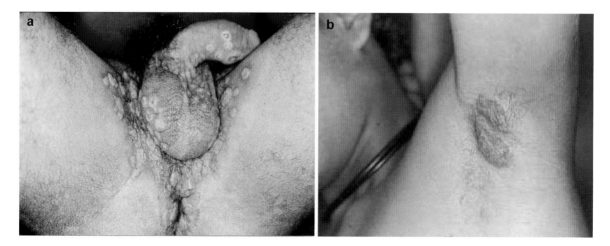

Fig. 3.29. (**a**) Syphilitic condylomata lata. (**b**) Syphilitic condylomata lata in the axilla

- Pruritus may be present.
- Follicular-like pattern with a regular distribution, shiny papules smaller than 1–2 mm, skin-colored to pink, dome shaped.

3.4.10 Syphilitic Condylomata Lata
(Fig. 3.29 a, b)

- Characteristic lesions of secondary syphilis
- Moist, raised nodules or plaques, often seen in warm, moist areas such as the buttocks, genitals, and upper thighs

- Highly infectious
- Distinguished by darkfield microscopy or serology

3.4.11 Verrucous carcinoma (Buschke-Löwenstein tumor)

Verrucous carcinoma (giant condylomata or Buschke-Löwenstein tumor) (Fig. 3.30) is considered a penile neoplastic lesion with a locally invasive behavior and it is usually associated with high-risk HPV 16.

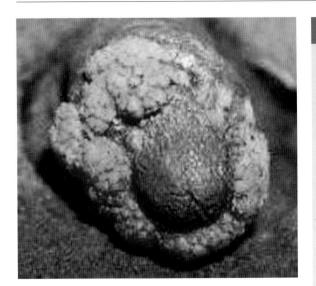

Fig. 3.30. Verrucous carcinoma (Buschke-Löwenstein tumor)

3.4.12 Squamous Intraepithelial Lesions (SILs)/ Penile Intraepithelial Neoplasia (PIN)/ Penile Squamous Cell Carcinomas (SCCs)

See Chap. 5, 6.

3.5 Detection Methods

3.5.1 Clinical Diagnosis

3.5.1.1 Physical Examination

Anogenital warts are primarily diagnosed by their characteristic appearance on clinical examination.

3.5.1.2 Acetic Acid Solution Test (Acetowhite Test)

The acetowhite test is associated with a high number of false-negative and false-positive results (Mansur, 2002). False-positive results are common when coexisting inflammatory conditions are present (i.e., candidiasis) (Fig. 3.31 a, b).

The acetowhite test sensitivity for hyperplastic warts is very high, but for pigmented papules the test sensitivity is very low.

Detection of unapparent subclinical HPV-infected areas using the acetowhite test is not simple (Kumar and Gupta, 2001); however, according to the CDC treatment guidelines (Workowski and Berman, 2007), the acetowhite test can be useful for identifying flat genital warts (Fig. 3.32 a, b).

3

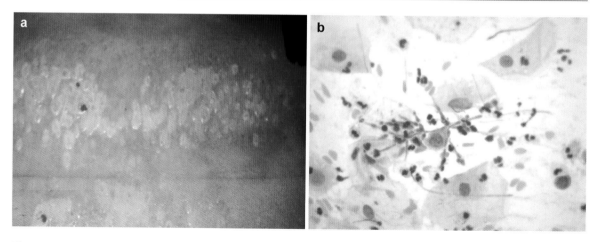

Fig. 3.31. (**a**) Candidal balanitis. (**b**) Candidal balanitis (histology). (Source: Photograph courtesy of Filomena Marino Carvalho MD, PhD, São Paulo, Brazil)

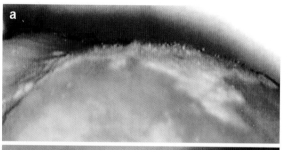

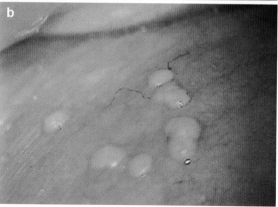

Fig. 3.32. (**a**) Flat condyloma (after acetowhite test). (**b**) Flat lesions after acetowhite test

How to Perform the Acetowhite Test

The warts and adjacent normal penile skin/mucosa (as well as scrotal, perineal, and perianal area) are wrapped in gauze soaked in 5% acetic acid solution for about 3–5 min (Fig. 3.33).

The whole area is subsequently examined with a magnifying hand lens or microscope/colposcope (between 8× and 40×) (Fig. 3.34 a–c).

- Highlighted HPV-related lesions develop a white color (Fig. 3.35 a–c), which is attributed to an overexpression of cytokeratin 10 in the HPV-infected suprabasal cells. These are undifferentiated cells rich in protein content and the whitening might be caused by protein denaturation.
- HPV lesions often exhibit well-demarcated punctuated capillary patterns.
- Acetowhite test in inflammatory conditions (i.e., Candida infection) usually presents with a more irregular and diffuse pattern (Fig. 3.31a).

Expert Advice

Although the acetowhite test is not recommended for screening purposes, it is useful for:

- Visualizing subclinical HPV-related anogenital lesions
- Identifying lesions for targeted biopsy
- Demarcating lesions during surgical therapy (Hadway et al., 2006; Bandieramonte et al., 2008)

See also Sects. 5.3.1 and 5.6.4.7 in Chap. 5.

3.5.2　Laboratory Diagnosis

See also Chap. 2.

3.5.2.1　Cytology

Bar-Am and Niv (2007) recently recommended that male sexual partners of females with CIN 3 (severe dysplasia) undergo peniscopy and cytology (Fig. 3.36 a, b) of abnormal areas detected on colposcopic examination.

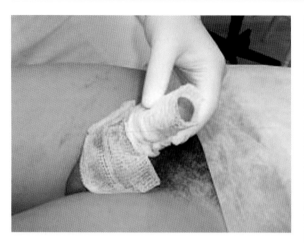

Fig. 3.33. Penile/scrotal area is wrapped in gauze soaked in 5% acetic acid solution

3.5.2.2 Histological Techniques

Histological techniques for the detection of HPV infection in men have low sensitivity and low specificity (Strand et al., 1996; Krebs and Schneider, 1987).

Pathological findings (Fig. 3.37 a, b):

- Papillomatosis
- Hyperkeratosis
- Acanthosis, associated with elongation and branching of the rete ridges into the underlying vascular dermis
- Large, vacuolated keratinocytes with an eccentric pyknotic nucleus surrounded by a perinuclear halo (koilocytes) (Fig. 3.38)

The presence of koilocytes (Fig. 3.39) is a morphological indication of HPV infection.
Each koilocyte contains approximately 50–100 virions, and Bryan and Brown (2001) showed that the desquamation of cornified cells shedding koilocytes successfully transmitted HPV type 11 infection.

Expert Advice

Flat penile warts reveal acanthosis and hyperkeratosis and do not contain parakeratosis or papillomatosis; however, these lesions usually exhibit an abundance of koilocytes.

When to Recommend Lesion Biopsy and Histological Evaluation

- Long-lasting penile lesion
- Lesions that are unresponsive to classic medical treatments

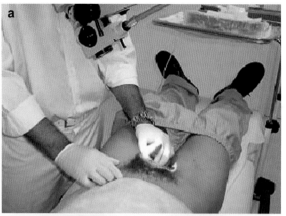

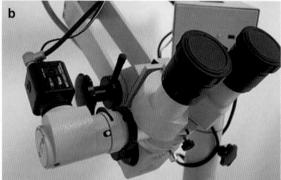

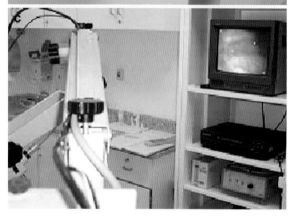

Fig. 3.34. (**a**) Area is examined with microscope/colposcope. (**b**) Video camera is attached to microscope. (**c**) Examination can be fully documented

- Lesions that undergo a sudden growth, ulcerate, or are fixed to underlying planes
- Sudden change in lesion pigmentation
- Atypical lesions in immunocompromised individuals

3

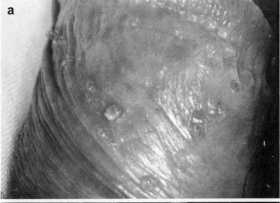

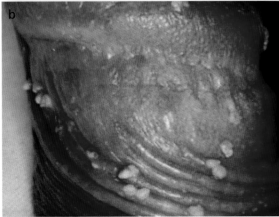

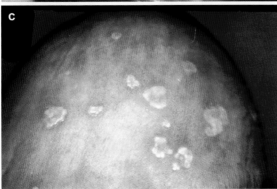

Fig. 3.35. (**a**) Warty lesions before acetic acid solution application. (**b**) Warty lesions develop a white color after solution use. (**c**) Acetowhite test of HPV-related glans lesions

3.5.2.3 Culture

HPV cannot be efficiently propagated in most culture systems.

3.5.2.4 Serological Testing

Serological testing for HPV antibodies has relatively low sensitivity (Dillner, 1999; Carter et al., 2000).

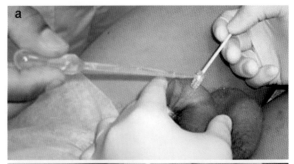

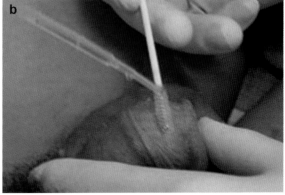

Fig. 3.36 (**a**) Penile brushing cytology. (**b**) Saline drops increase cellularity

Detection of antibody response to viral capsid proteins usually produces conflicting results and these tests are currently used only in research settings.

Antibody responses to HPV may persist for several years or resolve with the clearance of the infection.

Therefore, there is no current clinical indication for the use of HPV serology.

3.5.2.5 Molecular Tests

There are no currently accepted recommendations for HPV DNA testing of specimens obtained from men in clinical settings. Nevertheless, HPV infection in both genders can only be accurately confirmed using molecular detection methods for the presence of HPV DNA in the collected specimens (de Carvalho et al., 2006) (Fig. 3.40a, b).

> **Expert Advice**
>
> Flores et al. (2008) recently confirmed that male specimens collected with the swab method (i.e., using exfoliated skin cells) can be used for molecular HPV testing, and they concluded that PCR-based HPV detection is a reliable diagnostic method in men.

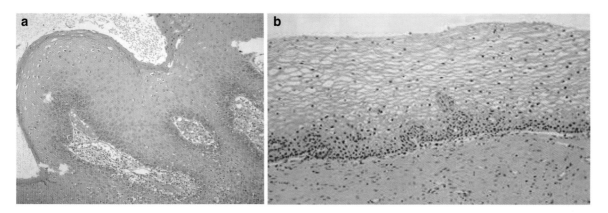

Fig. 3.37. (**a**) Condyloma acuminatum (Source: Photograph courtesy of Filomena Marino Carvalho MD, PhD, São Paulo, Brazil). (**b**) Normal epithelium

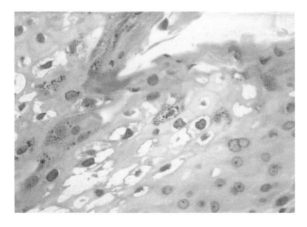

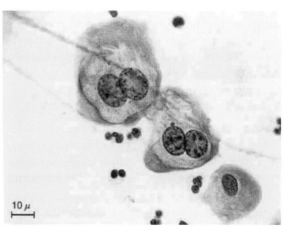

Fig. 3.38. Vacuolated keratinocytes exhibiting eccentric nucleus surrounded by a perinuclear halo (koilocytes) (Source: Photograph courtesy of Monica Stiepcich MD, PhD, São Paulo, Brazil)

Fig. 3.39. Koilocytes (Source: Photograph courtesy of Monica Stiepcich MD, PhD, São Paulo, Brazil)

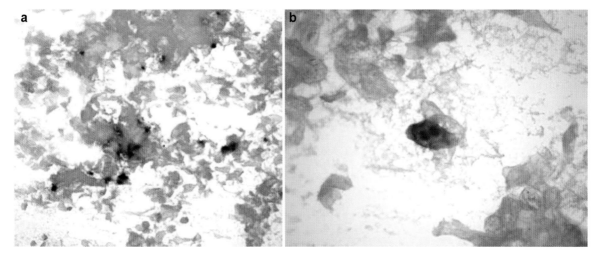

Fig. 3.40. (**a**) Glans brushing HPV DNA-positive (in situ hybridization 10×). (**b**) Glans brushing HPV DNA-positive (koilocyte) (in situ hybridization 40×) (Source: Photograph courtesy of Monica Stiepcich MD, PhD, São Paulo, Brazil)

3.6   Treatment

HPV-related lesions often inflict considerable psychological and psychosexual distress and frustration on patients. These negative emotional feelings occur not only because of the cosmetic problem but mainly because of the stigma of the lesions being sexually transmitted.

Studies show that HPV can persist latently in tissue that appears macroscopically normal (Ferenczy et al., 1985; Macnab et al., 1986). Therefore, because of this possible association with subclinical infection, every treatment method for HPV infection is associated with a high rate of recurrence.

The primary goal of treatment is to remove symptomatic visible lesions. Although there is no current evidence that treatment of genital warts has a favorable impact on the incidence of cervical and genital cancer, treatment of visible lesions may reduce HPV DNA tissue persistence and infectivity (Workowski and Berman, 2007).

> A thorough review of the literature through a database search of Medline and Lilacs has revealed innumerous controlled studies, historical reviews, and case reports evaluating distinct treatment modalities for genital warts and HPV-associated diseases. Reported results varied widely across studies, mainly because of the use of different analytical methods. Thus, great effort has been made in this book to mostly consider high-quality randomized controlled trials on which to base clinical decisions.

Therapy choice is based on lesion:

- Number
- Size and morphology
- Location

Additional factors that define therapy choice include:

- Physician experience
- Treatment cost (Table 3.1), efficacy (Table 3.1), convenience, and adverse effects
- Patient choice

Factors that might influence response to therapy include:

- Patient immunologic status
- Treatment compliance
- Age (de Sanjose et al., 2003)

Expert Advice

Pictures or schematic representations of HPV-associated lesions recorded at each visit are a useful tool for evaluating treatment response and follow-up.

Treatment methods (Table 3.1) are categorized according to their mode of action:

- Antimetabolic therapy (podophyllin, podophyllotoxin, and 5-fluorouracil (FU))
- Immunomodulation and antiviral therapy (imiquimod, interferons (IFNs), BCG, and polyphenon E)
- Cytodestructive methods (surgical excision, cryotherapy, laser therapy, trichloroacetic acid)

Recommended therapeutic modalities can also be classified as:

Home-Applied Therapy

- Podophyllotoxin solution or gel
- Imiquimod 5% cream
- 5-FU cream
- Polyphenon E

Physician-Applied Therapy

- Surgical excision and/or electrosurgery
- Cryotherapy
- Carbon dioxide (CO_2) laser
- Photodynamic therapy (ALA-PDT)
- IFN-α
- Bacille Calmette-Guérin (BCG)
- Podophyllin solution
- Trichloroacetic acid

Expert Advice

The treatment method should be changed if:

- Improvement is not documented after three physician-administered treatment sessions
- Already treated lesions reappear throughout the course of therapy
- Patient is not tolerating current treatment

However, no treatment change is required for patients whose original lesions have responded well to treatment but fresh lesions are occurring at new sites.

Table 3.1 Treatment methods currently available for external genital warts (see also text) (Adapted from: Kodner and Nasraty (2004). Reproduced with permission from *American Family Physician*. Copyright © 2004 American Academy of Family Physicians. All Rights Reserved)

Treatment	Clearance rates (%)	Risk of recurrence (%)	Cost (U.S. $)/(package)
Podophyllin	17–45[a] (Stone et al., 1990)	23–65 (Scheinfeld and Lehman, 2006)	385[b] (Alam and Stiller, 2001)
Podophyllotoxin	68–88 (Beutner and Ferenczy, 1997)	16–34	334[b] (Alam and Stiller, 2001)
5-Fluorouracil (5-FU)	30–95 (Beutner and Ferenczy, 1997)	0–8	40 (tube 15 g)
Surgical excision/ electrofulguration	61–94[c] (Wiley et al., 2002)	26–40 (Beutner and Ferenczy, 1997)	210–415[b] (Alam and Stiller, 2001)
Cryotherapy	79–88 (Scheinfeld and Lehman, 2006)	25–39[d] (Beutner and Ferenczy, 1997)	482[b] (Fine et al., 2007)
CO_2 laser	69–88 (Padilla-Ailhaud, 2006)	25–33[e]	200–535[b] (Alam and Stiller, 2001)
Trichloroacetic acid (TCA)	70–81[f] (Abdullah et al., 1993)	36	264[b] (Fine et al., 2007)
5-Aminolaevulinic acid photodynamic therapy (ALA-PDT)	95–100 (Chen et al., 2007)	NA	NA
Aldara (Imiquimod)	51[g] (Moore et al., 2001)	16[h] (Vexiau et al., 2005)	153–291[b] (12–24 sachets)
Interferon	36–53 (Beutner and Ferenczy, 1997)	21–25	2.744–5.083[b] (Alam and Stiller, 2001)
Bacille Calmette-Guérin (BCG)	80[i] (Metawea et al., 2005)	NA	140–160 (per vial)
Veregen/Polyphenon E (sinecatechins 15% ointment)	50 (Stockfleth et al., 2008)	10.6–11.8 (Gross et al., 2007)	227–250[b] (15 g)
Cidofovir	50[j] (Matteelli et al., 2001)	35.29 (Orlando et al., 2002)	NA

[a]At 3 months
[b]Total estimated costs
[c]Within 3–6 weeks
[d]Despite multiple sessions
[e]After 16 months' follow-up
[f]After six applications
[g]16-week therapy
[h]At 6 months (low recurrence risk after 3 months)
[i]Maximum of six applications
[j]Lesion reduction
NA Data not available

HPV treatment options in pregnant patients comprise:

- Surgical excision
- Cryotherapy
- Trichloroacetic acid

3.6.1 Antimitotic Therapy

3.6.1.1 Podophyllin

Podophyllin resin is derived from the rhizomes of the May apple or Mandrake plant (*Podophyllum peltatum Linné*), a perennial species of the northern and middle states of the United States. It is still used as first-line therapy in developing countries, but some authors suggest the drug should be removed from clinical treatment protocols because of its low efficacy, high toxicity, and a serious mutagenicity profile.

Mechanism of Action

Podophyllin is a cytotoxic agent that arrests mitosis in metaphase. The drug promotes local tissue necrosis and consequently disrupts viral activity. In 1944, Culp and Kaplan (1944) were the first to report the use of topical podophyllin resin for the treatment of HPV-related anogenital lesions.

How to Use

A thin layer of a 10–25% podophyllin suspension in tincture of benzoin should be applied to each lesion and allowed to air-dry completely.

Lesions covered by the prepuce should be allowed to dry for several minutes before the prepuce is returned to its usual position.

The treated area should be thoroughly washed 1–4 h after application to avoid local irritation.

Treatment may be repeated weekly, but if lesions persist after five weekly sessions, alternative therapy should be considered.

Important

- Uninvolved skin should be protected with petroleum jelly, such as Vaseline, to avoid irritation.
- Drug application should not exceed 0.5 ml per session or an area of warts >10 cm^2 per session.
- No open lesions or wounds should exist in the affected area.

Indications

- Moist warts with a large surface area and lesions with many surface projections

Podophyllin is not recommended for intraurethral warts.

Advantages

- Easily available
- Inexpensive in some geographical areas (at least when assessed by weight)
- Cost per treatment in the U.S. – U.S. $385 (approximate price of podophyllum resin 25% – U.S. $150 per 30 ml)
- Efficacy – Clearance rate of 17–45% at 3 months and 73% at 9 months, according to the comparative analysis using podophyllin, cryotherapy, and electrofulguration performed by Stone et al. (1990)

Disadvantages

- Unstandardized preparation
- Physician-applied treatment (highly recommended)
- Less effective than surgery (Khawaja, 1989; Jensen, 1985), podofilox (Lacey et al., 2003), and cryotherapy (Stone et al., 1990)
- High recurrence rates – 23–65%, according to a recent evidence-based review of medical and surgical treatments of genital warts performed by Scheinfeld and Lehman (2006)
- Mutagenic properties (Petersen and Weismann, 1995)

- Contraindicated in pregnancy

Adverse Effects

Local

- Burning sensation
- Pain
- Ulceration

Systemic

Podophyllin can be absorbed systemically and toxicity increases when it is applied to mucosal surfaces or areas greater than 110 mm^2.

Very rare side effects:

- Bone marrow suppression
- Liver dysfunction
- Neurological disturbances – podophyllin hallucinations, psychosis
- Gastrointestinal disturbances – nausea, vomiting, diarrhea, abdominal pain

Combination Therapy

*Podophyllin 25% Used in Combination
with Cryotherapy*

- Efficacy – 75% of patients required only two weekly treatments to become wart free, in the recent comparative study performed by Sherrard and Riddell (2007) that evaluated commonly used therapies for external genital warts

3.6.1.2 Podophyllotoxin (Podofilox Solution 0.5%; Condylox Gel and Solution 0.5%)

Podophyllotoxin is an antimitotic agent derivative of podophyllin.

Mechanism of Action

Podophyllotoxin, chemically synthesized or purified from the plant families Coniferae and Berberidaceae (species of *Juniperus* and *Podophyllum hexandrum*), acts primarily by binding to microtubule subunits and arresting cell division in mitosis (Wilson et al., 1974). The effect of the drug on HPV may also be related to local immunomodulating effects.

How to Use

Podophyllotoxin 0.5% Solution or Gel

The solution and gel should be applied with a cotton swab and with a finger, respectively, and allowed to air-dry. The involved area should be thoroughly washed if excessive pain, burning, itching, or swelling occurs.

Podophyllotoxin should be applied to warts twice daily for three consecutive days, and then discontinued for four consecutive days.

Alternative regimen – applied every other day for 3 weeks.

This 1-week cycle of treatment may be repeated until warts are no longer visualized or for a maximum of four cycles.

- If response to podophyllotoxin is incomplete after four weekly cycles, discontinue treatment and consider alternative therapy.

- Application to uninvolved skin should be minimized. Treatment should be limited to no more than 0.5 g of the gel per day.

Indications

- In a recent medical survey, it was elected as the treatment of choice for multiple small penile lesions (Sonnex and Vrotsou, 2007).

Podofilox is not recommended for anal or urethral warts.

Advantages

- Patient-applied solution and cream.
- Purified solution exhibits low clinical toxicity and is mutagenic free.
- Can be used as first-line therapy.
- Efficacy – More effective than podophyllin; in addition, podophyllotoxin *solution* is more effective than podophyllotoxin *cream* when both are compared with podophyllin (Lacey et al., 2003).
- Cost per treatment – Extensive warts: U.S. $334 (Alam and Stiller, 2001) (approximate price of Podofilox gel 0.5% – U.S. $234 per 3.0 g/tube).

Disadvantages

- Highly effective for short-term treatment but does not provide a long-term cure (Kirby et al., 1990)

- Contraindicated during pregnancy

3.6.1.3 5-Fluorouracil Cream (Efudex®)

5% Fluorouracil (5-FU) is an antimetabolite agent that has been used topically for HPV-related genital lesions.

Mechanism of Action

FU, a pyrimidine analog, is a widely used chemotherapeutic agent that belongs to a group of drugs known as antimetabolites. The drug is incorporated into RNA in preference to the natural substrate uracil, and it inhibits cell growth and promotes apoptosis by targeting the enzyme thymidylate synthetase.

3

How to Use

5-FU Cream

5-FU cream should be applied to the whole penile surface with clean fingertips and after 1–3 h the drug should be completely washed off the treated area. Treatment is repeated 3–5 days a week for a maximum of 4 weeks.

Hands should be washed immediately after contact with the cream.

Important

- The scrotum should be protected from the cream. In case of contact, the area should be washed with soap and water.

Indications

- 5-FU cream is more effective for intraurethral warts (see Chap. 4).
- Alternative option in recalcitrant external lesions.

Advantages

- Inexpensive – approximate price U.S. $40/15 g (generic)
- Patient-applied therapy (pretreatment orientation is highly advised to avoid treatment complications)
- Efficacy – reported cure rates of 30–95%

Disadvantages

- Severe local side effects can occur.

- Contraindicated during pregnancy (possible teratogenic risks).

Side Effects

- Pain
- Ulceration (Fig. 3.41 a, b)

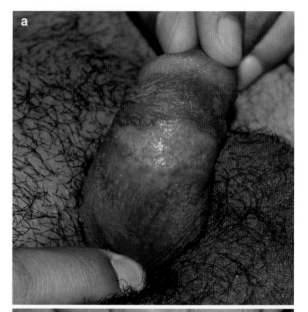
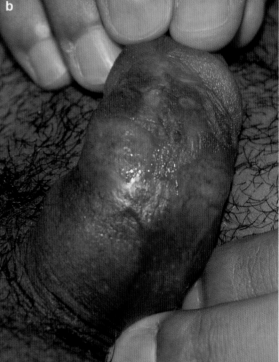

Fig. 3.41. (**a**) Severe penile ulceration caused by Efurix. (**b**) Ulceration nearly affecting the entire penile circumference

3.6.2 Destructive Therapy

3.6.2.1 Surgical Excision/Electrosurgery

Surgical excision alone or in combination with electrofulguration may be used in the treatment of genital warts. The heat that is produced in the tissue at the point of entry of high-frequency currents leads to the destruction of the lesion.

> **Surgical Technique**
>
> Simple lesion excision with a scalpel or scissors followed by electrocautery of the remaining affected tissue down to the skin surface, or alternatively, complete destruction of HPV-related lesions by means of electrofulguration.

> **Important**
>
> - Intensive coagulation should be avoided as it can result in slow wound healing, bleeding, and scarring.

> **Expert Advice**
>
> Use of a topical anesthetic is recommended. EMLA cream (a eutectic mixture of lidocaine 2.5% and prilocaine 2.5%) applied 30 min before the surgical procedure is indicated for patients who do not tolerate the pain of the 1% lidocaine injection.

> **Important**
>
> - A solution of 1% lidocaine without epinephrine should be used for procedures involving the penis and distal urethra.

Indications

- Small isolated warts on the shaft of the penis
- Large exophytic lesions in the anogenital area

Advantages

- The method produces immediate results.
- Efficacy – 61–94% clearance within 3–6 weeks of treatment, according to Wiley et al. (2002).

- Widely available and cost effective – Surgical excision of simple warts: U.S. $210; extensive lesions: U.S. $318; electrofulguration of extensive lesions: U.S. $415 (Alam and Stiller, 2001).

Disadvantages

- Office procedure for small lesions but larger lesions need an operating room setting.
- Local/regional or general anesthesia required depending on the size/location of the lesion and the patient's age.
- High recurrence rates when method is used against flat acetowhite HPV-associated lesions (Wikstrom and von Krogh, 1998).
- In a recent randomized study that compared ablation alone vs. imiquimod 5% cream and a combination of the two treatments, Schofer et al. (2006) found recurrences at 6 months in 26.4% of cases treated with excision and in 6.3% of patients treated with imiquimod monotherapy.
- Healing time – around 2 weeks.
- Electrosurgery plume hazards from released viral organisms (see Sect. 10.4.1.2 in Chap. 10).

Adverse Effects

- Postoperative pain
- Scarring

> **Expert Advice**
>
> Postectomy (circumcision) is not a treatment modality for extensive preputial warts and should not be recommended. However, the procedure can be performed, if necessary, after the complete clearance of HPV-associated genital lesions (Fig. 3.42).

3.6.2.2 Cryotherapy

Cryotherapy involves the application of nitrous oxide or liquid nitrogen ($-196\,°C$) to anogenital lesions.

Mechanism of Action

The freeze-thaw cycle produces dermal and vascular damage and edema, leading to both epidermal and dermal cytolysis.

3

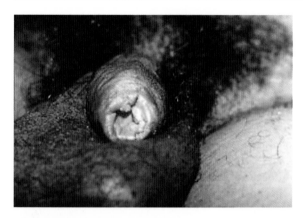

Fig. 3.42. Penile condyloma and associated phimosis

How to Use

Liquid nitrogen may be applied directly to the lesion with a cotton-tipped swab or sprayed onto it for about 20 s.

- Lesion turns white (frozen) and subsequent thaw produces cell damage.
- Two freeze-thaw cycles are usually performed.
- Safety margin is included by letting the white border extend approximately 1–2 mm beyond the periphery of the lesion.

Treatment can be repeated every 2–4 weeks, if necessary.

Indications

- Smaller, flatter genital lesions on the shaft of the penis
- Grouped lesions
- Lesions on hair-bearing areas (Scheinfeld and Lehman, 2006)

Advantages

- Anesthesia usually not required for small lesions (EMLA cream is recommended).
- Cost per successful treatment – approximately U.S. $482 (Fine et al., 2007).
- Ease of application.
- Rapid destructive effect.
- Efficacy – clearance rates range from 79 to 88%, according to the review of Scheinfeld and Lehman (2006). Most used method in a recent U.S. survey (cryotherapy employed in 38% of cases, no treatment in 21% and podophyllin in 17%) (Newman et al., 2008).

Disadvantages

- Office procedure.
- Optimal number of freeze–thaw cycles is not established.
- Healing time – usually 1–2 weeks following treatment.
- Recurrences – 25–39% despite multiple treatments.

Adverse Effects

- Mild discomfort, swelling, and erythema.
- Preputial lesions, particularly flat genital warts, are prone to scarring and fibrosis after treatment.
- Pigmentary changes in the short term.

Combination Therapies

Cryotherapy + Podophyllotoxin

A combination of cryotherapy and podophyllotoxin is the most common first-line treatment for HPV-related anogenital lesions in the United Kingdom, regardless of site (McClean and Shann, 2005).

3.6.2.3 CO_2 Laser

Mechanism of Action

Thermal tissue ablation (vaporization) using focused infrared light energy (Fig. 3.43a, b).

Laser Technique

See also Chap. 10.

Power Settings

- 4–10 W in continuous or pulsed mode (promotes tissue vaporization with a shallow penetration depth).

CO_2 laser is coupled to the operating microscope/colposcope for enhanced visualization (focal distance: 250 mm) and lesions are vaporized under direct colposcopic guidance.

It is important to focus the beam over the lesion and move the laser beam as quickly as possible.

Lesions are vaporized along with a 2–5-mm border of normal-appearing epithelium (Fig. 3.44 a–d).

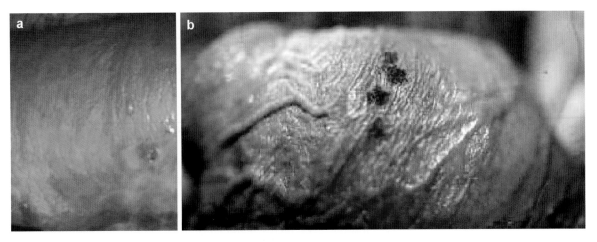

Fig. 3.43. (**a**) CO_2 laser vaporization of penile shaft lesions (see laser plume). (**b**) Final result

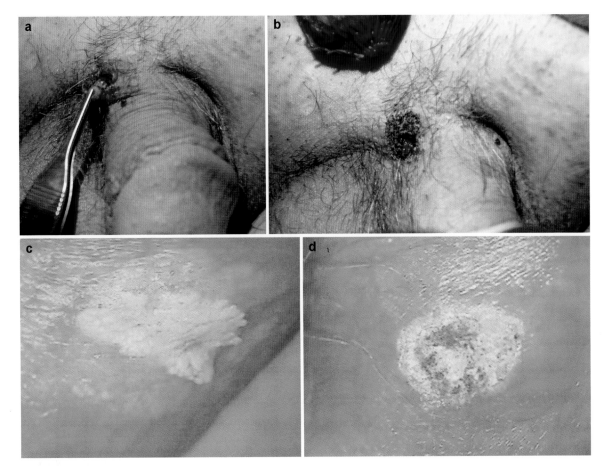

Fig. 3.44. (**a**) Laser excision of penis base lesion. (**b**) A 2–3-mm security margin around the lesion. (**c**) Penis shaft lesion. (**d**) A 2–3- mm security margin around the lesion

Indications

- Primary and recurrent HPV-related anogenital lesions
- Extensive and exophytic lesions

Advantages

- Fast and precise treatment modality.
- Bloodless surgical field.
- Safe – water is the endogenous target absorber.
- Efficacy – Padilla-Ailhaud (2006) showed clearance rates of 69% and 88% after first and second CO_2 laser sessions, respectively. Moreover, in a recent study evaluating persistence and recurrence rates of anogenital condyloma and HPV-related intraepithelial neoplasias after CO_2 laser treatment, Aynaud et al. (2008) reported that after 1.4 laser sessions 83% of patients were in remission at 6–month follow-up.
- Promotes rapid healing – usually 2 weeks following treatment.
- Minimal or no scar formation in most cases.
- Probable elimination of the infective agent.

Disadvantages

- Cost per treatment - approximately U.S. $200 (single lesions) to U.S. $535 (extensive lesions) (Alam and Stiller, 2001).
- Laser therapy training.
- Day clinic or office procedure under local anesthesia.
- Large lesions in female and pediatric patients may require general anesthesia.
- CO_2 laser plume hazards from released viral organisms (see Sect. 10.4.2.2 in Chap. 10).
- Recurrence rates ranged from 25 to 33%, with an average follow-up of 16 months in the study performed by Padilla-Ailhaud (2006).

Adverse Effects

- Postoperative pain
- Scarring less pronounced when compared with electrofulguration

Combination Therapy

Laser therapy followed by postoperative systemic INF-α-2b in patients presenting with recalcitrant genital warts.

- Efficacy – complete clearance of warts was reported in 52% of patients treated with laser and INF-α-2b subcutaneously vs. clearance of 22% among patients treated with laser and placebo (Petersen et al., 1991).

3.6.2.4   Photodynamic Therapy

Photodynamic therapy (PDT) was introduced in the 1990s. In this technique, light of a specific wavelength is absorbed by certain photosensitizing molecules that are exogenously administered to a target tissue. The agent commonly used is 5-aminolaevulinic acid (ALA), a prodrug that is selectively absorbed by tumor cells and rapidly proliferating cells and that stimulates porphyrin accumulation in the tissue (Casas and Batlle, 2002). Porphyrins will then act as the photosensitizing agent.

Mechanism of Action

Following activation by red light, ALA is transformed to protoporphyrin IX (PpIX). This induces the formation of singlet oxygen, which leads to the death or destruction of the involved cells (Loh et al., 1993). Furthermore, Smetana et al. (1997) demonstrated that ALA–PDT could also inactivate viral particles.

How to Use (Chen et al., 2007)

20% ALA solution is prepared by dissolving ALA in sterile saline immediately prior to its application.

- An absorbent cotton ball is soaked in the solution and is applied over the lesions and adjacent healthy skin (5-mm border).
- Small amounts of the solution are dropped onto the surface of the cotton ball every 30 min and, after a 3-h interval, the lesions are occluded with cling film and thick gauze for light protection. Light irradiation of the involved area is performed using a cylindrical helium-neon laser fiber.
- If lesions are not totally eradicated, treatment can be repeated once a week for a maximum of 3 weeks.

Indications

Lesions in sensitive mucosal tissues (penis and urethra)

Advantages

- Efficacy – Chen et al. (2007) have found complete response rates of 95 and 100% after one and two sessions of ALA-PDT treatment, respectively.
- Compared with conventional CO_2 laser therapy, topical application of ALA-PDT is more effective and has a lower recurrence rate (Chen et al., 2007).
- Minimal or absent scarring.
- The photosensitizers have fluorescence properties, assisting in the pretreatment visualization of the lesions.

Disadvantages

- Physician-applied therapy
- Expensive, although probably cost-effective when multiple lesions are treated in one irradiation field

Adverse Effects

- Mild burning and/or stinging sensation during irradiation

3.6.3 Immunotherapy

3.6.3.1 Interferons (INF-α)

IFN-α, the most widely used INF, is a cytokine produced primarily by leukocytes and it is approved by the U.S. Food and Drug Administration (FDA) for the treatment of condyloma acuminata in patients 18 years of age or older.

Mechanism of Action

The main functions of IFN-α are immunomodulatory and antiproliferative, and it also has the ability to interfere with viral replication (Isaacs and Lindenmann, 1987).

Indications

- Recurrent or recalcitrant lesions

INF use for the management of HPV-associated lesions can be administered:

- Intralesionally
- Topically

3.6.3.2 Intralesional Injection of -INF-α

How to Use

Intralesional INF Injection

INF-α-n3 (Alferon N injection; available in 1-ml vials).

- 0.05 ml per lesion administered twice a week for up to 8 weeks.

INF-α-2b, recombinant (Intron-A; vial of 10 million IU should be used for HPV lesions).

- 0.1 ml of reconstituted Intron-A vial is injected into each lesion three times a week on alternate days for 3 weeks.

Advantages

- Efficacy – Friedman-Kien et al. (1988) reported complete clearance of lesions in 62% of INF-α-treated patients compared to 21% of placebo-treated patients.
- Reduced systemic side effects with intralesional treatment.

Disadvantages

- Physician-applied therapy
- High-cost treatment – simple warts: U.S. $2,744; extensive warts: U.S. $5,803 (Alam and Stiller, 2001)
- Not recommended for routine clinical practice
- Not effective in immunosuppressed individuals

Side Effects

Local

- Painful injections (Trizna et al., 1998)
- Hyperemia and edema at the injection site

3

Systemic

- Influenza-like symptoms (usually clear within 24 h of treatment)
- Autoimmune reactions
- Cardiovascular symptoms
- Depression

Combination Treatment

Intralesional INF-a-2b (1.5 × 10⁶ IU) plus topical 25% podophyllin resin compared to topical podophyllin resin alone (Douglas et al., 1990)

- Efficacy – complete clearance of lesions in 67% of patients receiving combination therapy vs. 42% in those receiving monotherapy with podophyllin
- Recurrence rate – 67% in the combination treatment arm, and 65% in the podophyllin-only arm after 11 weeks of follow-up

3.6.3.3   Topical INF Ointment

Topical INF treatment is tolerated much better than the injections, although it is less effective (Syed et al., 1994).

3.6.3.4   Imiquimod 5% Cream (Aldara®)

Aldara cream is the first topical FDA-approved immunomodulator for the treatment of external anogenital warts.

Mechanism of Action

The topically applied drug imidazoquinoline is an immunomodulator that acts stimulating toll-like receptors (i.e., TLR 7) on antigen-presenting cells, which enhances the local production of Th1 cytokines and T cell-mediated cytotoxic immune response.

Imiquimod also showed an antiangiogenic effect through a possible promotion of INF-γ production, an effect mediated by IL-18 (Majewski et al., 2005).

How to Use

Imiquimod cream comes in single-use packets. Open packets with unused cream should be discarded.

A thin layer of imiquimod 5% cream should be applied and rubbed to external visible warts at bedtime. The area is then washed with soap and water 6–10 h after application. Treatment is executed every other day three times per week, and the weekly cycles can be repeated until all of the warts disappear, up to a maximum of 16 weeks.

Important

- Imiquimod may weaken condoms and diaphragms, and sexual contact is not recommended while the cream is on the skin.

Indications

- Not suitable for the treatment of long-standing, fibrotic warts (von Krogh, 2001).
- Circumcised men have better responses than uncircumcised men (Carrasco et al., 2002).
- In a recent medical survey, it was elected predominantly for large or bulky lesions (Sonnex and Vrotsou, 2007).

Advantages

- Patient-applied cream.
- Efficacy – Complete clearance of warts occurred in 51% of patients within 16 weeks of therapy, according to the review performed by Moore et al. (2001). Moreover, in a recent meta-analysis of 5% imiquimod and 0.5% podophyllotoxin, Yan et al. (2006) reported clinical cure rates of 50.34% with imiquimod and 56.41% with the podophyllotoxin treatment, but more serious adverse effects were associated with the latter.

Disadvantages

- Expensive – Approximate cost U.S. $153,99 (12 sachets) and U.S. $291,99 (24 sachets).

- Average treatment length – 9.5 weeks.
- Recurrence rate – In a recent study, Vexiau et al. (2005) observed recurrences at 6 months in 16% of the patients. In addition, the investigators reported that most of the recurrences (86.6%) were already present at 3 months, suggesting that after this period the recurrence risk is low.

Adverse Effects

Local

Mild and transient local inflammatory reaction reported in 31% of patients.

- Hyperemia, swelling, pruritus, bleeding
- Blisters, flaking, scaling, dryness, or thickening of the skin
- Burning, stinging, pain in the treated area

Systemic

- Headache
- Diarrhea
- Back pain
- Fatigue
- Fever

Expert Advice

If response to imiquimod is less than 50% by 6 weeks of treatment, discontinue use and consider alternative therapy.

Combination Treatment

Imiquimod use following laser treatment:

- Effective in reducing recurrences (Hoyme et al., 2002).
- Cream should only be applied when wound healing is completed.

3.6.3.5 Bacille Calmette-Guérin

Application of viable bacille Calmette-Guérin (BCG) induces a cytotoxic immune response against malignant and virally transformed cells, and may also increase the immunological ability to eliminate HPV in men. However, the exact mechanism of the immune response to HPV infection has not been elucidated.

How to Use

Topical BCG (81 mg/ml suspension containing viable bacteria of the BCG Connaught strain) applied weekly to the lesions for six consecutive weeks.

- Exposure to healthy penile skin should be avoided and areas in contact with the BCG mixture should be washed thoroughly 2 h after treatment.

Advantages

- Efficacy – Metawea et al. (2005) reported that complete response was achieved in 80% of the patients after a maximum of six applications.

Disadvantages

- High cost (U.S. $140–160 per vial)
- Physician-applied therapy

Adverse Effects

- Transient erythema
- Mild fever

Combination Treatment

Laser vaporization and adjuvant BCG
- Efficacy – the annual recurrence rate in patients with refractory/recurrent HPV-related genital lesions decreased significantly after BCG therapy, according to Bohle et al. (1998).

3.7 Other Treatment Modalities

3.7.1 Chemical Destruction

3.7.1.1 Trichloroacetic Acid

Trichloroacetic acid (TCA) produces protein coagulation, leading to cell lysis and destruction of the affected tissue.

3

TCA in a Solution Concentration of 60–90%

Lidocaine gel (and not EMLA, to avoid mucosal edema) is initially spread over the involved area. A small amount of TCA is then applied to each lesion with a cotton tip applicator and is allowed to dry until a white frosting develops.

Usual regimen – once a week for four consecutive weeks.

- The dry end of the cotton tip can be used to remove the destroyed tissue.
- Application to uninvolved skin should be minimized, but if it occurs the area should be washed with liquid soap or a neutralizing agent should be used (talcum powder or sodium bicarbonate).

Indications

- Particularly effective for treating small, moist, acuminate or papular lesions.
- Recommended for post-treatment control of small papular warts (Fig. 3.45 a–d).
- Less efficacious for keratinized or large lesion.
- In the medical survey performed by Sonnex and Vrotsou (2007), TCA was infrequently chosen as a treatment option (<6% of respondents).

Advantages

- Easily available.
- Efficacy – In a comparative study that evaluated cryotherapy (liquid nitrogen) and TCA, Abdullah et al. (1993) reported clearance rates of 70–81% after six applications.

Disadvantages

- Physician-applied therapy
- Recurrence rates of 36%
- Longer time to wart clearance and increased lesion persistence when used as single therapy (Sherrard and Riddell, 2007)
- Cost per successful treatment –approximately U.S. $264 (Fine et al., 2007)

Adverse Effects

- Burning sensation following TCA application that may last for up to 10 min
- Pain
- Ulceration
- Crust formation

3.7.2 Novel Therapies

3.7.2.1 Cidofovir

Cidofovir is a nucleotide analog of deoxycytidine monophosphate (dCMP), which is converted to the active cidofovir diphosphate that inhibits viral DNA polymerases (Ho et al., 1992). Cidofovir is an antiviral agent currently FDA approved for the treatment of cytomegalovirus (CMV) retinitis in HIV patients, but the topical formulation has been effective in treating refractory HPV-related anogenital lesions (Hengge and Tietze, 2000; Schurmann et al., 2000).

Cidofovir 1.5% gel and 1% cidofovir cream is topically applied to the lesions once daily, and repeated 3–5 days a week for 2 weeks followed by 2 weeks of observation.

Indications

- Recurring or recalcitrant anogenital warts, particularly in HIV-infected patients

Advantages

- Patient-applied therapy.
- Efficacy – Recent data reported by Matteelli et al. (2001) showed a reduction of more than 50% of lesions in 58% of HIV-infected patients.
- Recurrence – 35.29% in the study performed by Orlando et al. (2002) using topical 1% cidofovir gel.

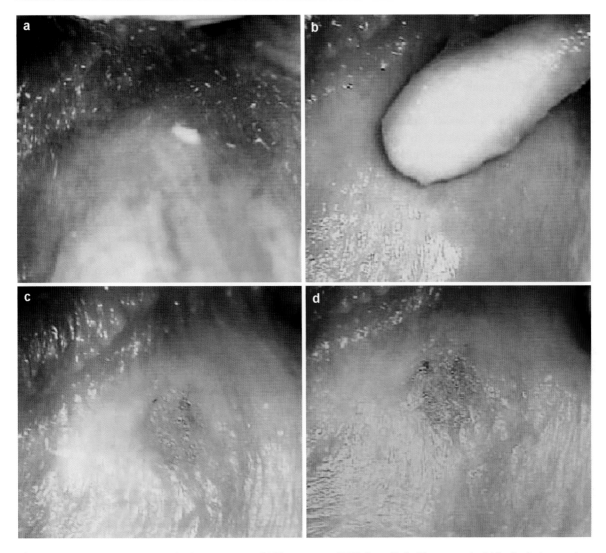

Fig. 3.45 (**a**) Small wart 6 weeks after laser treatment. (**b**) Tiny amount of TCA is applied with a cotton tip. (**c**) Lesion is destroyed — immediate result. (**d**) Visual aspect 1 day after TCA use

Disadvantages

- Expensive
- Not FDA approved for this indication
- Unstandardized preparation

Adverse Effects

- Local mucosal erosion is a common and sometimes severe event.
- Pain.

- No systemic side effects.

Combination Treatment

Cidofovir vs. electrocautery excision vs. combination of both treatments:
- Efficacy – complete resolution observed in 100% of HIV-infected patients treated with combination therapy (Orlando et al., 2002)
- Recurrence – 27% with electrocautery-cidofovir combination treatment

3.7.2.2 Veregen™ (Sinecatechins 15% Ointment)

Veregen was originally developed under the name of Polyphenon E ointment.[1]

Sinecatechins 15% ointment is a proprietary extract of green tea (*Camellia sinensis*) leaves, and green tea catechins have demonstrated antiviral, antioxidative, antiproliferative, and immunostimulatory activity.

Mechanism of Action

The exact mechanism of action of sinecatechins ointment is unknown, although epigallocatechin gallate (a major component of both green tea and sinecatechins ointment) has been shown to suppress the growth of HPV-infected cervical cancer cell lines (Ahn et al., 2003).

How to Use

Veregen 15% ointment is applied to all warts three times daily up to a maximum of 16 weeks.

Important

- Sinecatechins may weaken condoms and diaphragms, and sexual contact is not recommended while the cream is on the skin.

Indications

- Veregen is FDA approved for the topical treatment of external genital and perianal warts.

Further clinical studies are recommended to evaluate use of sinecatechins in intra-anal, intravaginal, and cervical condylomas, as well as other intraepithelial lesions.

Advantages

- Safe.
- Patient-applied therapy.

- Efficacy – Stockfleth et al. (2008) showed clearance rates of 50% or higher in 78% of patients enrolled in the randomized controlled trial that evaluated topical Polyphenon E efficacy on external genital and perianal warts.
- Better responses reported in women (complete wart clearance in 60% of women vs. 45% of men) (Stockfleth et al., 2008).

Disadvantages

- Recurrence rates – 10.6% and 11.8% for Polyphenon E 15% or 10% cream, respectively, 12 weeks after end of treatment, according to Gross et al. (2007)
- Expensive – approximate monthly cost: US $227–250/ 15 g tube (based on 2008 average wholesale price)

Adverse Effects

- Mild or moderate local site reactions, with a reported decline during continued use

3.8 Management of Latent and Subclinical HPV Infection

Expert Advice

Management of Latent and Subclinical HPV Infection

Asymptomatic Patients

- Observation alone is recommended, mainly because currently there are no treatments available that can completely eliminate HPV from infected cells.

Symptomatic Patients with Predominance of Balanoposthitis Symptoms

- Short treatment course of a systemic and/or topical antifungal therapy.
- Short course of a topical cicatrizant and/or antibiotic ointment application.

Symptomatic Patients with Predominance of Flat Visible Lesions

- Should be managed by the same treatment methods used for external lesions.

[1]Approval of the drug in Europe under the name of Polyphenon® E ointment is expected from the second half of 2008 (MediGene AG, http://www.medigene.com/englisch/ProjektPE.php).

3.9 Circumcision and HPV

The studies assessing HPV infection risk and circumcision status yield conflicting results (Shin et al., 2004; Castellsague et al., 2002).

However, recent data from a randomized controlled trial that evaluated male circumcision for the prevention of HIV and other sexually transmitted infections in Africa showed a significantly reduced prevalence of high- and low-risk HPV genotypes among the circumcised group of men (Tobian et al., 2009).

Moreover, in another recent study Hernandez et al. (2008a) showed that uncircumcised men have an increased risk of HPV infection, including with oncogenic (high risk) as well as multiple HPV types.

The prevalence of any HPV infection in the glans/corona was significantly higher in uncircumcised men, possibly due to the close contact with the foreskin, a putative vulnerable site for HPV infection.

3.10 Follow-Up

Follow-up evaluation 3 months after topical therapies is indicated, since external genital wart recur most frequently during this period and can be difficult to identify. Earlier follow-up visits may be beneficial in relapsing and immunosuppressed patients.

Following surgical treatments, patients return on postoperative day 12 for monitoring of the cicatrization, treatment of possible complications, and checking for any early signs of recurrence (Workowski and Berman, 2007). Subsequently, follow-up evaluation 3–4 weeks after the end of treatment is recommended, and then every 2–3 months for half a year if control examinations yield negative results.

Patients should be oriented to self-refer if lesions reappear.

3.11 Prevention

Strategies should be aimed at reducing the risk of acquiring HPV infection.

- Abstinence from sexual activity, including skin-to-skin contact – the most reliable prevention method.
- Delay the onset of sexual activity.
- Reduce the number of sex partners (Kjaer et al., 2005).
- Promote condom use on a regular basis – Condoms may not provide complete protection against HPV transmission, yet Bleeker et al. (2003) reported that condom use promoted regression of HPV-related flat penile lesions in male sexual partners of women with CIN.
- Circumcision – according to Tobian et al. (2009), the procedure can significantly reduce the incidence of several STIs and confer partial protection against HPV infection.
- Immunization with prophylactic HPV vaccines.

According to a recent phase-III study that evaluated the efficacy of the prophylactic quadrivalent HPV vaccine in preventing HPV-related lesions in men naïve to all four vaccine HPV types (6, 11, 16, and 18), Gardasil was 89.4% effective in preventing external anogenital warts (Giuliano and Palefsky, 2008). Efficacy against individual vaccine HPV types 6 and 11 (usually responsible for the development of genital warts) was 84.3 and 90.9%, respectively, and against high-risk types 16 and 18 it was 100%. Furthermore, persistent viral infection and HPV DNA detection rates were reduced in 85.6% and in 44.7% of the vaccinated individuals, respectively (Palefsky and Giuliano, 2008) (see Sect. 11.8 in Chap. 11).

References

Abdullah AN, Walzman M, Wade A (1993) Treatment of external genital warts comparing cryotherapy (liquid nitrogen) and trichloroacetic acid. Sex Transm Dis 20: 344–345

Ahn WS, Huh SW, Bae SM, Lee IP, Lee JM, Namkoong SE, Kim CK, Sin JI (2003) A major constituent of green tea, EGCG, inhibits the growth of a human cervical cancer cell line, CaSki cells, through apoptosis, G(1) arrest, and regulation of gene expression. DNA Cell Biol 22: 217–224

Alam M, Stiller M (2001) Direct medical costs for surgical and medical treatment of condylomata acuminata. Arch Dermatol 137: 337–341

Aynaud O, Buffet M, Roman P, Plantier F, Dupin N (2008) Study of persistence and recurrence rates in 106 patients with condyloma and intraepithelial neoplasia after CO_2 laser treatment. Eur J Dermatol 18: 153–158

Baken LA, Koutsky LA, Kuypers J, Kosorok MR, Lee SK, Kiviat NB, Holmes KK (1995) Genital human papillomavirus infection among male and female sex partners: prevalence and type-specific concordance. J Infect Dis 171: 429–432

Baldwin SB, Wallace DR, Papenfuss MR, Abrahamsen M, Vaught LC, Kornegay JR, Hallum JA, Redmond SA, Giuliano AR (2003) Human papillomavirus infection in men attending a sexually transmitted disease clinic. J Infect Dis 187: 1064–1070

Bandieramonte G, Colecchia M, Mariani L, Lo Vullo S, Pizzocaro G, Piva L, Nicolai N, Salvioni R, Lezzi V, Stefanon B, De Palo G (2008) Peniscopically controlled CO_2 laser excision for conservative treatment of in situ and T1 penile carcinoma: report on 224 patients. Eur Urol 54: 875–882

Bandyopadhyay D, Sen S (2003) Perianal verrucous epidermal naevus mimicking perianal warts. Sex Transm Infect 79: 424

Bar-Am A, Niv J (2007) The role of HPV DNA in the evaluation and follow-up of asymptomatic male sexual partners of females with CIN3. Eur J Gynaecol Oncol 28: 207–210

Barrasso R, Gross GE (1997) External genitalia: diagnosis. In: Gross GE, Barrasso R (eds) Human papillomavirus infection, a clinical atlas. Ullstein Mosby, Berlin, pp 296–331

Beutner KR, Ferenczy A (1997) Therapeutic approaches to genital warts. Am J Med 102: 28–37

Bleeker MC, Hogewoning CJ, Berkhof J, Voorhorst FJ, Hesselink AT, van Diemen PM, van den Brule AJ, Snijders PJ, Meijer CJ (2005a) Concordance of specific human papillomavirus types in sex partners is more prevalent than would be expected by chance and is associated with increased viral loads. Clin Infect Dis 41: 612–620

Bleeker MC, Hogewoning CJ, Voorhorst FJ, van den Brule AJ, Berkhof J, Hesselink AT, Lettink M, Starink TM, Stoof TJ, Snijders PJ, Meijer CJ (2005b) HPV-associated flat penile lesions in men of a non-STD hospital population: less frequent and smaller in size than in male sexual partners of women with CIN. Int J Cancer 113: 36–41

Bleeker MC, Hogewoning CJ, Voorhorst FJ, van den Brule AJ, Snijders PJ, Starink TM, Berkhof J, Meijer CJ (2003) Condom use promotes regression of human papillomavirus-associated penile lesions in male sexual partners of women with cervical intraepithelial neoplasia. Int J Cancer 107: 804–810

Bleeker MC, Snijders PF, Voorhorst FJ, Meijer CJ (2006) Flat penile lesions: the infectious "invisible" link in the transmission of human papillomavirus. Int J Cancer 119: 2505–2512

Bohle A, Doehn C, Kausch I, Jocham D (1998) Treatment of recurrent penile condylomata acuminata with external application and intraurethral instillation of bacillus calmette-guerin. J Urol 160: 394–396

Boxman IL, Hogewoning A, Mulder LH, Bouwes Bavinck JN, ter Schegget J (1999) Detection of human papillomavirus types 6 and 11 in pubic and perianal hair from patients with genital warts. J Clin Microbiol 37: 2270–2273

Brown DR, Schroeder JM, Bryan JT, Stoler MH, Fife KH (1999a) Detection of multiple human papillomavirus types in Condylomata acuminata lesions from otherwise healthy and immunosuppressed patients. J Clin Microbiol 37: 3316–3322

Brown TJ, Yen-Moore A, Tyring SK (1999b) An overview of sexually transmitted diseases. Part II. J Am Acad Dermatol 41: 661–677; quiz 678–680

Bryan JT, Brown DR (2001) Transmission of human papillomavirus type 11 infection by desquamated cornified cells. Virology 281: 35–42

Buechner SA (2002) Common skin disorders of the penis. BJU Int 90: 498–506

Carrasco D, van der Straten M, Tyring SK (2002) Treatment of anogenital warts with imiquimod 5% cream followed by surgical excision of residual lesions. J Am Acad Dermatol 47: S212–S216

Carter JJ, Koutsky LA, Hughes JP, Lee SK, Kuypers J, Kiviat N, Galloway DA (2000) Comparison of human papillomavirus types 16, 18, and 6 capsid antibody responses following incident infection. J Infect Dis 181: 1911–1919

Casas A, Batlle A (2002) Rational design of 5-aminolevulinic acid derivatives aimed at improving photodynamic therapy. Curr Med Chem Anticancer Agents 2: 465–475

Castellsague X, Bosch FX, Munoz N, Meijer CJ, Shah KV, de Sanjose S, Eluf-Neto J, Ngelangel CA, Chichareon S, Smith JS, Herrero R, Moreno V, Franceschi S (2002) Male circumcision, penile human papillomavirus infection, and cervical cancer in female partners. N Engl J Med 346: 1105–1112

Chen K, Chang BZ, Ju M, Zhang XH, Gu H (2007) Comparative study of photodynamic therapy vs. CO_2 laser vaporization in treatment of condylomata acuminata: a randomized clinical trial. Br J Dermatol 156: 516–520

Coleman N, Birley HD, Renton AM, Hanna NF, Ryait BK, Byrne M, Taylor-Robinson D, Stanley MA (1994) Immunological events in regressing genital warts. Am J Clin Pathol 102: 768–774

Cook LS, Koutsky LA, Holmes KK (1993) Clinical presentation of genital warts among circumcised and uncircumcised heterosexual men attending an urban STD clinic. Genitourin Med 69: 262–264

Culp OS, Kaplan IW (1944) Condylomata acuminata: Two hundred cases treated with podophyllin. Ann Surg 120: 251–256

de Carvalho JJ, Syrjanen KJ, Jacobino M, Rosa NT, Carvalho LZ (2006) Prevalence of genital human papillomavirus infections established using different diagnostic techniques among males attending a urological clinic. Scand J Urol Nephrol 40: 138–143

de Sanjose S, Bosch FX, Tafur LA, Nascimento CM, Izarzugaza I, Izquierdo A, Barricarte A, Shah KV, Meijer CJ, Munoz N (2003) Clearance of HPV infection in middle aged men and women after 9 years' follow up. Sex Transm Infect 79: 348

Dillner J (1999) The serological response to papillomaviruses. Semin Cancer Biol 9: 423–430

Doorbar J, Sterling JC (2001) The biology of human papillomaviruses. In: Sterling JC, Tyring SK (eds) Human papillomaviruses: Clinical and scientific advances. Arnold, London, pp 10–23

Douglas JM, Jr., Eron LJ, Judson FN, Rogers M, Alder MB, Taylor E, Tanner D, Peets E (1990) A randomized trial of combination therapy with intralesional interferon alpha 2b and podophyllin versus podophyllin alone for the therapy of anogenital warts. J Infect Dis 162: 52–59

Ferenczy A, Mitao M, Nagai N, Silverstein SJ, Crum CP (1985) Latent papillomavirus and recurring genital warts. N Engl J Med 313: 784–788

Fine P, Ball C, Pelta M, McIntyre C, Momtaz M, Morfesis J, Cullins V, Rash RM (2007) Treatment of external genital warts at Planned Parenthood Federation of America centers. J Reprod Med 52: 1090–1096

Fleischer AB, Jr., Parrish CA, Glenn R, Feldman SR (2001) Condylomata acuminata (genital warts): Patient demographics and treating physicians. Sex Transm Dis 28: 643–647

Flores R, Abalos AT, Nielson CM, Abrahamsen M, Harris RB, Giuliano AR (2008) Reliability of sample collection and laboratory testing for HPV detection in men. J Virol Methods 149: 136–143

Franceschi S, Castellsague X, Dal Maso L, Smith JS, Plummer M, Ngelangel C, Chicharoen S, Eluf-Neto J, Shah KV, Snijders PJ, Meijer CJ, Bosch FX, Munoz N (2002) Prevalence and determinants of human papillomavirus genital infection in men. Br J Cancer 86: 705–711

Franco EL (1996) Epidemiology of anogential warts and cancer. In: Reid R, Lorincz A (eds) Human papillomaviruses I. W.B. Saunders, Philadelphia, pp 597–623

Friedman-Kien AE, Eron LJ, Conant M, Growdon W, Badiak H, Bradstreet PW, Fedorczyk D, Trout JR, Plasse TF (1988) Natural interferon alfa for treatment of condylomata acuminata. JAMA 259: 533–538

Gillison ML, Shah KV (2003) Chapter 9: Role of mucosal human papillomavirus in nongenital cancers. J Natl Cancer Inst Monogr: 57–65

Giovannelli L, Bellavia C, Capra G, Migliore MC, Caleca M, Giglio M, Perino A, Matranga D, Ammatuna P (2007) HPV group- and type-specific concordance in HPV infected sexual couples. J Med Virol 79: 1882–1888

Giuliano A, Palefsky J (2008) The efficacy of quadrivalent HPV (types 6/11/16/18) vaccine in reducing the incidence of HPV infection and HPV-related genital disease in young men In: European Research Organization on Genital Infection and Neoplasia – EUROGIN Nice, France

Giuliano AR, Nielson CM, Flores R, Dunne EF, Abrahamsen M, Papenfuss MR, Markowitz LE, Smith D, Harris RB (2007) The optimal anatomic sites for sampling heterosexual men for human papillomavirus (HPV) detection: The HPV detection in men study. J Infect Dis 196: 1146–1152

Goncalves MA, Donadi EA (2004) Immune cellular response to HPV: Current concepts. Braz J Infect Dis 8: 1–9

Greer CE, Wheeler CM, Ladner MB, Beutner K, Coyne MY, Liang H, Langenberg A, Yen TS, Ralston R (1995) Human papillomavirus (HPV) type distribution and serological response to HPV type 6 virus-like particles in patients with genital warts. J Clin Microbiol 33: 2058–2063

Gross G, Meyer KG, Pres H, Thielert C, Tawfik H, Mescheder A (2007) A randomized, double-blind, four-arm parallel-group, placebo-controlled Phase II/III study to investigate the clinical efficacy of two galenic formulations of Polyphenon E in the treatment of external genital warts. J Eur Acad Dermatol Venereol 21: 1404–1412

Hadjivassiliou M, Stefanaki C, Nicolaidou E, Bethimoutis G, Anyfantakis V, Caroni C, Katsambas A (2007) Human papillomavirus assay in genital warts-correlation with symptoms. Int J STD AIDS 18: 329–334

Hadway P, Corbishley CM, Watkin NA (2006) Total glans resurfacing for premalignant lesions of the penis: initial outcome data. BJU Int 98: 532–536

Hengge UR, Tietze G (2000) Successful treatment of recalcitrant condyloma with topical cidofovir. Sex Transm Infect 76: 143

Hernandez BY, Wilkens LR, Zhu X, McDuffie K, Thompson P, Shvetsov YB, Ning L, Goodman MT (2008a) Circumcision and human papillomavirus infection in men: a site-specific comparison. J Infect Dis 197: 787–794

Hernandez BY, Wilkens LR, Zhu X, Thompson P, McDuffie K, Shvetsov YB, Kamemoto LE, Killeen J, Ning L, Goodman MT (2008b) Transmission of human papillomavirus in heterosexual couples. Emerg Infect Dis 14: 888–894

Hippelainen M, Syrjanen S, Koskela H, Pulkkinen J, Saarikoski S, Syrjanen K (1993) Prevalence and risk factors of genital human papillomavirus (HPV) infections in healthy males: a study on Finnish conscripts. Sex Transm Dis 20: 321–328

Ho HT, Woods KL, Bronson JJ, De Boeck H, Martin JC, Hitchcock MJ (1992) Intracellular metabolism of the anti-herpes agent (S)-1-[3-hydroxy-2-(phosphonylmethoxy)propyl]cytosine. Mol Pharmacol 41: 197–202

Hoyme UB, Hagedorn M, Schindler AE, Schneede P, Hopfenmuller W, Schorn K, Eul A (2002) Effect of adjuvant imiquimod 5% cream on sustained clearance of anogenital warts following laser treatment. Infect Dis Obstet Gynecol 10: 79–88

Insinga RP, Dasbach EJ, Myers ER (2003) The health and economic burden of genital warts in a set of private health plans in the United States. Clin Infect Dis 36: 1397–1403

Isaacs A, Lindenmann J (1987) Virus interference. I. The interferon. By A. Isaacs and J. Lindenmann, 1957. J Interferon Res 7: 429–438

Jensen SL (1985) Comparison of podophyllin application with simple surgical excision in clearance and recurrence of perianal condylomata acuminata. Lancet 2: 1146–1148

Kataoka A, Claesson U, Hansson BG, Eriksson M, Lindh E (1991) Human papillomavirus infection of the male diagnosed by Southern-blot hybridization and polymerase chain reaction: Comparison between urethra samples and penile biopsy samples. J Med Virol 33: 159–164

Khawaja HT (1989) Podophyllin versus scissor excision in the treatment of perianal condylomata acuminata: a prospective study. Br J Surg 76: 1067–1068

Kirby P, Dunne A, King DH, Corey L (1990) Double-blind randomized clinical trial of self-administered podofilox solution versus vehicle in the treatment of genital warts. Am J Med 88: 465–469

Kjaer SK, Munk C, Winther JF, Jorgensen HO, Meijer CJ, van den Brule AJ (2005) Acquisition and persistence of human papillomavirus infection in younger men: a prospective follow-up study among Danish soldiers. Cancer Epidemiol Biomarkers Prev 14: 1528–1533

Koshiol JE, Laurent SA, Pimenta JM (2004) Rate and predictors of new genital warts claims and genital warts-related healthcare utilization among privately insured patients in the United States. Sex Transm Dis 31: 748–752

Krebs HB, Schneider V (1987) Human papillomavirus-associated lesions of the penis: colposcopy, cytology, and histology. Obstet Gynecol 70: 299–304

Kumar B, Gupta S (2001) The acetowhite test in genital human papillomavirus infection in men: what does it add? J Eur Acad Dermatol Venereol 15: 27–29

Lacey CJ, Goodall RL, Tennvall GR, Maw R, Kinghorn GR, Fisk PG, Barton S, Byren I (2003) Randomised controlled trial and economic evaluation of podophyllotoxin solution, podophyllotoxin cream, and podophyllin in the treatment of genital warts. Sex Transm Infect 79: 270–275

Lajous M, Mueller N, Cruz-Valdez A, Aguilar LV, Franceschi S, Hernandez-Avila M, Lazcano-Ponce E (2005) Determinants of prevalence, acquisition, and persistence of human papillomavirus in healthy Mexican military men. Cancer Epidemiol Biomarkers Prev 14: 1710–1716

Lazcano-Ponce E, Herrero R, Munoz N, Hernandez-Avila M, Salmeron J, Leyva A, Meijer CJ, Walboomers JM (2001) High prevalence of human papillomavirus infection in Mexican males: comparative study of penile-urethral swabs and urine samples. Sex Transm Dis 28: 277–280

Li HX, Zhu WY, Xia MY (1995) Detection with the polymerase chain reaction of human papillomavirus DNA in condylomata acuminata treated with CO_2 laser and microwave. Int J Dermatol 34: 209–211

Loh CS, MacRobert AJ, Bedwell J, Regula J, Krasner N, Bown SG (1993) Oral versus intravenous administration of 5-aminolaevulinic acid for photodynamic therapy. Br J Cancer 68: 41–51

Macnab JC, Walkinshaw SA, Cordiner JW, Clements JB (1986) Human papillomavirus in clinically and histologically normal tissue of patients with genital cancer. N Engl J Med 315: 1052–1058

Majewski S, Marczak M, Mlynarczyk B, Benninghoff B, Jablonska S (2005) Imiquimod is a strong inhibitor of tumor cell-induced angiogenesis. Int J Dermatol 44: 14–19

Mansur CP (2002) Human papillomaviruses. In: Tyring SK, Yen-Moore A (eds) Mucocutaneous manifestations of viral diseases. Marcel Dekker, New York, pp 247–294

Mao C, Hughes JP, Kiviat N, Kuypers J, Lee SK, Adam DE, Koutsky LA (2003) Clinical findings among young women with genital human papillomavirus infection. Am J Obstet Gynecol 188: 677–684

Matteelli A, Beltrame A, Graifemberghi S, Forleo MA, Gulletta M, Ciravolo G, Tedoldi S, Casalini C, Carosi G (2001) Efficacy and tolerability of topical 1% cidofovir cream for the treatment of external anogenital warts in HIV-infected persons. Sex Transm Dis 28: 343–346

McClean H, Shann S (2005) A cross-sectional survey of treatment choices for anogenital warts. Int J STD AIDS 16: 212–216

Metawea B, El-Nashar AR, Kamel I, Kassem W, Shamloul R (2005) Application of viable bacille calmette-guerin topically as a potential therapeutic modality in condyloma acuminata: A placebo-controlled study. Urology 65: 247–250

Moore RA, Edwards JE, Hopwood J, Hicks D (2001) Imiquimod for the treatment of genital warts: a quantitative systematic review. BMC Infect Dis 1: 3

Narang T, Kanwar A (2006) Verrucous epidermal naevus on penis. In: Indian J Dermatol vol 51, pp 222–223

Newman L, Datta D, Ahrens K, Bissette J, Kerani R, Klinger E, Kohn R, Rietmeijer K, Weinstock H (2008) Monitoring genital wart disease in STD clinics through the STD Surveillance Network (SSuN). In: National STD Prevention Conference, Illinois, Chicago

Nicolau SM, Camargo CG, Stavale JN, Castelo A, Dores GB, Lorincz A, de Lima GR (2005) Human papillomavirus DNA detection in male sexual partners of women with genital human papillomavirus infection. Urology 65: 251–255

Nielson CM, Flores R, Harris RB, Abrahamsen M, Papenfuss MR, Dunne EF, Markowitz LE, Giuliano AR (2007) Human papillomavirus prevalence and type distribution in male anogenital sites and semen. Cancer Epidemiol Biomarkers Prev 16: 1107–1114

Orlando G, Fasolo MM, Beretta R, Merli S, Cargnel A (2002) Combined surgery and cidofovir is an effective treatment for genital warts in HIV-infected patients. AIDS 16: 447–450

Padilla-Ailhaud A (2006) Carbon dioxide laser vaporization of condyloma acuminata. J Low Genit Tract Dis 10: 238–241

Palefsky J, Giuliano A (2008) Efficacy of the quadrivalent HPV vaccine against HPV 6/11/16/18-related genital infection in young men In: European Research Organization on Genital Infection and Neoplasia – EUROGIN, Nice, France

Pao CC, Tsai PL, Chang YL, Hsieh TT, Jin JY (1993) Possible non-sexual transmission of genital human papillomavirus infections in young women. Eur J Clin Microbiol Infect Dis 12: 221–222

Partridge JM, Koutsky LA (2006) Genital human papillomavirus infection in men. Lancet Infect Dis 6: 21–31

Persson G, Andersson K, Krantz I (1996) Symptomatic genital papillomavirus infection in a community. Incidence and clinical picture. Acta Obstet Gynecol Scand 75: 287–290

Petersen CS, Bjerring P, Larsen J, Blaakaer J, Hagdrup H, From E, Obergaard L (1991) Systemic interferon alpha-2b increases the cure rate in laser treated patients with multiple persistent genital warts: a placebo-controlled study. Genitourin Med 67: 99–102

Petersen CS, Weismann K (1995) Quercetin and kaempherol: an argument against the use of podophyllin? Genitourin Med 71: 92–93

Pierson D, Bandel C, Ehrig T, Cockerell CJ (2003) Benign epithelial tumors and proliferations. In: Bolognia JL, Jorizzo JL, Rapini RP (eds) Dermatology. Mosby, Edinburgh, pp 1697–1720

Scheinfeld N, Lehman DS (2006) An evidence-based review of medical and surgical treatments of genital warts. Dermatol Online J 12: 5

Schofer H, Van Ophoven A, Henke U, Lenz T, Eul A (2006) Randomized, comparative trial on the sustained efficacy of topical imiquimod 5% cream versus conventional ablative methods in external anogenital warts. Eur J Dermatol 16: 642–648

Schurmann D, Bergmann F, Temmesfeld-Wollbruck B, Grobusch MP, Suttorp N (2000) Topical cidofovir is effective in treating extensive penile condylomata acuminata. AIDS 14: 1075–1076

Sherrard J, Riddell L (2007) Comparison of the effectiveness of commonly used clinic-based treatments for external genital warts. Int J STD AIDS 18: 365–368

Shin HR, Franceschi S, Vaccarella S, Roh JW, Ju YH, Oh JK, Kong HJ, Rha SH, Jung SI, Kim JI, Jung KY, van Doorn LJ, Quint W (2004) Prevalence and determinants of genital infection with papillomavirus, in female and male university students in Busan, South Korea. J Infect Dis 190: 468–476

Smetana Z, Malik Z, Orenstein A, Mendelson E, Ben-Hur E (1997) Treatment of viral infections with 5-aminolevulinic acid and light. Lasers Surg Med 21: 351–358

Smith JS, Moses S, Hudgens MG, Agot K, Franceschi S, Maclean IW, Ndinya-Achola JO, Parker CB, Pugh N, Meijer CJ, Snijders PJ, Bailey RC (2007) Human papillomavirus detection by penile site in young men from Kenya. Sex Transm Dis 34: 928–934

Sonnex C, Strauss S, Gray JJ (1999) Detection of human papillomavirus DNA on the fingers of patients with genital warts. Sex Transm Infect 75: 317–319

Sonnex C, Vrotsou K (2007) Treatment of ano-genital warts: the effect of an educational event on practitioner choice. Int J STD AIDS 18: 531–537

Stockfleth E, Beti H, Orasan R, Grigorian F, Mescheder A, Tawfik H, Thielert C (2008) Topical Polyphenon E in the treatment of external genital and perianal warts: a randomized controlled trial. Br J Dermatol 158: 1329–1338

Stone KM, Becker TM, Hadgu A, Kraus SJ (1990) Treatment of external genital warts: a randomised clinical trial comparing podophyllin, cryotherapy, and electrodesiccation. Genitourin Med 66: 16–19

Strand A, Rylander E, Wilander E, Zehbe I, Kraaz W (1996) Histopathologic examination of penile epithelial lesions is of limited diagnostic value in human papillomavirus infection. Sex Transm Dis 23: 293–298

Syed TA, Lundin S, Cheema KM, Kahlon BM, Cheema R, Ahmad SA, Ahmad M (1994) Human leukocyte interferon-alpha in cream, for the treatment of genital warts in Asian women: a placebo-controlled, double-blind study. Clin Investig 72: 870–873

Tay SK, Ho TH, Lim-Tan SK (1990) Is genital human papillomavirus infection always sexually transmitted? Aust N Z J Obstet Gynaecol 30: 240–242

Tobian AA, Serwadda D, Quinn TC, Kigozi G, Gravitt PE, Laeyendecker O, Charvat B, Ssempijja V, Riedesel M, Oliver AE, Nowak RG, Moulton LH, Chen MZ, Reynolds SJ, Wawer MJ, Gray RH (2009) Male circumcision for the prevention of HSV-2 and HPV infections and syphilis. N Engl J Med 360: 1298-1309

Trizna Z, Evans T, Bruce S, Hatch K, Tyring SK (1998) A randomized phase II study comparing four different interferon therapies in patients with recalcitrant condylomata acuminata. Sex Transm Dis 25: 361–365

Tseng CJ, Pao CC, Lin JD, Soong YK, Hong JH, Hsueh S (1999) Detection of human papillomavirus types 16 and 18 mRNA in peripheral blood of advanced cervical cancer patients and its association with prognosis. J Clin Oncol 17: 1391–1396

Van Doornum GJ, Prins M, Juffermans LH, Hooykaas C, van den Hoek JA, Coutinho RA, Quint WG (1994) Regional distribution and incidence of human papillomavirus infections among heterosexual men and women with multiple sexual partners: a prospective study. Genitourin Med 70: 240–246

Vexiau D, Decuypere L, Moyse D, Aractingi S (2005) [Efficacy and safety of 5% imiquimod cream in external genital warts: a 6 month follow-up evaluation]. Ann Dermatol Venereol 132: 845–851

von Krogh G (2001) Management of anogenital warts (condylomata acuminata). Eur J Dermatol 11: 598–603; quiz 604

Weaver BA, Feng Q, Holmes KK, Kiviat N, Lee SK, Meyer C, Stern M, Koutsky LA (2004) Evaluation of genital sites and sampling techniques for detection of human papillomavirus DNA in men. J Infect Dis 189: 677–685

Wikstrom A, Popescu C, Forslund O (2000) Asymptomatic penile HPV infection: a prospective study. Int J STD AIDS 11: 80–84

Wikstrom A, von Krogh G (1998) Efficacy of surgical and/or podophyllotoxin treatment against flat acetowhite penile human papillomavirus associated lesions. Int J STD AIDS 9: 537–542

Wiley DJ, Douglas J, Beutner K, Cox T, Fife K, Moscicki AB, Fukumoto L (2002) External genital warts: diagnosis, treatment, and prevention. Clin Infect Dis 35: S210–S224

Wilson L, Bamburg JR, Mizel SB, Grisham LM, Creswell KM (1974) Interaction of drugs with microtubule proteins. Fed Proc 33: 158–166

Workowski KA, Berman SM (2007) Centers for Disease Control and Prevention sexually transmitted diseases treatment guidelines. Clin Infect Dis 44 Suppl 3: S73–S76

Yan J, Chen SL, Wang HN, Wu TX (2006) Meta-analysis of 5% imiquimod and 0.5% podophyllotoxin in the treatment of condylomata acuminata. Dermatology 213: 218–223

Yun K, Joblin L (1993) Presence of human papillomavirus DNA in condylomata acuminata in children and adolescents. Pathology 25: 1–3Fig. 3.20. (Continued)

Human Papillomavirus-Associated Lesions of the Urinary Tract

4

Alberto Rosenblatt and Homero Gustavo de Campos Guidi

Contents

A. Rosenblatt (✉)
Albert Einstein Jewish Hospital, Sao Paulo, Brasil
e-mail: albrose1@gmail.com

4.1   Introduction

Human papillomavirus (HPV) infection can affect the urethra of male and female individuals causing symptoms and concern. Urethral lesions (warts) may occasionally develop and the urethra can also be a source of HPV infection, contributing to the spread of infection between partners.

This chapter reviews updated concepts concerning urethral HPV, including new detection methods, treatment options, and prevention. In addition, the role of HPV in the development of urethral, bladder, prostate, and kidney cancer is also discussed.

4.2   Overview

The prevalence of urethral involvement among genital HPV-associated lesions is 4–25% (von Krogh, 2001) and the prevalence of HPV detection in the urethra, in the absence of clinical lesions, ranges from 3 to 50% (Rosemberg et al., 1988; Katelaris et al., 1988; Cecchini et al., 1988; Aynaud et al., 2003).

Chuang et al. (1984) reported that the male urethra is affected more often than the female urethra, and recent analysis by von Krogh (2001) reported HPV-related meatal lesions in 20–25% of male and 4–8% of female individuals. Meatal warts have also been observed in children, and Takatsuki et al. (1993) described a relapsing meatal condyloma in a 4-year-old boy.

A. Rosenblatt, H. G. de Campos Guidi, *Human Papillomavirus*,
DOI: 10.1007/978-3-540-70974-9-4, © Springer-Verlag Berlin Heidelberg 2009

HPV-related lesions are usually found at the distal 2–3 cm of the urethra, and the proximal urethra is usually not involved without previous or simultaneous lesions in the distal portion (Culp and Kaplan, 1944; Gartman, 1956; von Krogh, 2001). Rothman et al. (1994) showed that of 90 men with external meatal warts, 15 (16.7%) also had more proximal lesions and only 5 (5.6%) had lesions at or beyond the pendulous urethra.

Detection studies using cytological analysis of urethral brushings as well as hybridization techniques applied to urethral brushings have shown evidence to support the urethra as a reservoir for HPV (Cecchini et al., 1988; Zderic et al., 1989).

The association of HPV and urethral carcinoma in both sexes has been described by several investigators (Wiener et al., 1992; Wiener and Walther, 1994; Sumino et al., 2006). However, bladder involvement is rare in immunocompetent individuals and although high- and low-risk HPV types can be detected in bladder specimens, there is ongoing controversy on the role of HPV in bladder carcinogenesis (Noel et al., 1994; Olsen et al., 1995; Aynaud et al., 1998; Griffiths and Mellon, 2000; Chrisofos et al., 2004; Youshya et al., 2005).

4.3   Clinical Manifestations

4.3.1   Symptoms

● Asymptomatic in the majority of cases

4.3.1.1   Less Frequent

● Itching sensation usually preceding the appearance of the lesion
● Light bleeding or spotting following masturbation or coitus
● Hemospermia (Jones, 1991)
● Urethral discharge and dysuria
● Urethritis (significantly associated with HPV detection, according to recent data presented by de Carvalho et al. (2006)
● Secondary infection resulting in pyuria

4.3.1.2   Atypical Occurrence

● Urinary retention due to meatal obstruction (Kilciler et al., 2007) (Fig. 4.1)

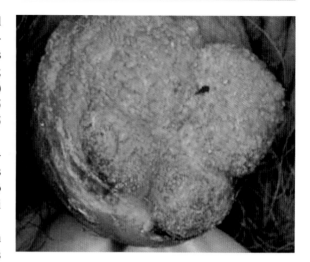

Fig. 4.1. HPV-related lesion obstructing the urethral meatus

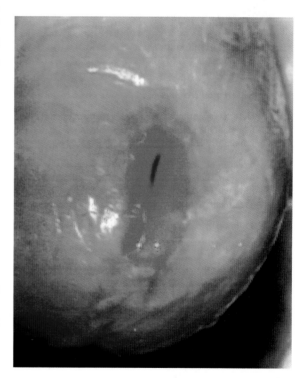

Fig. 4.2. Meatal "rouge lips"

4.3.2   Presentation

● Meatal lips can exhibit hyperemia and edema ("rouge lip" appearance) (Fig. 4.2). Fralick et al. (1994) reported that "rouge lip" was associated with urethral HPV infection in 30% of cases.

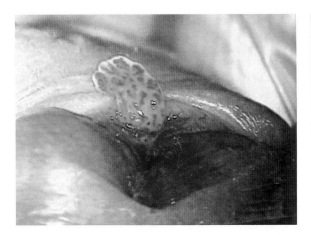

Fig. 4.3. Urethral lesion extending through the meatus

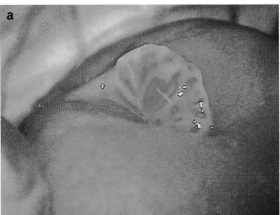

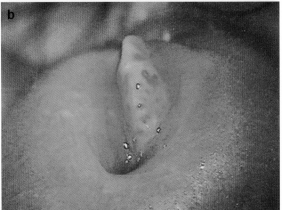

Fig. 4.5. (**a**) Fleshy appearance of urethral condyloma. (**b**) Broad-based lesion, friable and vascular

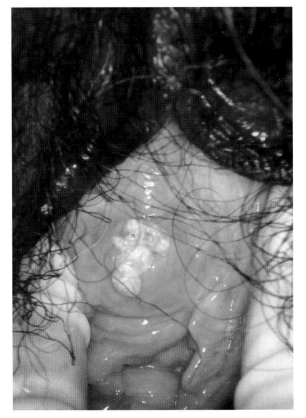

Fig. 4.4. HPV-related lesion protruding through the female meatus

- Lesions are usually found on the moist surface of the fossa navicularis and extend through the meatus (Fig. 4.3).

- HPV-associated lesions can rarely extend to the proximal urethra and bladder in immunosuppressed individuals.
- Lesions are usually single and rarely multiple (Fig. 4.4).
- Classic flesh appearance, soft, friable, and vascular (Fig. 4.5a, b).
- Meatal sentinel lesions may indicate presence of urethral involvement (Fig. 4.6a–c).
- Urethral lesions can coexist with external warts (in up to 36% of cases, according to Huguet Perez et al., 1996) (Fig. 4.7a, b).
- HPV-related urethral lesions can exhibit a hyperpigmented appearance (Fig. 4.8).

4

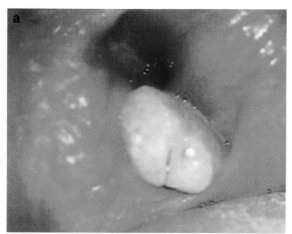

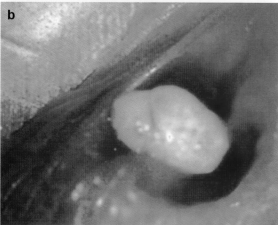

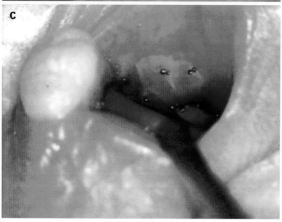

Fig. 4.6 (**a**) Sentinel lesion. (**b**) Meatal sentinel lesion. (**c**) Meatal sentinel and urethral lesion

115 **4.3.2.1 Lesion Base**

116 ● Individually on a stalk
117 ● Broad-based and coalescent (Fig. 4.9)

4.4 Differential Diagnosis

● Normal anatomic variance
● Urethral caruncle
● Urethral polyp in young female patients
● Other sexually transmitted diseases (STDs), if urethral discharge is the main symptom
● Urethral malignancy (may also be associated with HPV-related lesions)

Expert Advice

If urethral discharge is the only symptom, further investigation is necessary to determine the exact etiology of the discharge, because different STDs may coexist.

4.5 Detection Methods

4.5.1 Clinical Diagnosis

4.5.1.1 Physical Examination of the Meatus and Fossa Navicularis

Despite its reduced sensitivity, clinical examination is the reference standard for detecting HPV infection of the male urethra (Aynaud et al., 2003).

● Gentle manual eversion of the meatal lips allows for the visual inspection of the urethral meatus and fossa navicularis (Fig. 4.10).

Expert Advice

Meatal lip eversion should be performed on every patient and particularly in those presenting with genital condyloma (Fig. 4.11a, b).

Expert Advice

Urethral malformations (hypospadias and epispadias) (Fig. 4.12a–c) and anatomic variance (Fig. 4.13) should be carefully examined for genital warts.

● Visual inspection using a magnifying glass, surgical microscope, or an articulated microscope (Fig. 4.14a, b), and using three magnifications (3.5×, 5.4×, 8×) or five magnifications (2×, 3.5×, 5.4×, 8×, 13.3×).

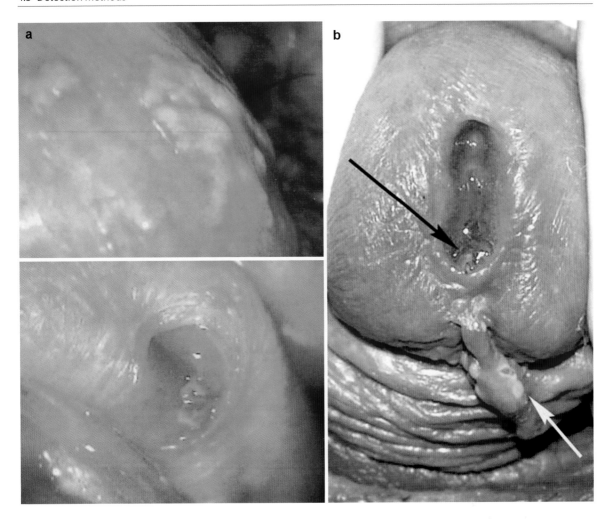

Fig. 4.7. (**a**) Flat condyloma (glans penis) associated with urethral lesion. (**b**) Urethral lesion (*black arrow*) and frenular lesion (*white arrow*)

- Meatoscopy.
  - The use of a meatal spreader (Hartmann nasal speculum) allows visualization of the first 2 cm of the urethra (Aynaud, 1992).
  - An otoscope is useful for the adequate visualization of lesions in the fossa navicularis and first 3 cm of urethra (Fig. 4.15).

How to Perform Meatoscopy Using the Otoscope

Aqueous chlorhexidine solution is used to clean the glans and urethral meatus, and a small amount of lidocaine gel is applied to the meatal area. A sterile and disposable otoscope cone is gently introduced through the meatus while the patient exerts penile traction.

- The procedure is asymptomatic.

Expert Advice

Thin (1992) recommends that meatoscopy should be performed on all patients with meatal warts to correctly assess the lesion base and extension.

4.5.2 Laboratory Diagnosis

4.5.2.1 Brushing Cytology

- To improve the quality of the specimen, saline solution drops are instilled into the meatus before "brushing" of the fossa navicularis and meatal area (Fig. 4.16).
  - The weak adherence of HPV-related lesions in the urethra usually yields high cellularity samples.
  - Lubricant or anesthetic gel is usually not used as it might influence smear quality.

4

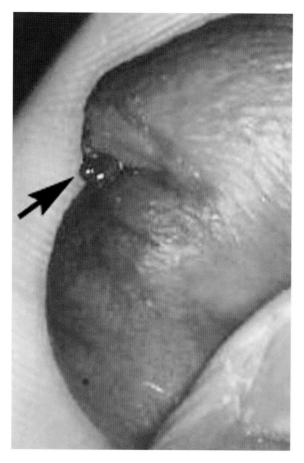

Fig. 4.8. Hyperpigmented HPV-related urethral lesion (*arrow*)

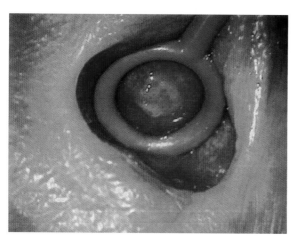

Fig. 4.9. Broad-based lesion

– The use of a soft plastic bacteriological loop (Fig. 4.16) is preferred to avoid urethral trauma and pain during specimen collection.

According to Aynaud et al. (2003):

● In the absence of clinical lesions in the urethra, cytology is nonspecific for urethral HPV infection.

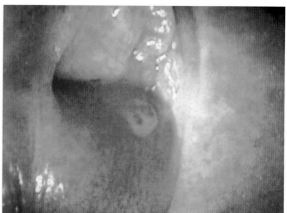

Fig. 4.10 Meatal lip eversion

● Urethral cytology as a single screening method may lead to a high number of false-positive findings.

4.5.2.2 Biopsy and Histopathological Evaluation

Specimens can be removed for histopathological evaluation with:

● Cold cup biopsy using a suitable instrument for meatal warts (Fig. 4.17a, b)
● Endoscopic resection for urethral and bladder lesions

Histopathological Findings

● Koilocytosis (Fig. 4.18), the hallmark histopathological feature of HPV infection, can lead to false-positive and false-negative results and its use as a pathognomonic sign of HPV infection is not recommended (Strand et al., 1996).
● HPV DNA can be detected in biopsy specimens that lack the classic histological features of HPV infection, although the detection rate is much lower than for condylomata (Nuovo et al., 1990).

Biopsy Indications

● If lesion appearance is equivocal or atypical
● To rule out malignancy, particularly in immunocompromised patients
● If lesion is unresponsive or worsens during clinical treatment
● If lesion exhibits irregular dyschromia

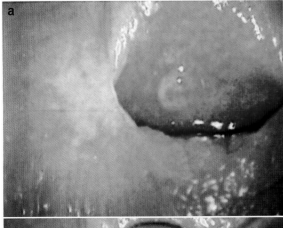

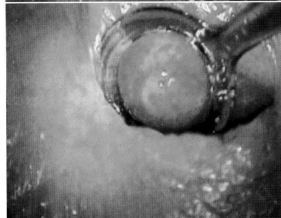

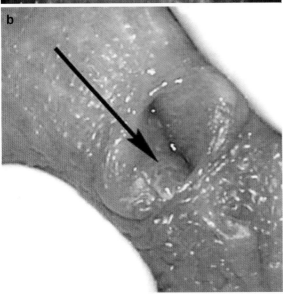

Fig. 4.11. (**a**) Meatal lip eversion disclosing small fossa navicular lesion. (**b**) Small fossa navicular lesion (*arrow*)

4.5.2.3 Molecular Tests

See also Chap. 2.

Urethral Meatus/Fossa Navicularis (Fig. 4.19)

1. Specimens are collected by brushing the urethral meatus and fossa navicularis.
   - In a survey evaluating HPV prevalence in Mexican soldiers performed by Aguilar et al. (2006), HPV DNA was detected more frequently in external genitalia samples (46.4%) than in the urethra (20.8%) or meatus samples (12.1%).

Can HPV Detection Be Improved by Adding Urethral Samples?

Although urethral sampling provides adequate cell counts, the HPV DNA testing does not markedly increase overall HPV positivity beyond that found in the glans penis and coronal sulcus due to its low sensitivity for HPV detection.

Furthermore, the discomfort caused by the collection method could be a barrier for its generalized use (Aguilar et al., 2006).

Urine/Semen

- HPV DNA is present in the urine of patients with urethral condylomata, as urine may wash infected cells from the urethral epithelium (Iwasawa et al., 1997). However, in a recent study evaluating the presence of HPV DNA in first-voided urine (FVU) and urethroglandular brushed samples, D'Hauwers et al. (2007) reported that HPV-PCR tested positive in 60% of the male brushed samples and negative in all of the male FVU specimens.
- High-risk HPV DNA has been detected at variable percentages in semen (8–64%), but the consequences of this finding are yet unknown (Green et al., 1991).
- HPV DNA has been found in samples from the vas deferens (possibly eliminating the issue of urethral contamination), and thus raising the question of HPV transmission through sperm donation (Rintala et al., 2002).

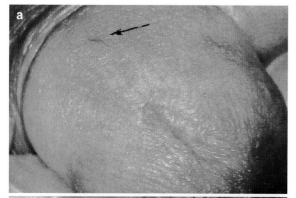

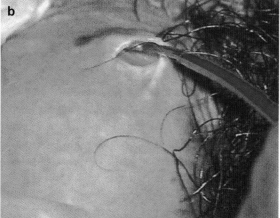

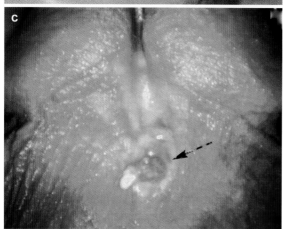

Fig. 4.12. (**a**) Balanic epispadia (*arrow*). (**b**) Careful examination of epispadic urethral meatus. (**c**) HPV-related lesion (*arrow*) protruding through the hypospadiac meatus

- However, Rintala et al. (2004) found no significant associations between seminal HPV DNA and altered semen parameters in HPV-positive semen, except for borderline lower pH values.

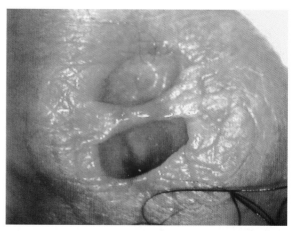

Fig. 4.13. Lacuna magna (also known as Guérin's sinus)

- At present, there is no consensus about the real value of urethral and semen samples when the overall HPV male infection is considered. In a recent HPV detection study, Giuliano et al. (2007) reported that the exclusion of these two sites, plus the scrotal and perianal areas, resulted in a prevalence reduction of less than 5%.

4.5.2.4 Urethroscopy

- Urethroscopy using a 0-degree lens should be performed on all patients with distal penile (glans, corona, or frenulum) or meatal lesions (Kaplinsky et al., 1995).

Urethroscopy – When to Perform

- Urethroscopy should not be performed until all meatal condylomata have been eradicated to avoid the potential risk of seeding disease into the proximal urethra, prostate, or bladder during retrograde passage of the cystoscope (Sumino et al., 2004).
- Urethral instillation of 5-fluorouracil (5-FU) prior to instrumentation of the involved distal urethra is recommended.

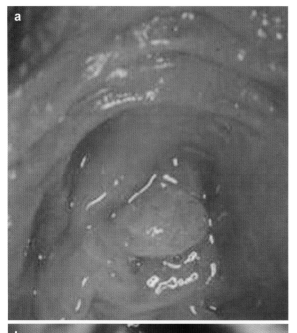

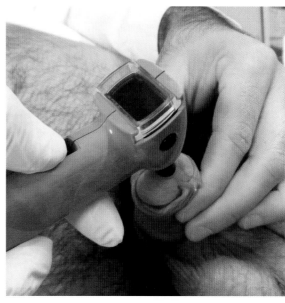

Fig. 4.15. An otoscope is used for distal urethra inspection

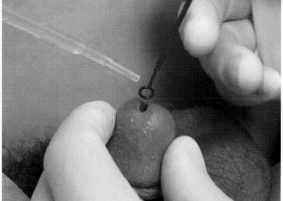

Fig. 4.14. (**a**) HPV-related lesion protruding through the female urethral meatus. (**b**) Condyloma located in the female urethra

Fig. 4.16. Meatal and fossa navicularis cytology using a plastic bacteriological loop and saline drops

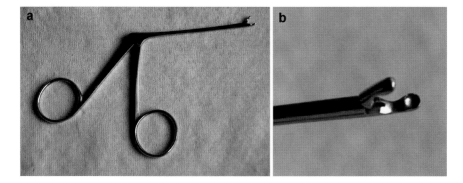

Fig. 4.17. (**a**) Hartman-Herzfeld Ear Forceps. (**b**) Cup-shaped jaws

4

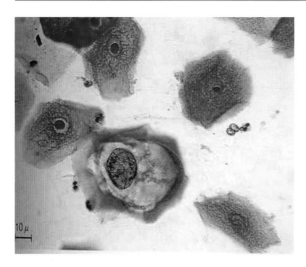

Fig. 4.18. Koilocyte (detailed in *blue*) (Source: Photograph courtesy of Monica Stiepcich MD, PhD, São Paulo, Brazil)

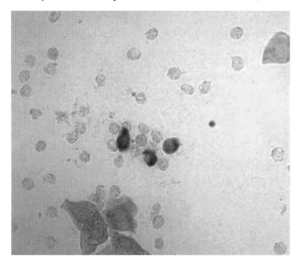

Fig. 4.19. Urethral brushing HPV DNA-positive (in situ hybridization 40×) (Source: Photograph courtesy of Monica Stiepcich MD, PhD, São Paulo, Brazil)

> **Expert Advice**
>
> A simplified "waterless" urethroscopy can be performed using a pediatric cystoscope with a 0-degree lens and lidocaine 2% gel as an alternative to conventional urethroscopy.

4.5.2.5   Image Diagnosis

Antegrade and Retrograde Urethrography

● Sawczuk et al. (1983) recommended the use of antegrade and retrograde urethrography as an alternative

to urethroscopy to screen for and follow the treatment response of urethral HPV, minimizing the risk of virus dissemination.

● Antegrade and retrograde urethrography are useful examinations in cases of multiple condylomata and large lesions, but false-negative results are common in small or flat urethral lesions.

 – The use of catheters for radiological contrast medium instillation is contraindicated to prevent retrograde seeding of disease into the proximal urethra or bladder.

Ultrasonography and Computed Tomography

Pelvic US and CT Can Be Performed

● To rule out bladder involvement in immunosuppressed patients presenting with distal urethral lesions
● As a screening examination prior to cystoscopy

4.6   Treatment (Table 4.1)

Therapy choice is based on lesion:

● Number
● Size and morphology
● Location

Additional factors that define therapy choice:

● Physician experience
● Treatment cost, convenience, and adverse effects
● Patient choice
● Meatal anatomy

> **Expert Advice**
>
> Pictures or a schematic representation of lesions at each visit is a useful tool for evaluating treatment response and follow-up.

4.6.1   Medical Therapies

4.6.1.1   Cytotoxic Agents

Podophyllotoxin

Podophyllotoxin contains purified podophyllin in a standardized concentration in cream (not available in the United States), gel, or solution preparation.

Table 4.1 Treatments for urethral warts (Adapted from: Kodner and Nasraty (2004). Reproduced with permission from *American Family Physician*. Copyright © 2004 American Academy of Family Physicians. All Rights Reserved)

Treatment	Clearance rates (%)	Risk of recurrence (%)	Adverse effects
Cryotherapy	Female proximal urethra: 75 with one treatment and 25 with two treatments (Sand et al., 1987)	25–39 (Beutner and Ferenczy, 1997)	Pain or blisters at application site
Imiquimod (Aldara) Contra-indicated in urethral lesions	‡	‡	Erythema; irritation, ulceration, and pain; burning, erosion, flaking, edema, induration, and pigmentary changes at application site; minimal systemic absorption
Interferon	64 (Levine et al., 1996)	‡	None
CO_2 laser treatment	50–86.6 (Rosemberg et al., 1982; Graversen et al., 1990; Krogh et al., 1990)	5–50	Similar to surgical excision; risk of spreading HPV via smoke plumes; low risk of urethral stricture, meatal stenosis and frequency (Krogh et al., 1990)
Nd:YAG laser treatment	30–40 (Volz et al., 1994); 100 (Bloiso et al., 1988)	35.7 (Zaak et al., 2003)	Reduced risk of meatal stenosis; less plumes with reduced risk of HPV spreading
Podofilox (condylox) Contra-indicated in urethral lesions	‡	‡	Burning at application site, pain, meatitis; low risk of systemic toxicity
Podophyllin resin Contra-indicated in urethral lesions	‡	‡	Local irritation, erythema, burning, and soreness at application site; possibly mutagenicity, oncogenicity
Endoscopic electrocoagulation	‡	14–35.2 (Gonzalvo Perez et al., 1994; Huguet Perez et al., 1996)	Pain, bleeding, scarring and meatal stenosis; risk of burning and allergic reaction from local anesthetic
5-FU cream and solution	25–95 (Dyment, 1996)	53 (Carpiniello et al., 1990)	Risk of severe local side effects (scrotal irritation or meatitis)
BCG	‡	Reduced from 3.2 with standard therapy to 0.75 (Bohle et al., 1998)	Mild dysuria, penile edema, fever of short duration
5-ALA photodynamic therapy	95 (Wang et al., 2004)	6.3 (Chen et al., 2007)	Mild burning and/or stinging sensation; erythema, mild edema, and skin erosion following treatment
Transurethral resection	‡	‡	Bleeding, dysuria, frequency; risk of urethral stricture, meatal stenosis

Time until recurrence varied across studies, but recurrence rates typically are measured at 3 months after treatment. ‡- insufficient data; *5-FU* 5-fluorouracil; *BCG* bacille Calmette-Guérin

4

Expert Advice

Podofilox is not recommended for intraurethral warts. Although it can be used to treat meatal lesions (Clinical Effectiveness Group, 2007), caution should be taken with the urethral mucosa.

How to Use

Podophyllotoxin 0.15% cream is applied once daily with a cotton-tipped swab for 3–4 days, and then discontinued for four consecutive days (von Krogh, 2001).

The 1-week cycle of treatment may be repeated until there is no visible wart tissue or for a maximum of four cycles.

● Stop use if signs of local irritation persist.

Advantages

● Patient-applied medication.
● Cream or gel formulations are easier to use for perimeatal and meatal lesions.
● Inexpensive.

Disadvantages

● Limited data evaluating use of podophyllotoxin for the treatment of meatal warts
● Recurrence rate for meatal warts: Insufficient evidence-based data
● Contraindicated during pregnancy

Adverse Effects

● Pain and burning sensation at application site
● Meatitis
● Low risk of systemic toxicity

Podophyllin

Expert Advice

Podophyllin is not recommended for intraurethral warts. Although it can be used to treat meatal lesions (Workowski and Berman, 2007), caution should be taken with the urethral mucosa.

How to Use

Podophyllin 10–25% in a compound tincture of benzoin should be applied to meatal lesions with a cotton-tipped swab once weekly.

The affected area should be clean and dry before application and, after use, podophyllin should be allowed to air dry. The involved area should be thoroughly washed 1–4 h after application.

● Stop use if signs of local irritation persist.

Advantages

● Efficacy – data for meatal warts: No evidence-based data available

Disadvantages

● Recurrence rate: No evidence-based data available

Adverse Effects

● Meatitis
● Burning and pain at application site
● Meatal stenosis and adhesions
● Systemic side effects due to higher absorption of podophyllin by moist surface of urethral mucosa

● Contraindicated during pregnancy (potential risk of mutagenicity and oncogenicity)

5-Fluorouracil Cream (Efudex®)

Fluorouracil, a fluoropyrimidine, is a widely used chemotherapeutic agent that belongs to a group of drugs known as antimetabolites. It is incorporated into RNA in preference to the natural substrate uracil and the drug inhibits cell growth and promotes apoptosis by targeting the enzyme thymidylate synthetase.

Advantages

● Patient-applied medication.
● Inexpensive: U.S. $40.99/15 g (generic).
● Painless.
● Efficacy: 5-FU efficacy ranged from 25 to 95%, according to the study performed by Dyment (1996).

Disadvantages

● Risk of severe local side effects (scrotal irritation or meatitis (Fig. 4.20)) if not correctly used.
● Recurrence rate: Carpiniello et al. (1990) reported recurrences in 53% of the patients in a long-term follow-up of subclinical HPV infection treated with 5-FU.

How to Use

5-FU cream is applied with a cotton swab or injected (1 ml) into the urethra 3–4 times a week and washed away after 30–60 min.
    Treatment duration is approximately 3–4 weeks.

Important

The scrotum should be protected to avoid possible skin erosion.

Expert Advice

In a recent case report of an HIV-infected patient presenting with pan-urethral warts, Wen et al. (2006) demonstrated good results using intraurethral instillation of 5-FU solution (500 mg in normal saline 50 ml) once a week for 7 weeks, and then once a month until urethral lesions were no longer detected at urethroscopy.

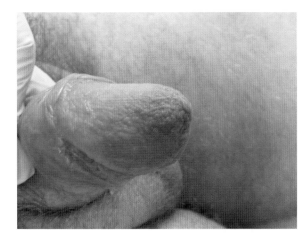

Fig. 4.20. Meatitis after intraurethral 5-FU application

4.6.1.2 Immune-Response Modifiers

Imiquimod (Aldara®)

Expert Advice

Not approved for use against cervical, vaginal, intraurethral, or rectal warts (3M Pharmaceuticals, Aldara, package insert), although treatment can be recommended in selected patients with recurring disease.
    Imiquimod use for urethral meatal lesions can be recommended if the lesion base is visualized (Clinical Effectiveness Group, 2007).

How to Use

Imiquimod is applied to urethral meatal warts at bedtime and washed off in the morning.
    It should be repeated three times per week for 16 weeks.
● Stop use if signs of local irritation persist.

Advantages

● Patient-applied medication
● May stimulate a cell-mediated immune response against HPV
● Efficacy rate: Insufficient data for urethral warts

Disadvantages

● Expensive: U.S. $153.99 (12 sachets) and U.S. $291.99 (24 sachets) (2008-based costs)
● No direct antiviral activity
● Therapeutic effects may take up to 4 weeks to occur
● Limited data evaluating use of imiquimod for the treatment of urethral meatal warts (Workowski and Berman, 2007)
● Prolonged treatment duration
● Contraindicated during pregnancy

Adverse Effects

Frequent

● Mild to severe erythema
● Localized erosions
● Itching or burning sensations

Less Frequent

- Local irritation
- Induration
- Crust formation
- Tenderness

4.6.2 Surgical Therapies

4.6.2.1 Excision

Excision of meatal warts can be performed using scissors, scalpel, or electrocautery.

Indications

- Usually recommended for large lesions that involve the urethral meatus and cause obstruction (Scheinfeld and Lehman, 2006).
- Excision is the preferred option when histopathological examination is needed to rule out malignancy.

Advantages

- Efficacy rate: 35–70% for urethral meatal lesions

Disadvantages

- Anesthesia is required (local, regional, or general).
- Scarring.
- Pain.
- Meatotomy may be required for fossa navicular lesions (Gartman, 1956) (Fig. 4.21).
- Recurrence rate: 20% for urethral meatal lesions.

Complications

- Excessive bleeding can occur as urethral warts are highly vascular.
- Allergic reaction risk from local anesthetic.

Expert Advice

Use of a topical anesthetic is recommended. EMLA cream (AstraZeneca, Wilmington, Delaware), a eutectic mixture of lidocaine 2.5% and prilocaine 2.5%, should be applied in the urethral meatus for a minimum of 15 min before the procedure to minimize pain from local anesthetic injection (a solution of 1% lidocaine *without epinephrine* should be used for procedures involving the penis and distal urethra) (see also Sect. 10.6.3.4 in Chap. 10).

4.6.2.2 Endoscopic Electrosurgical Techniques

Advantages

- Widely available and cost effective.
- Office procedure.
- Bleeding can be easily controlled.
- Efficacy rate: Huguet Perez et al. (1996) reported clearance of lesions after two sessions in nearly all of the 24 patients treated with the method.

Disadvantages

- Anesthesia is required (local, regional, or general).
- Development of meatal stenosis resulting from circumferential thermal injury of the meatus (McKenna and McMillan, 1990; Zheng et al., 2000). However, a novel technique to avoid meatal stenosis described by Shaw and Payne (2007) reported good short-term results.

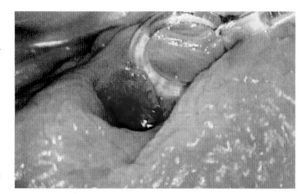

Fig. 4.21. Urethral lesion and a difficult meatus

- Postoperative pain (usually controlled with simple analgesics).
- Recurrence rate: Available data report recurrences in 14–35.2% of patients (Gonzalvo Perez et al., 1994; Huguet Perez et al., 1996), with no differences observed between subjects submitted to electrocoagulation and those patients treated by Nd:YAG laser photocoagulation (Huguet Perez et al., 1996).

Complications

- Pain
- Bleeding
- Scarring
- Burning risk
- Risk of allergic reaction from local anesthetic

4.6.2.3 Cryotherapy

Cryotherapy involves application of nitrous oxide or liquid nitrogen (−196°C) to HPV-related lesions. It induces dermal and vascular damage and edema, causing cellular destruction by thermal-induced cytolysis.

> **How to Use**
>
> Liquid nitrogen is applied directly to meatal warts with a cotton-tipped swab for about 10–20 s until a white halo appears around the circumference of the lesion (indicating that it is frozen). Subsequent thaw produces cell lysis.
>   Treatment is repeated every 2 weeks until the lesion disappears.
> - According to Dyment (1996), it is important to treat a small margin of normal-appearing tissue surrounding the lesion because HPV DNA has been found as far out as 5-10 mm from the visible wart.

Advantages

- Relatively inexpensive.
- Ease of application.
- Rapid destructive effect.
- Injected anesthesia is not usually required, but topical anesthesia with lidocaine (spray or gel) or EMLA cream may facilitate therapy.

- Can be used for any meatal wart that is accessible to treatment.
- Efficacy for proximal urethral lesions in female patients: 75% with one treatment session and 25% with two sessions, according to the study performed by Sand et al. (1987).
- Healing usually occurs 1–2 weeks after treatment.

Disadvantages

- Recurrence rate: 25–39% (Beutner and Ferenczy, 1997)

Adverse Effects

- Pain or blisters at application site

4.6.2.4 CO_2 Laser Vaporization

See Chap. 10.

Indications

- Lesions located in the urethral meatus and fossa navicularis

> **CO_2 Laser Technique**
>
> See Chap. 10.
>
> - Carbon dioxide (CO_2) laser is coupled to the operating microscope for enhanced visualization.
> - Lesions are vaporized under direct colposcopic guidance.
> - Power settings of 4–5 W in continuous or pulsed mode are used in urethral meatus and fossa navicularis for depth destruction not exceeding 1 mm.
> - It is important to focus the beam over the lesion and move the laser beam as quickly as possible.
> - Lesions are vaporized along with a 2–3-mm border of normal-appearing epithelium (Fig. 4.22a. b).

> Following vaporization of the lesion(s), the unfocused laser beam should be quickly "flashed" over the remaining epithelium of the urethral meatus and fossa navicularis. The brief thermal effect created will likely destroy any latent virus contained within the area.
> - Bleeding is controlled with the unfocused laser beam.

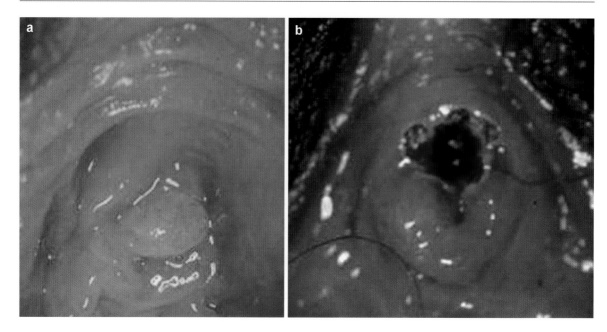

Fig. 4.22. (**a**) Laser treatment of female meatal lesion. (**b**) A 2–3-mm safety margin

Expert Advice

Urologists are frequently consulted for the diagnosis and treatment of female urethral lesions associated with HPV. Gentle traction exerted on the lesion exposes its pedicle, and the urethral mucosa around the lesion is minimally affected in the majority of cases.

Important

Urethroscopy should be performed at a later stage to avoid the potential risk of seeding disease into the proximal urethra and bladder.

(See above, *Urethroscopy – When to Perform*)

Advantages

- Sharply precise
- Shallow depth of penetration with above settings
- Fast and usually bloodless technique
- Good cosmetic results
- Office procedure
- Efficacy: 86.6% after single treatment (Rosemberg et al., 1982); 50% after single treatment, and 86% after three treatments (Graversen et al., 1990); 78% after single treatment of isolated meatal lesion (Krogh et al., 1990)

Disadvantages

- Expensive and not widely available.
- Experience with the technique required.
- Recurrence rate: 5–50%, usually developing within 3 months after treatment.
- HPV DNA may be released during the procedure and a smoke evacuation system must always be used (see Sect. 10.4.1.2 in Chap. 10).

Complications

- Urethral stricture (less than 2%), meatal stenosis (8%), and frequency (3%) (Krogh et al., 1990)

4.6.2.5   Neodymium:YAG Laser/Holmium: YAG Laser

Mechanism of Action

Photothermic mechanism causing protein denaturation, coagulative necrosis, and a minimal amount of carbonization and vaporization

- Zone of thermal injury: 0.5–1.0 mm

Indications

- External lesions
- Intraurethral lesions located proximally of the fossa navicularis
- Bladder lesions

Intraurethral 5-FU cream application following laser procedures to prevent recurrence is highly recommended (see *5% Fluorouracil Cream* above).

4.6.2.6 Transurethral Resection of HPV-Related Lesions of the Urethra and Bladder

See also Sect. 4.6.2.2.

Technique

"Side fire" or "end fire" laser fibers are introduced through the urethrocystoscope when treatment is directed to anterior urethral and bladder lesions.
- Neodymium (Nd):YAG laser settings: Power: 10–20 W
- Holmium (Ho):YAG laser settings: Pulse rate: 13–15 W/Pulse energy 1.0–1.5 J

Indications

- Isolated intraurethral lesions proximal to the fossa navicularis
- Bladder lesions

Advantages

- Nd:YAG and Ho:YAG lasers can be used to treat intraurethral and bladder lesions.
- Coagulates tissue causing less plume.
- Outpatient procedure.
- Efficacy: Among the 20 cases of meatal and/or urethral condyloma treated with Nd:YAG laser, Volz et al. (1994) reported cure rates of 30% after one treatment and 40% after up to five separate treatments. However, Bloiso et al. (1988) found 100% efficacy with no recurrences with an average follow-up of 13 months.
- Recurrences following Nd:YAG laser: Zaak et al. (2003) detected recurrences in 35.7% of 168 patients presenting with urethral condylomata (recurrences were mainly on the meatus and in the distal urethra).
- Reduced incidence of urethral stricture.
- Meatotomy is not required in most cases.

Complications

- Risk of urethral stricture, particularly for lesions affecting the whole urethral circumference
- Bladder and urethral perforation

4.6.2.7 5-Aminolaevulinic Acid Photodynamic Therapy

5-Aminolaevulinic acid photodynamic therapy (ALA-PDT) is a new technique introduced in the 1990s for the treatment of superficial epithelial skin tumors. Wang et al. (2004) recently described the method for the treatment of urethral condylomata.

Mechanism of Action

- Following the exogenous application of the photosensitizer ALA to HPV-related lesions, it is selectively absorbed by the hyperplastic tissue and transformed to endogenous protoporphyrin IX (PpIX).
- The PpIX is then activated by red light leading to the formation of singlet oxygen, causing necrosis and apoptosis of the HPV-infected cells.
- Smetana et al. (1997) postulated that ALA-PDT could also inactivate viral particles by binding to virion surface glycoproteins and preventing the early steps of the HPV infection cycle.

Disadvantages

- Laser experience required.
- Eye protection is needed.
- Cost.
- Not worldwide applicable.

Complications

- Bladder and urethra perforation (laser fiber tip should not touch lesion to avoid perforation risk).

4

Advantages

- Chen et al. (2007) reported that the application of ALA-PDT is simpler, more effective, and safer compared with conventional CO_2 laser therapy.
- Efficacy: 95% after a follow-up of 6–24 months (Wang et al., 2004).
- Recurrence: 6.3% in the comparative study of PDT vs. CO_2 laser vaporization performed by Chen (2007).
- No scarring or urethral stricture.
- Fluorescence of the photosensitizers can assist in the localization of lesions.

Adverse Effects

- Mild burning and/or stinging sensation during treatment
- Erythema, mild edema, and skin erosion following treatment

How to Use (Chen et al., 2007)

20% ALA solution under occlusive dressing for 3 h, followed by irradiation with helium-neon laser at a dose of 100 J cm^2 and a power of 100 mW.

A cotton swab soaked in the solution is gently inserted into the meatus or, alternatively, a cotton ball is placed over the glans penis covering the meatus and adjacent normal mucosa (5-mm border). The solution is dropped over the cotton ball every 30 min. Lesions are then occluded with food-grade cling film and covered with thick gauze for light protection.

After a 3-h interval, irradiation with helium-neon laser is performed.

Treatment can be repeated once a week for a maximum of 3 weeks.

ALA Solution Preparation

20% ALA (Fudan Zhangjiang Bio-Pharm, Shanghai, China) is dissolved in sterile saline immediately before its application.

4.6.3 Treatment Failures – What to do?

4.6.3.1 Immune-Response Modifiers

Bacille Calmette-Guérin

The combination of surgical ablative methods and immunomodulative agents seems to be a promising treatment modality for recurrent HPV infection. Bohle et al. (1998) demonstrated that local application of bacille Calmette-Guérin (BCG) is effective in the adjuvant treatment of recurrent urethral condylomata acuminate.

How to Use (Bohle et al., 1998)

BCG Preparation

81 mg Connaught strain is dissolved in 2 ml sterile saline for direct instillation into the urethra at low pressure.

- Solution is instilled once a week for 6 weeks and is maintained intraurethrally for a minimum of 2 h (a dressing can be taped over the meatus to avoid inadvertent emptying).
- After 2 h the dressing is removed and the patient is allowed to void spontaneously.

Advantages

- Office procedure.
- Efficacy: It is suggested that the annual recurrence rate is decreased using intraurethral BCG instillation as an adjuvant to laser therapy. According to Bohle et al. (1998), recurrence rate was reduced from 3.2 with standard therapy to 0.75 with BCG therapy.

Disadvantages

- High cost (U.S. $140–$160 per vial) may prevent extended treatment.

Adverse Effects

- Mild dysuria
- Penile edema
- Fever of short duration

Interferon

How to Use (Levine et al., 1996)

Interferon

25 millions units of interferon-α-2b (Intron A, Schering-Plough, Kennilworth, NJ) in 5–7 cm³ sterile saline

- The solution is instilled intraurethrally once a week for 6 weeks.
- In case of recurrence, retreatment with an additional 6-week course of 50 million units of interferon-α-2b is recommended.

Advantages

- Interferon appears to eradicate subclinical disease by antiviral (Friedman-Kien et al., 1988; Agarwal et al., 1994), antiproliferative (Salmon et al., 1983), and immunomodulative activity (Herberman et al., 1982).
- Efficacy rate: 9 of 14 (64%) patients were disease-free for an average of 11.8 months, in the study performed by Levine et al. (1996).
- No adverse effects were described in the same study.

Disadvantages

- Expensive
- Prolonged treatment duration

4.7 Follow-Up

Recurrences occur most frequently during the first 3 months following treatment.

Closer follow-up is advisable for patients with intraurethral warts, particularly for those harboring high-risk HPV and/or those who have not responded to other treatment modalities.

Following laser treatment, patients return on postoperative day 12 to monitor cicatrization, treat possible complications, and check for early recurrences. A follow-up evaluation is advised 3–4 weeks after the end of treatment, and every 2–3 months thereafter for half a year if control examinations yield negative results.

Patients should be instructed to watch for recurrences and self-refer whenever lesions reappear.

Follow-up tests for urethral lesions:

- Urethral brushing polymerase chain reaction (PCR) 2 months after treatment.
- Urethrocystoscopy is performed 3 months after treatment and every 3 months thereafter for a period of 1 year.
- US/CT is performed 4 weeks after therapy for HPV-related lesions in the proximal urethra or bladder.

4.8 Prevention

See also Chap. 3.

A recent phase-I/II clinical trial using a therapeutic vaccine for male intraurethral flat condyloma showed promising results (Albarran et al., 2007). The vaccine was administered into the urethra once a week over a 4-week period. The immune response after MVA E2 treatment was determined by measuring the antibodies against the MVA E2 virus and by analyzing the lymphocyte cytotoxic activity against cancer cells bearing oncogenic papillomavirus. Lesion changes were monitored by colposcopy and brush histological analysis, whereas viral presence was determined by the Hybrid capture® method. In 28 of 30 patients that received the MVA E2 vaccine, the flat condyloma in the urethra was completely eliminated and absence of the papillomavirus was confirmed by brush histologic examination. In addition, patients treated with MVA E2 did not show any lesion recurrence after 1 year of treatment and all patients developed antibodies against the MVA E2 vaccine and E2 viral protein, generating a specific cytotoxic response against papilloma-transformed cells.

4.9 The Role of HPV in Urethral, Bladder, Renal, and Prostate Cancer Development

4.9.1 Urethral Cancer

Detection studies using cytological analysis of urethral brushings as well as hybridization techniques applied to urethral brushings showed evidence to support the urethra as a reservoir for HPV (Cecchini et al., 1988; Zderic et al., 1989).

Moreover, several studies have shown that HPV is associated with urethral carcinoma in both sexes (Wiener et al., 1992; Wiener and Walther, 1994; Sumino et al., 2006; Mevorach et al., 1990).

Tumors of the anterior urethra are mostly squamous cell carcinoma (SCC) arising in the bulbar and penile portion. Although transitional cell carcinoma (TCC) usually occurs in the posterior urethra, Sumino et al. (2006) recently reported TCC of the navicular fossa that was associated with low-risk and high-risk HPV infection.

Youshya et al. (2005) suggested that HPV is unlikely to play an etiological role in the development of TCC but, according to Noel et al. (1994), the virus could act as an oncogenic agent in immunosuppressed patients.

In addition, the iatrogenic seeding of HPV into the urethral lumen could also play a role in the development of urethral SCC and TCC in immunocompromised or elderly patients (Steele et al., 1997; Bans et al., 1983).

4.9.2 Bladder Cancer

The majority of bladder cancers detected in the Western world are TCCs, while SCCs represent the second most common morphological type identified (Young, 1996).

HPV-related papillomatous lesions are commonly found on the anogenital mucosa (zur Hausen, 1996), and in immunosuppressed patients these benign lesions may involve the urothelial mucosa (Fig. 4.23) (Benoit

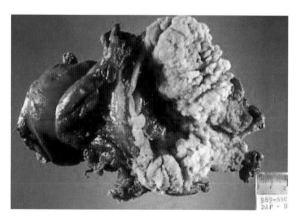

Fig. 4.23. Vulvar neoplasia (virology HPV 16/18) invading urethra and bladder in immunosuppressed patient

et al., 1988). This finding prompted investigators to explore a link between HPV colonization of the urinary tract and the development of urothelial malignancy.

However, methods used to detect the virus have often been associated with false-positive results and although condylomatous bladder lesions attributable to HPV infection have been described in immunocompetent and immunosuppressed patients, the etiological role of HPV in bladder TCC is still a matter of discussion (Chetsanga et al., 1992; Anwar et al., 1992a; Shibutani et al., 1992; Knowles, 1992; Furihata et al., 1993; Sinclair et al., 1993; Agliano et al., 1994; Chang et al., 1994; Sano et al., 1995; Olsen et al., 1995; Mvula et al., 1996).

Furthermore, immunohistochemical assay (IHA) and PCR tests were used to investigate HPV in TCC, with very different results (Aynaud et al., 1998; Chetsanga et al., 1992; Chan et al., 1997; De Gaetani et al., 1999).

The disparity of theses results suggests that the association of HPV with bladder TCC may be influenced by geographical location, owing to the fact that most studies reporting a high incidence of HPV-positive samples were performed in Asia (Yu et al., 1999; Barghi et al., 2005; Wiwanitkit, 2005; Smetana et al., 1995), in strong contrast to the extremely low rate of HPV positivity that was found in northern European, American, and even African studies (Aynaud et al., 1998; Simoneau et al., 1999; Sur et al., 2001). In addition, the highly sensitive PCR technique was unable to disclose HPV DNA sequences in most studies.

In contrast, data from a preliminary study performed by Moonen et al. (2007) that recently evaluated an association between HPV DNA, p53 status, and clinical outcome in bladder cancer patients suggest a likely correlation between tumor grade/stage and infection with oncogenic HPV types.

Therefore, while available data appear not to support the etiological role of HPV in the development of TCC and SCC of the bladder in immunocompetent patients (Maloney et al., 1994; Lu et al., 1997; Gutierrez et al., 2006), further studies are definitely required.

4.9.3 Prostate Cancer

Owing to the fact that HPV is sexually transmitted and is commonly detected in anogenital cancers, many studies investigate the possible etiologic role of HPV in prostate cancer.

Rabkin et al. (1992) reported that the risk of prostate cancer is increased in men who develop anal cancer, an HPV-related tumor.

According to Choo et al. (1999), HPV E6 and E7 proteins can affect human prostate cells in vitro through their effects on the cellular tumor suppressor gene products p53 and Rb, respectively. However, studies on the detection of the virus in prostate tissues have yielded conflicting results (McNicol and Dodd, 1990; Anwar et al., 1992b; McNicol and Dodd, 1991; Ibrahim et al., 1992; Dodd et al., 1993; Wideroff et al., 1996; Masood et al., 1991; Effert et al., 1992).

Strickler et al. (1998) suggested that HPV DNA is uncommon in the prostates of older men and is not associated with prostate cancer.

In contrast, several studies also suggest that HPV type 16 antibodies may predict the development of future prostate cancer (Hisada et al., 2000; Dillner et al., 1998), and seropositivity against HPV 18 has been associated with a 2.6-fold increased risk of developing prostate cancer (Dillner et al., 1998).

In conclusion, the association between HPV and/or other viral infections has not been substantiated by current studies and yet, if validated, the association would likely account for a small subset of prostate cancers (Strickler and Goedert, 2001).

4.9.4 Renal Cancer

There are few studies and conflicting results regarding the influence of HPV in the development of renal cell carcinoma (RCC) (Rotola et al., 1992; Kamel et al., 1994).

Grce et al. (1997) using snap-frozen samples and PCR technology failed to detect HPV in both RCC specimens and samples of corresponding normal renal tissue.

However, Kuwahara et al. (1998) analyzed the presence of HPV DNA and overexpression of the p53 protein in 31 patients with carcinoma of the renal pelvis and ureter. The investigators reported that HPV DNA 16 or 18 was present in 9 of 28 patients with renal/ureteral TCC and p53 expression was found in 7 of the TCC cases, suggesting that high-risk HPV types and p53 protein are involved in the pathogenesis of urothelial tumors.

Additional research is needed before any causal relationship can be defined.

References

Agarwal C, Hembree JR, Rorke EA, Eckert RL (1994) Interferon and retinoic acid suppress the growth of human papillomavirus type 16 immortalized cervical epithelial cells, but only interferon suppresses the level of the human papillomavirus transforming oncogenes. Cancer Res 54: 2108–2112

Agliano AM, Gradilone A, Gazzaniga P, Napolitano M, Vercillo R, Albonici L, Naso G, Manzari V, Frati L, Vecchione A (1994) High frequency of human papillomavirus detection in urinary bladder cancer. Urol Int 53: 125–129

Aguilar LV, Lazcano-Ponce E, Vaccarella S, Cruz A, Hernandez P, Smith JS, Munoz N, Kornegay JR, Hernandez-Avila M, Franceschi S (2006) Human papillomavirus in men: Comparison of different genital sites. Sex Transm Infect 82: 31–33

Albarran YCA, de la Garza A, Cruz Quiroz BJ, Vazquez Zea E, Diaz Estrada I, Mendez Fuentez E, Lopez Contreras M, Andrade-Manzano A, Padilla S, Varela AR, Rosales R (2007) MVA E2 recombinant vaccine in the treatment of human papillomavirus infection in men presenting intraurethral flat condyloma: A phase I/II study. BioDrugs 21: 47–59

Anwar K, Naiki H, Nakakuki K, Inuzuka M (1992a) High frequency of human papillomavirus infection in carcinoma of the urinary bladder. Cancer 70: 1967–1973

Anwar K, Nakakuki K, Shiraishi T, Naiki H, Yatani R, Inuzuka M (1992b) Presence of ras oncogene mutations and human papillomavirus DNA in human prostate carcinomas. Cancer Res 52: 5991–5996

Aynaud O (1992) Meatal spreader. J Urol 147: 409

Aynaud O, Ionesco M, Barrasso R (2003) Cytologic detection of human papillomavirus DNA in normal male urethral samples. Urology 61: 1098–1101

Aynaud O, Tranbaloc P, Orth G (1998) Lack of evidence for a role of human papillomaviruses in transitional cell carcinoma of the bladder. J Urol 159: 86–89; discussion 90

Bans LL, Eble JN, Lingeman JE, Maynard BR (1983) Transitional cell carcinoma of the fossa navicularis of the male urethra. J Urol 129: 1055–1056

Barghi MR, Hajimohammadmehdiarbab A, Moghaddam SM, Kazemi B (2005) Correlation between human papillomavirus infection and bladder transitional cell carcinoma. BMC Infect Dis 5: 102

Benoit G, Orth G, Vieillefond A, Sinico M, Charpentier B, Jardin A, Fries D (1988) Presence of papilloma virus type 11 in condyloma acuminatum of bladder in female renal transplant recipient. Urology 32: 343–344

Beutner KR, Ferenczy A (1997) Therapeutic approaches to genital warts. Am J Med 102: 28–37

Bloiso G, Warner R, Cohen M (1988) Treatment of urethral diseases with neodymium:YAG laser. Urology 32: 106–110

Bohle A, Doehn C, Kausch I, Jocham D (1998) Treatment of recurrent penile condylomata acuminata with external application and intraurethral instillation of bacillus Calmette Guerin. J Urol 160: 394–396

Carpiniello VL, Schoenberg M, Malloy TR (1990) Long-term followup of subclinical human papillomavirus infection treated with the carbon dioxide laser and intraurethral 5-fluorouracil: A treatment protocol. J Urol 143: 726–728

Cecchini S, Cipparrone I, Confortini M, Scuderi A, Meini L, Piazzesi G (1988) Urethral cytology of Cytobrush specimens. A new technique for detecting subclinical human papillomavirus infection in men. Acta Cytol 32: 314–317

Chan KW, Wong KY, Srivastava G (1997) Prevalence of six types of human papillomavirus in inverted papilloma and papillary transitional cell carcinoma of the bladder: an evaluation by polymerase chain reaction. J Clin Pathol 50: 1018–1021

Chang F, Lipponen P, Tervahauta A, Syrjanen S, Syrjanen K (1994) Transitional cell carcinoma of the bladder: Failure to demonstrate human papillomavirus deoxyribonucleic acid by in situ hybridization and polymerase chain reaction. J Urol 152: 1429–1433

Chen K, Chang BZ, Ju M, Zhang XH, Gu H (2007) Comparative study of photodynamic therapy vs CO2 laser vaporization in treatment of condylomata acuminata: A randomized clinical trial. Br J Dermatol 156: 516–520

Chetsanga C, Malmstrom PU, Gyllensten U, Moreno-Lopez J, Dinter Z, Pettersson U (1992) Low incidence of human papillomavirus type 16 DNA in bladder tumor detected by the polymerase chain reaction. Cancer 69: 1208–1211

Choo CK, Ling MT, Chan KW, Tsao SW, Zheng Z, Zhang D, Chan LC, Wong YC (1999) Immortalization of human prostate epithelial cells by HPV 16 E6/E7 open reading frames. Prostate 40: 150–158

Chrisofos M, Skolarikos A, Lazaris A, Bogris S, Deliveliotis C (2004) HPV 16/18-associated condyloma acuminatum of the urinary bladder: First international report and review of literature. Int J STD AIDS 15: 836–838

Chuang TY, Perry HO, Kurland LT, Ilstrup DM (1984) Condyloma acuminatum in Rochester, Minn., 1950–1978. I. Epidemiology and clinical features. Arch Dermatol 120: 469–475

Clinical Effectiveness Group BAfSHaHB (2007) United Kingdom national guideline on the management of anogenital warts. In: British Association for Sexual Health and HIV (BASHH), London (UK)

Culp OS, Kaplan IW (1944) Condylomata acuminata: Two hundred cases treated with podophyllin. Ann Surg 120: 251–256

de Carvalho JJ, Syrjanen KJ, Jacobino M, Rosa NT, Carvalho LZ (2006) Prevalence of genital human papillomavirus infections established using different diagnostic techniques among males attending a urological clinic. Scand J Urol Nephrol 40: 138–143

De Gaetani C, Ferrari G, Righi E, Bettelli S, Migaldi M, Ferrari P, Trentini GP (1999) Detection of human papillomavirus DNA in urinary bladder carcinoma by in situ hybridisation. J Clin Pathol 52: 103–106

D'Hauwers K, Depuydt C, Bogers JP, Stalpaert M, Vereecken A, Wyndaele JJ, Tjalma W (2007) Urine versus brushed samples in human papillomavirus screening: Study in both genders. Asian J Androl 9: 705–710

Dillner J, Knekt P, Boman J, Lehtinen M, Af Geijersstam V, Sapp M, Schiller J, Maatela J, Aromaa A (1998) Seroepidemiological association between human-papillomavirus infection and risk of prostate cancer. Int J Cancer 75: 564–567

Dodd JG, Paraskevas M, McNicol PJ (1993) Detection of human papillomavirus 16 transcription in human prostate tissue. J Urol 149: 400–402

Dyment PG (1996) Human papillomavirus infection. Adolesc Med 7: 119–130

Effert PJ, Frye RA, Neubauer A, Liu ET, Walther PJ (1992) Human papillomavirus types 16 and 18 are not involved in human prostate carcinogenesis: Analysis of archival human prostate cancer specimens by differential polymerase chain reaction. J Urol 147: 192–196

Fralick RA, Malek RS, Goellner JR, Hyland KM (1994) Urethroscopy and urethral cytology in men with external genital condyloma. Urology 43: 361–364

Friedman-Kien AE, Eron LJ, Conant M, Growdon W, Badiak H, Bradstreet PW, Fedorczyk D, Trout JR, Plasse TF (1988) Natural interferon alfa for treatment of condylomata acuminata. JAMA 259: 533–538

Furihata M, Inoue K, Ohtsuki Y, Hashimoto H, Terao N, Fujita Y (1993) High-risk human papillomavirus infections and overexpression of p53 protein as prognostic indicators in transitional cell carcinoma of the urinary bladder. Cancer Res 53: 4823–4827

Gartman E (1956) Intraurethral verruca acuminata in men. J Urol 75: 717–718

Giuliano AR, Nielson CM, Flores R, Dunne EF, Abrahamsen M, Papenfuss MR, Markowitz LE, Smith D, Harris RB (2007) The optimal anatomic sites for sampling heterosexual men for human papillomavirus (HPV) detection: The HPV detection in men study. J Infect Dis 196: 1146–1152

Gonzalvo Perez V, Ramada Benlloch F, Blasco Alfonso JE, Donderis Guastavino C, Pallas Costa Y, Navalon Verdejo P, Zaragoza Orts J (1994) [Endoscopic electrofulguration of intraurethral condylomata acuminata]. Actas Urol Esp 18: 234–236

Graversen PH, Bagi P, Rosenkilde P (1990) Laser treatment of recurrent urethral condylomata acuminata in men. Scand J Urol Nephrol 24: 163–166

Grce M, Furcic I, Hrascan R, Husnjak K, Krhen I, Marekovic Z, Zeljko Z, Pavelic K (1997) Human papillomaviruses are not associated with renal carcinoma. Anticancer Res 17: 2193–2196

Green J, Monteiro E, Bolton VN, Sanders P, Gibson PE (1991) Detection of human papillomavirus DNA by PCR in semen from patients with and without penile warts. Genitourin Med 67: 207–210

Griffiths TR, Mellon JK (2000) Human papillomavirus and urological tumours: II. Role in bladder, prostate, renal and testicular cancer. BJU Int 85: 211–217

Gutierrez J, Jimenez A, de Dios Luna J, Soto MJ, Sorlozano A (2006) Meta-analysis of studies analyzing the relationship between bladder cancer and infection by human papillomavirus. J Urol 176: 2474–2481; discussion 2481

Herberman RB, Ortaldo JR, Mantovani A, Hobbs DS, Kung HF, Pestka S (1982) Effect of human recombinant interferon on cytotoxic activity of natural killer (NK) cells and monocytes. Cell Immunol 67: 160–167

Hisada M, Rabkin CS, Strickler HD, Wright WE, Christianson RE, van den Berg BJ (2000) Human papillomavirus antibody and risk of prostate cancer. JAMA 283: 340–341

Huguet Perez J, Errando Smet C, Regalado Pareja R, Rosales Bordes A, Salvador Bayarri J, Vicente Rodriguez J (1996) [Urethral condyloma in the male: Experience with 48 cases]. Arch Esp Urol 49: 675–680

Ibrahim GK, Gravitt PE, Dittrich KL, Ibrahim SN, Melhus O, Anderson SM, Robertson CN (1992) Detection of human papillomavirus in the prostate by polymerase chain reaction and in situ hybridization. J Urol 148: 1822–1826

Iwasawa A, Hiltunen-Back E, Reunala T, Nieminen P, Paavonen J (1997) Human papillomavirus DNA in urine specimens of men with condyloma acuminatum. Sex Transm Dis 24: 165–168

Jones DJ (1991) Haemospermia: A prospective study. Br J Urol 67: 88–90

Kamel D, Turpeenniemi-Hujanen T, Vahakangas K, Paakko P, Soini Y (1994) Proliferating cell nuclear antigen but not p53 or human papillomavirus DNA correlates with advanced clinical stage in renal cell carcinoma. Histopathology 25: 339–347

Kaplinsky RS, Pranikoff K, Chasan S, DeBerry JL (1995) Indications for urethroscopy in male patients with penile condylomata. J Urol 153: 1120–1121

Katelaris PM, Cossart YE, Rose BR, Thompson CH, Sorich E, Nightingale B, Dallas PB, Morris BJ (1988) Human papillomavirus: The untreated male reservoir. J Urol 140: 300–305

Kilciler M, Bedir S, Erdemir F, Coban H, Erten K, Ors O, Ozgok Y (2007) Condylomata acuminata of external urethral meatus causing infravesical obstruction. Int Urol Nephrol 39: 107–109

Knowles MA (1992) Human papillomavirus sequences are not detectable by Southern blotting or general primer-mediated polymerase chain reaction in transitional cell tumours of the bladder. Urol Res 20: 297–301

Krogh J, Beuke HP, Miskowiak J, Honnens de Lichtenberg M, Nielsen OS (1990) Long-term results of carbon dioxide laser treatment of meatal condylomata acuminata. Br J Urol 65: 621–623

Kuwahara M, Fujisaki N, Kagawa S, Furihata M, Ohtsuki Y (1998) Determination of p53 protein and high-risk human papillomavirus DNA in carcinomas of the renal pelvis and ureter. Int J Mol Med 1: 703–707

Levine LA, Elterman L, Rukstalis DB (1996) Treatment of subclinical intraurethral human papilloma virus infection with interferon alfa-2b. Urology 47: 553–557

Lu QL, Lalani el N, Abel P (1997) Human papillomavirus 16 and 18 infection is absent in urinary bladder carcinomas. Eur Urol 31: 428–432

Maloney KE, Wiener JS, Walther PJ (1994) Oncogenic human papillomaviruses are rarely associated with squamous cell carcinoma of the bladder: Evaluation by differential polymerase chain reaction. J Urol 151: 360–364

Masood S, Rhatigan RM, Powell S, Thompson J, Rodenroth N (1991) Human papillomavirus in prostatic cancer: No evidence found by in situ DNA hybridization. South Med J 84: 235–236

McKenna JG, McMillan A (1990) Management of intrameatal warts in men. Int J STD AIDS 1: 259–263

McNicol PJ, Dodd JG (1990) Detection of papillomavirus DNA in human prostatic tissue by Southern blot analysis. Can J Microbiol 36: 359–362

McNicol PJ, Dodd JG (1991) High prevalence of human papillomavirus in prostate tissues. J Urol 145: 850–853

Mevorach RA, Cos LR, di Sant'Agnese PA, Stoler M (1990) Human papillomavirus type 6 in grade I transitional cell carcinoma of the urethra. J Urol 143: 126–128

Moonen PM, Bakkers JM, Kiemeney LA, Schalken JA, Melchers WJ, Witjes JA (2007) Human papilloma virus DNA and p53 mutation analysis on bladder washes in relation to clinical outcome of bladder cancer. Eur Urol 52: 464–468

Mvula M, Iwasaka T, Iguchi A, Nakamura S, Masaki Z, Sugimori H (1996) Do human papillomaviruses have a role in the pathogenesis of bladder carcinoma. J Urol 155: 471–474

Noel JC, Thiry L, Verhest A, Deschepper N, Peny MO, Sattar AA, Schulman CC, Haot J (1994) Transitional cell carcinoma of the bladder: Evaluation of the role of human papillomaviruses. Urology 44: 671–675

Nuovo GJ, Hochman HA, Eliezri YD, Lastarria D, Comite SL, Silvers DN (1990) Detection of human papillomavirus DNA in penile lesions histologically negative for condylomata. Analysis by in situ hybridization and the polymerase chain reaction. Am J Surg Pathol 14: 829–836

Olsen S, Marcussen N, Jensen KM, Lindeberg H (1995) Urethral condylomata, due to human papilloma virus (HPV) type 6/11., associated with transitional cell tumors in the bladder and ureter. A case report. Scand J Urol Nephrol Suppl 172: 51–55

Rabkin CS, Biggar RJ, Melbye M, Curtis RE (1992) Second primary cancers following anal and cervical carcinoma: Evidence of shared etiologic factors. Am J Epidemiol 136: 54–58

Rintala MA, Grenman SE, Pollanen PP, Suominen JJ, Syrjanen SM (2004) Detection of high-risk HPV DNA in semen and its association with the quality of semen. Int J STD AIDS 15: 740–743

Rintala MA, Pollanen PP, Nikkanen VP, Grenman SE, Syrjanen SM (2002) Human papillomavirus DNA is found in the vas deferens. J Infect Dis 185: 1664–1667

Rosemberg SK, Jacobs H, Fuller T (1982) Some guidelines in the treatment of urethral condylomata with carbon dioxide laser. J Urol 127: 906–908

Rosemberg SK, Reid R, Greenberg M, Lorincz AT (1988) Sexually transmitted papillomaviral infection in the male: II. The urethral reservoir. Urology 32: 47–49

Rothman I, Berger RE, Kiviat N, Navarro AL, Remington ML (1994) Urethral meatal warts in men: results of urethroscopy and biopsy. J Urol 151: 875–877

Rotola A, Monini P, Di Luca D, Savioli A, Simone R, Secchiero P, Reggiani A, Cassai E (1992) Presence and physical state of HPV DNA in prostate and urinary-tract tissues. Int J Cancer 52: 359–365

Salmon SE, Durie BG, Young L, Liu RM, Trown PW, Stebbing N (1983) Effects of cloned human leukocyte interferons in the human tumor stem cell assay. J Clin Oncol 1: 217–225

Sand PK, Shen W, Bowen LW, Ostergard DR (1987) Cryotherapy for the treatment of proximal urethral condyloma acuminatum. J Urol 137: 874–876

Sano T, Sakurai S, Fukuda T, Nakajima T (1995) Unsuccessful effort to detect human papillomavirus DNA in urinary bladder cancers by the polymerase chain reaction and in situ hybridization. Pathol Int 45: 506–512

Sawczuk I, Badillo F, Olsson CA (1983) Condylomata acuminata: Diagnosis and follow-up by retrograde urethrography. Urol Radiol 5: 273–274

Scheinfeld N, Lehman DS (2006) An evidence-based review of medical and surgical treatments of genital warts. Dermatol Online J 12: 5

Shaw MB, Payne SR (2007) A simple technique for accurate diathermy destruction of urethral meatal warts. Urology 69: 975–976

Shibutani YF, Schoenberg MP, Carpiniello VL, Malloy TR (1992) Human papillomavirus associated with bladder cancer. Urology 40: 15–17

Simoneau M, LaRue H, Fradet Y (1999) Low frequency of human papillomavirus infection in initial papillary bladder tumors. Urol Res 27: 180–184

Sinclair AL, Nouri AM, Oliver RT, Sexton C, Dalgleish AG (1993) Bladder and prostate cancer screening for human papillomavirus by polymerase chain reaction: Conflicting results using different annealing temperatures. Br J Biomed Sci 50: 350–354

Smetana Z, Keller T, Leventon-Kriss S, Huszar M, Lindner A, Mitrani-Rosenbaum S, Mendelson E, Smetana S (1995) Presence of human papilloma virus in transitional cell carcinoma in Jewish population in Israel. Cell Mol Biol (Noisy-le-grand) 41: 1017–1023

Smetana Z, Malik Z, Orenstein A, Mendelson E, Ben-Hur E (1997) Treatment of viral infections with 5-aminolevulinic acid and light. Lasers Surg Med 21: 351–358

Steele GS, Fielding JR, Renshaw A, Loughlin KR (1997) Transitional cell carcinoma of the fossa navicularis. Urology 50: 792–795

Strand A, Rylander E, Wilander E, Zehbe I, Kraaz W (1996) Histopathologic examination of penile epithelial lesions is of limited diagnostic value in human papillomavirus infection. Sex Transm Dis 23: 293–298

Strickler HD, Burk R, Shah K, Viscidi R, Jackson A, Pizza G, Bertoni F, Schiller JT, Manns A, Metcalf R, Qu W, Goedert JJ (1998) A multifaceted study of human papillomavirus and prostate carcinoma. Cancer 82: 1118–1125

Strickler HD, Goedert JJ (2001) Sexual behavior and evidence for an infectious cause of prostate cancer. Epidemiol Rev 23: 144–151

Sumino Y, Emoto A, Satoh F, Nakagawa M, Mimata H (2006) Transitional cell carcinoma of the navicular fossa detected human papillomavirus 16. Int J Urol 13: 645–647

Sumino Y, Mimata H, Nomura Y (2004) Urethral condyloma acuminata following urethral instrumentation in an elderly man. Int J Urol 11: 928–930

Sur M, Cooper K, Allard U (2001) Investigation of human papillomavirus in transitional cell carcinomas of the urinary bladder in South Africa. Pathology 33: 17–20

Takatsuki K, Kamiyama Y, Sato S, Amemiya H, Iizumi T, Yazaki T, Umeda T (1993) [A case report of condyloma acuminatum of urethral meatus in a boy]. Hinyokika Kiyo 39: 479–481

Thin RN (1992) Meatoscopy: A simple technique to examine the distal anterior urethra in men. Int J STD AIDS 3: 21–23

Volz LR, Carpiniello VL, Malloy TR (1994) Laser treatment of urethral condyloma: A five-year experience. Urology 43: 81–83

von Krogh G (2001) Management of anogenital warts (condylomata acuminata). Eur J Dermatol 11: 598–603; quiz 604

Wang XL, Wang HW, Wang HS, Xu SZ, Liao KH, Hillemanns P (2004) Topical 5-aminolaevulinic acid-photodynamic therapy for the treatment of urethral condylomata acuminata. Br J Dermatol 151: 880–885

Wen YC, Wu HH, Chen KK (2006) Pan-urethral wart treated with 5-fluorouracil intraurethral instillation. J Chin Med Assoc 69: 391–392

Wideroff L, Schottenfeld D, Carey TE, Beals T, Fu G, Sakr W, Sarkar F, Schork A, Grossman HB, Shaw MW (1996) Human papillomavirus DNA in malignant and hyperplastic prostate tissue of black and white males. Prostate 28: 117–123

Wiener JS, Liu ET, Walther PJ (1992) Oncogenic human papillomavirus type 16 is associated with squamous cell cancer of the male urethra. Cancer Res 52: 5018–5023

Wiener JS, Walther PJ (1994) A high association of oncogenic human papillomaviruses with carcinomas of the female urethra: Polymerase chain reaction-based analysis of multiple histological types. J Urol 151: 49–53

Wiwanitkit V (2005) Urinary bladder carcinoma and human papilloma virus infection, an appraisal of risk. Asian Pac J Cancer Prev 6: 217–218

Workowski KA, Berman SM (2007) Centers for Disease Control and Prevention sexually transmitted diseases treatment guidelines. Clin Infect Dis 44(Suppl 3): S73–S76

Young R (1996) Usual variants of primary bladder lesions and secondary tumours of the bladder. In: Pathology of bladder cancer. Williams and Wilkins, Baltimore, pp 326–337

Youshya S, Purdie K, Breuer J, Proby C, Sheaf MT, Oliver RT, Baithun S (2005) Does human papillomavirus play a role in the development of bladder transitional cell carcinoma? A comparison of PCR and immunohistochemical analysis. J Clin Pathol 58: 207–210

Yu Z, Xia T, Xue Z (1999) [The detection of high risk human papillomaviruses in papillary transitional cell carcinoma of urinary bladder]. Zhonghua Wai Ke Za Zhi 37: 369–371; 322

Zaak D, Hofstetter A, Frimberger D, Schneede P (2003) Recurrence of condylomata acuminata of the urethra after conventional and fluorescence-controlled Nd:YAG laser treatment. Urology 61: 1011–1015

Zderic SA, Carpiniello VL, Malloy TR, Rando RF (1989) Urological applications of human papillomavirus typing using deoxyribonucleic acid probes for the diagnosis and treatment of genital condyloma. J Urol 141: 63–65

Zheng W, Vilos G, McCulloch S, Borg P, Denstedt JD (2000) Electrical burn of urethra as cause of stricture after transurethral resection. J Endourol 14: 225–228

zur Hausen H (1996) Papillomavirus infections - a major cause of human cancers. Biochim Biophys Acta 1288: F55–F78

Human Papillomavirus and Penile Intraepithelial Neoplasia

5

Alberto Rosenblatt and Homero Gustavo de Campos Guidi

Contents

A. Rosenblatt (✉)
Albert Einstein Jewish Hospital, Sao Paulo, Brasil
e-mail: albrose1@gmail.com

5.1 Introduction

Following the increase in the investigation of the male partner for human papillomavirus (HPV), along with novel detection methods and organ-confined nomenclature, a multitude of diagnoses of penile intraepithelial neoplasias (PINs) are now being presented to medical practitioners involved in the treatment of HPV-related diseases.

PIN is the term presently used to describe a precancerous lesion of the penis.

HPV infection is associated with PIN development, and PIN progression to penile invasive disease is an uncommon but possible event.

A. Rosenblatt, H. G. de Campos Guidi, *Human Papillomavirus*,
DOI: 10.1007/978-3-540-70974-9-5, © Springer-Verlag Berlin Heidelberg 2009

This chapter reviews current concepts of PINs, including distinctive clinical findings, grading and terminology, diagnosis, and therapeutic options.

5.2   Terminology

The generic term "penile intraepithelial neoplasia" ("Tis" in the TNM classification) is a histological entity equivalent to penile dysplasia. Squamous intraepithelial lesion (SIL) is another recommended term to describe atypical lesions of the penile epithelium.

According to the level of dysplastic abnormalities (i.e., morphologic criteria and tissue architecture, where the level of epithelial involvement by disorderly growth and cytologic atypia are analyzed), penile squamous intraepithelial lesions (or PIN) may be divided into low-grade (PIN 1) (Fig. 5.1a, b) and high-grade (PIN 3/in situ) lesions (Fig. 5.2a–c) (see also Chaps. 7 and 8).

What Happened to PIN 2?

The categorization of SILs into low- and high-grade depends mainly on the degree of koilocytosis[a] found, since koilocytosis translates into significant cellular differentiation (albeit associated with HPV infection). Like cervical intraepithelial neoplasia 2 (CIN 2), vaginal intraepithelial neoplasia 2 (VaIN 2), and anal intraepithelial neoplasia 2 (AIN 2), PIN 2 constitutes a group of lesions exhibiting variable degrees of koilocytosis, and therefore subjected to different interobserver interpretations (Fig. 5.3a, b). Therefore, the utilization of a Bethesda-type categorization (low- and high-grade) is recommended until more sensitive and less subjective risk markers for grading are available (Carvalho, personal communication, 31 October 2008).

---

[a]The presence of koilocytes (Fig. 5.4) is a morphological indication of HPV infection.

Moreover, according to Cubilla et al. (2000), low- and high-grade SILs can be further classified into:

- Squamous or simplex (the most frequent types)
- Warty (condylomatous) (Fig. 5.5) and basaloid (Fig. 5.6a, b)

Both warty and basaloid types are associated with HPV infection, whereas the typical squamous type is not related to HPV.

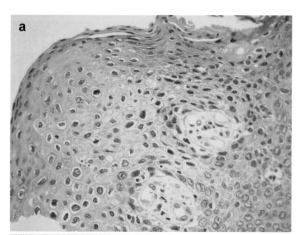

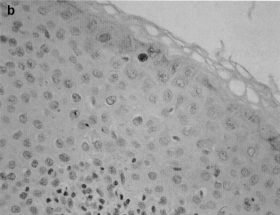

Fig. 5.1. (a) Penile intraepithelial neoplasia 1 (PIN 1). (b) PIN 1 with HPV-positive cell stained in *red* (immunohistochemistry) (Source: Photograph courtesy of Monica Stiepcich MD, PhD, São Paulo, Brazil)

PIN and vulvar intraepithelial neoplasia (VIN) share clinical and histological similarities and, according to Aynaud and Bergeron (2004), PIN can be categorized according to the same criteria recommended by the International Society for the Study of Vulvar Disease (ISSVD) (Bergeron, 2008). Based on the etiology and natural history of the penile lesion, PIN can be characterized as differentiated and undifferentiated (Aynaud and Bergeron, 2004).

5.2.1   Differentiated PIN

The atypia of differentiated PIN is confined to the inferior layers of the epithelium and usually originates from chronic benign balanopreputial lesions, such as penile lichen sclerosus (LS), extramammary Paget's disease (EMPD) involving the genital region, and Kaposi's sarcoma (KS).

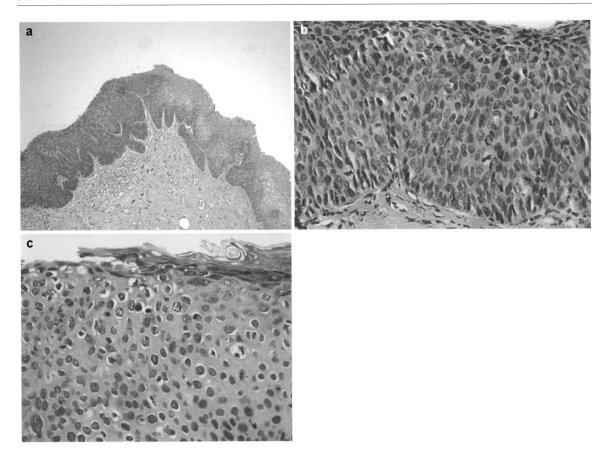

Fig. 5.2. (**a**) Transition PIN 3 and normal epithelium (Source: Photograph courtesy of Filomena Marino Carvalho MD, PhD, São Paulo, Brazil). (**b**) PIN 3 – severe dysplasia (Source: Photograph courtesy of Rubens Pianna de Andrade MD, PhD/ Monica Stiepcich MD, PhD São Paulo, Brazil). (**c**) PIN 3 detailed (Source: Photograph courtesy of Monica Stiepcich MD, PhD, São Paulo, Brazil)

5.2.2   Undifferentiated PIN

Undifferentiated PIN is currently been used to describe the premalignant conditions of the penis formerly referred to as Bowen's disease (BD) and erythroplasia of Queyrat (EQ). The dysplasia found in undifferentiated PIN involves more than two-thirds of the mucosa thickness and the lesions usually present a higher histological grade (PIN 3/in situ). High-risk HPV infection is usually associated with undifferentiated PIN (Fig. 5.7), but koilocytosis (the pathognomonic feature of HPV infection) is not frequently observed.

5.3   Overview

The classification of bowenoid papulosis (BP) is still a matter of debate among authors. According to Solsona et al. (2004), BP is a disorder that is sporadically associated with squamous cell carcinoma (SCC) of the penis. However, Porter et al. (2002) describe BP as a low-grade SCC in situ, although clinically distinct from BD and EQ.

Furthermore, BP can also be categorized as a form of cutaneous dysplasia (Micali et al., 2006).

BD and EQ are probably the same entity, as they share similar clinicopathological features.

- SCC in situ presenting on the shaft of the penis is known as BD.
- SCC in situ presenting on the mucous membranes of the glans penis, prepuce, coronal sulcus, frenulum, and urethral meatus is referred to as EQ.

These premalignant skin disorders display the same microscopic features of SCC in situ, such as epithelial proliferation, hyperkeratosis, and marked parakeratosis. The cell nuclei are hyperchromatic, clumped, and show lack of organization, maturation, and cohesion. Mitotic figures are prominent throughout the layers and abnormal forms are regularly found.

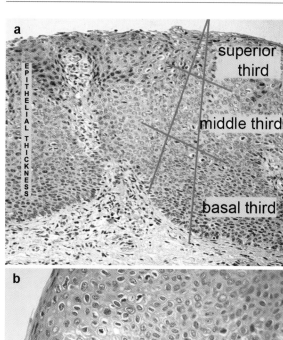

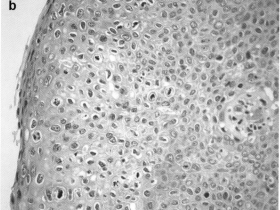

Fig. 5.3. (**a**)(**b**) Moderate dysplasia. (Source: Photograph courtesy of Monica Stiepcich MD, PhD, São Paulo, Brazil)

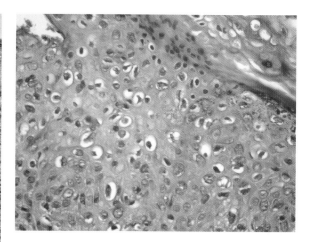

Fig. 5.5. Warty (condylomatous) type. (Source: Photograph courtesy of Filomena Marino Carvalho MD, PhD, São Paulo, Brazil)

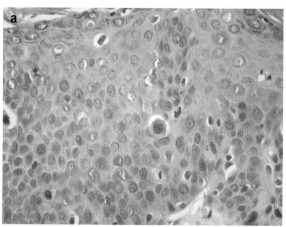

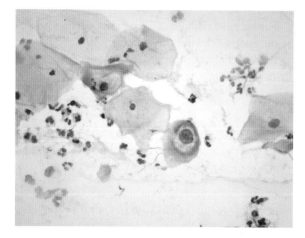

Fig. 5.4. Koilocytes. (Source: Photograph courtesy of Filomena Marino Carvalho MD, PhD, São Paulo, Brazil)

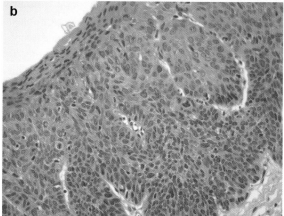

Fig. 5.6. (**a**)(**b**) Basaloid type. (Source: Photograph courtesy of Filomena Marino Carvalho MD, PhD, São Paulo, Brazil)

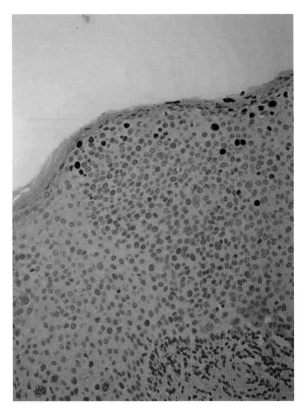

Fig. 5.7. PIN 3 – in situ hybridization showing HPV 16. (Source: Photograph courtesy of Monica Stiepcich MD, PhD, São Paulo, Brazil)

Progression to frankly invasive SCC can occur if lesions are left untreated, but it is a rare event.

PINs comprising BD, EQ, and BP are considered precursor lesions of basaloid and warty carcinomas of the penis, which are frequently associated with HPV infection (Gross and Pfister, 2004).

5.3.1 Natural History of PINs

The majority of PINs are completely asymptomatic. These premalignant penile disorders generally appear as clinically suspicious flat acetowhite lesions that mandate biopsy; hence, the correct diagnosis is made histologically. Furthermore, oncogenic HPV types 16, 18, and 33 are usually associated with these lesions.

In a preliminary analysis that evaluated the natural history of PIN lesions, Guidi et al. (2007) reported no malignant progression in all 17 patients with untreated PIN 1/2. In addition, no evidence of disease was found in six patients with PIN 3 treated with CO_2 laser during a mean follow-up of 51 months. Therefore, according

> **Expert Advice**
>
> The importance of the acetowhite test in the diagnosis and treatment of PIN is paramount. It allows for the exact location of the lesion and delimitates the area to be excised. Although the correlation between peniscopic images and histology is still not well defined (Horenblas, 2008), the execution of the acetowhite test during laser surgery performed with the operating microscope has been shown to increase the efficacy of conservative approaches for the treatment of in situ and superficial penile cancers (Bandieramonte et al., 2008). Moreover, it is also used as an adjunct to modern surgical techniques employed for the treatment of premalignant lesions of the penis (Hadway et al., 2006) (see Sect. 5.6.4.8). (See also *How to Perform the Acetowhite Test* in Chap. 3).

to these results, the investigators recommend that patients presenting with low-grade PIN should be reassured of the benign behavior of these lesions. The same affirmative attitude should be given to patients presenting with PIN 3, although treatment and surveillance are required in these cases.

Bandieramonte et al. (2008) recently performed a retrospective analysis of 106 patients with penile carcinoma in situ treated with CO_2 laser excision under peniscopic control. The authors reported that in only three cases could the resection margins not be clearly evaluated because of thermal artifacts. Lesion recurrences (22 in 12 patients) were in situ mostly and occurred in both treated and untreated areas.

The distinct epidemiology and the variable clinical characteristics presented by premalignant penile entities must be fully understood so as to avoid diagnostic inaccuracies that may impact on prognosis.

> **Expert Advice**
>
> Any long-lasting penile lesion that is unresponsive to classic medical treatments should be biopsied and sent for histological examination to exclude a possible SCC in situ (PIN) or invasive SCC.

5.3.2 Incidence

PIN is considered a rare disorder, although its real incidence is unknown.

The association of PIN with distinct HPV types that carry oncogenic potential may possibly influence future epidemiologic data, but evidence-based prospective studies are still needed to correctly define the natural history of this disorder.

5.3.3   Risk Factors

- Lack of circumcision – According to Schoen et al. (2000), circumcision at birth has a protective effect for SCC in situ, but protection is less evident than for invasive SCC.
- Chronic inflammatory dermatologic diseases of the penis such as lichen sclerosus (LS) (Nasca et al., 2003; Barbagli et al., 2006).
- HPV infection.
- Immunosuppression.

5.3.4   Differential Diagnosis

- Pigmented warts (see *Expert Advice* below (Fig. 5.14a, b))
- Seborrheic keratosis
- Nevi (Fig. 5.8) and melanoma
- Lentigo (Fig. 5.9)
- Angiokeratoma (Fig. 5.10)
- Lichen planus (Fig. 5.11)
- Psoriatic lesions (Fig. 5.18)

5.4   Multifocal Intraepithelial Neoplasia (Bowenoid Papulosis)

Bowenoid papulosis (BP) is a dermatological term coined by Wade, Kopf, and Ackerman (Wade et al.) in 1978. BP lesions have been described in young men and women (usually at the vulva), and gynecologists still refer to the disease as multifocal VIN.

- BP is considered a low-grade SCC in situ, although it can also be categorized as a form of cutaneous dysplasia.
- BP, BD, and EQ can occur concurrently (Porter et al., 2002).

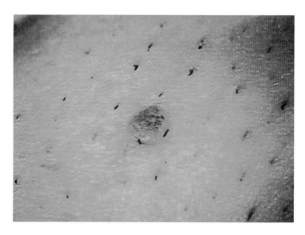

Fig. 5.8. Nevus at the penile shaft

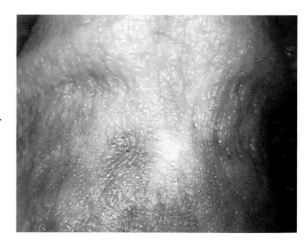

Fig. 5.9. Penile lentigo

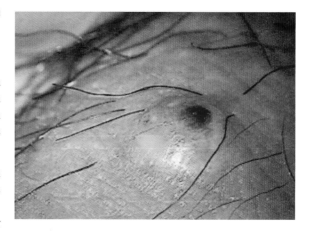

Fig. 5.10. Penile shaft angiokeratoma

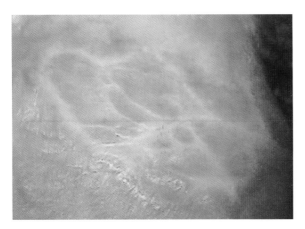

Fig. 5.11. Lichen planus – white geographical annular plaques

- BP mainly occurs in sexually active young men (average age – 30 years).
- It is highly prevalent in uncircumcised patients (Porter et al., 2002), despite the original report by Wade et al. (1978) of a higher BP prevalence in circumcised patients.
- Several HPV DNA genotypes have been detected by Hama et al. (2006), particularly high-risk type 16.
- Female sexual partners of affected men have a higher risk of developing cervical neoplasia (Obalek et al., 1986).
- The full-blown lesion may evolve over a period of weeks or months.
- Spontaneous regression of the lesions may occur within several months and, according to Yoneta et al. (2000), progression to invasive disease is an uncommon event.
- However, immunocompromised individuals and elderly patients are at higher risk of disease progression (Schwartz and Janniger, 1991).
- Feldman et al. (1989) recommend that the immunologic status should always be evaluated in patients with persistent BP lesions.

5.4.1 Clinical Manifestations

5.4.1.1 Symptoms

- Mostly asymptomatic.
- Pruritus (usually present in 30–50% of women).
- BP lesions may occasionally show inflammatory signs.

5.4.1.2 Presentation

- Multiple, small, darkly pigmented flat papules (Fig. 5.12) or patches mainly located on the penis shaft (Fig. 5.13), but glans penis, foreskin, and perianal area can also be affected.
- Lesions range in color from brown to pink (flesh-colored) and red.
- Lesions sometimes may coalesce and form large plaques.

Expert Advice

BP lesions are less papillomatous than common genital viral condyloma lesions and usually present a smooth-topped brown aspect (Fig. 5.14a, b).

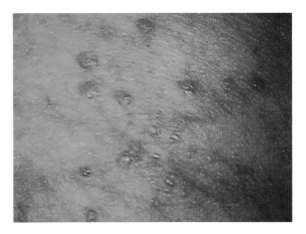

Fig. 5.12. Bowenoid papulosis – multiple, small, darkly pigmented flat papules

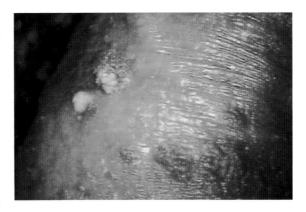

Fig. 5.13. Bowenoid papulosis located on the penis shaft

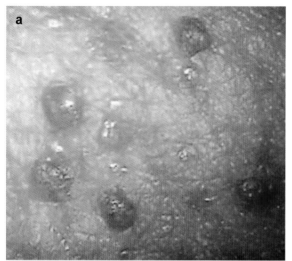

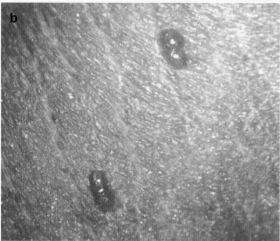

Fig. 5.14. (**a**) Bowenoid papulosis lesions – smooth-topped *brown* aspect. (**b**) Keratotic shaft papules, HPV-related

5.4.2 Diagnosis

● Physical examination
● Biopsy and histopathological examination

5.4.2.1 Histological Findings

● Epidermal thickening.
● Small and scattered atypical basaloid keratinocytes with large, hyperchromatic, pleomorphic nucleus, and frequent mitoses.
● The dermal-epidermal border is preserved.
● Inclusion-like bodies may be found in the stratum corneum and granular cell layer.

> **Expert Advice**
>
> The finding of inclusion-like bodies associated with the presence of innumerous mitoses in metaphase ("star-shaped" figures) may help differentiate BP from BD. However, correlation with clinical findings is essential for the correct diagnosis of BP.

5.4.3 Treatment

The main objective is the complete destruction of the lesions without the need for wide surgical margins. BP lesions can be adequately treated by surgical removal, electrosurgery, and cryosurgery, in much the same way as HPV-related lesions (see Chap. 3).

5.4.3.1 CO$_2$ Laser

Advantages

● Recurrence rate: 0–33%, according to a study performed by von Krogh and Horenblas (2000)

5.4.3.2 5-Fluorouracil Cream

There are few evidence-based reports using 5-fluorouracil (5-FU) for the treatment of BP.
Therapeutic regimen – 5-FU cream applied twice daily for 3 weeks (Porter et al., 2002).

5.4.3.3 Imiquimod Cream (Aldara®)

Advantages

● Efficacy – Complete clearance of the lesions reported on a small number of patients (Wigbels et al., 2001; Goorney and Polori, 2004). Additional studies are required to assess efficacy.

Therapeutic regimen – Imiquimod cream is applied on alternate days for up to 3 months (Porter et al., 2002).

5.4.4 Follow-Up

Patients should be instructed for self-examination and self-referral if a suspicious lesion is found.

A routine follow-up visit 3–6 months after treatment is recommended to check for recurrences, but immuno-suppressed patients should be carefully screened for possible progression to penile SCC.

5.5 Bowen's Disease

SCC in situ presenting on the shaft of the penis is known as Bowen's disease (BD).

BD of the penis most often affects elderly (>50 years) uncircumcised white men and, if untreated, progression to invasive disease has been reported in approximately 5% of cases (Cox et al., 2007; Lucia and Miller, 1992).

5.5.1 Risk Factors

- Presence of foreskin
- Poor genital hygiene
- Lichen sclerosus
- Preceding or concurrent papillomavirus infection (HPV types 16, 18, and 57b), according to studies performed by Ikenberg et al. (1983) and Ohnishi et al. (1999)

5.5.2 Clinical Manifestations

5.5.2.1 Symptoms

- Asymptomatic
- Pruritus (the most common reason to seek medical care and usually present in about 50% of women)
- Pain
- Crusting, scaling, or bleeding
- Difficulty in retracting the foreskin

5.5.2.2 Presentation

- Isolated and well-defined reddish scaly plaque with surface fissures and sometimes presenting foci of pigmentation located on the shaft of the penis.
- BD lesions grow slowly and may eventually ulcerate or develop a nodular appearance (Fig. 5.15), suggesting progression to malignant disease.

5.5.3 Diagnosis

- Physical examination
- Biopsy and histopathological examination

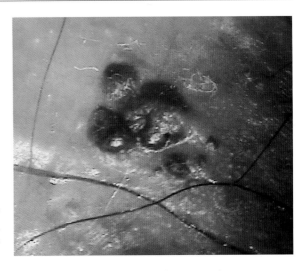

Fig. 5.15. Bowen's disease - nodular presentation

BD diagnosis is usually delayed for weeks or months because of the insidious onset and gradual progression of the lesion.

5.5.3.1 Histological Findings

- Epidermal acanthosis and parakeratosis.
- Replacement of mature keratinocytes with dysplastic cells showing nuclear atypia.
- Involvement of follicle-bearing epithelium by atypical cells.
- The dermis presents an inflammatory infiltrate but basal cells are normal.

5.5.4 Treatment

Surgical excision is the best treatment option for small lesions, according to von Krogh and Horenblas (2000).

BD recurrences from secondary progression of atypical cells in the epidermal lining of the hair follicle occur frequently, particularly when using treatment modalities such as topical 5-FU or electrosurgery.

Treatment should be applied to the visible lesion and to the bordering normal tissue, but a penis-preserving strategy is strongly recommended.

5.5.4.1 Surgical Excision and Electrosurgery

Indication

- Small lesions

Advantages

- Efficacy – regarded by Cox et al. (2007) as an effective treatment with low recurrence rates, although evidence-based results are limited

5.5.4.2 Cryotherapy

Advantages

- Good evidence of efficacy (Cox et al., 2007; Dawber and Colver, 1992)

Disadvantages

- Prolonged healing time

Side Effects

- Pain
- Inflammation
- Spontaneous bleeding
- Infection
- Meatal stenosis

5.5.4.3 5-Fluorouracil Cream

Indications

- Noninvasive lesions in unhairy locations (Tolia et al., 1976; Porter et al., 2002)
- Large and multiple lesions (in the latter case, Cox et al. (2007) recommended that 5-FU should be used for disease control, rather than for cure)

Therapeutic regimen – 5-FU cream may be applied twice a day for 3 weeks (Porter et al., 2002), but ideal regimen has not been established.

Side Effects

- Irritative symptoms may limit efficacy because of treatment interruption.
- Erosion and superficial necrosis.

5.5.4.4 Imiquimod Cream (Aldara®)

Indication

- Large lesions

Therapeutic regimen – Topical imiquimod can be applied on alternate days for up to 3 months, according to Porter et al. (2002).

Advantages

- Efficacy – complete response in few reported cases with short follow-up (3–18 months) (Schroeder and Sengelmann, 2002; Arlette, 2003; de Diego Rodriguez et al., 2005; Taliaferro and Cohen, 2008)

Disadvantages

- Expensive
- Not FDA-licensed for this indication
- Ideal regimen not yet established

5.5.4.5 CO_2 Laser

Advantages

- Excellent cosmetic and functional results
- Considered an acceptable indication for both initial treatment and disease recurrences (van Bezooijen et al., 2001)
- Efficacy – good long-term results (follow-up up to 24 months) for PIN associated with HPV infection (Malek, 1992)

Disadvantages

- van Bezooijen et al. (2001) reported a high incidence of recurrences
- Patient compliance for follow-up control required

5.5.4.6 Photodynamic Therapy with Methyl Aminolevulinate

Indication

- Large lesions

Advantages

- Excellent cosmetic and functional results.
- Efficacy – Photodynamic therapy (PDT) has demonstrated superior efficacy when compared to topical 5-FU or cryotherapy, according to a study performed by Morton et al. (2006).
- European Medicines Authority-approved therapy for BD.

Disadvantages

- Residual disease – In the study that evaluated PDT with methyl aminolevulinate (MAL) for atypical carcinoma in situ of the penis, Axcrona et al. (2007) reported histological residual disease in 30% of patients after median follow-wup of 20 months.

Side Effects

- Pain in the immediate week following treatment

5.5.4.7   Circumcision

Indication

- Lesions limited to the foreskin (Mikhail, 1980)

5.5.5   Follow-Up

Patients should be instructed for self-examination and self-referral if a suspicious lesion is found.

Routine follow-up visits 3–6 months following treatment are advised to check for early recurrences.

Since clinical inspection can be unreliable, biopsies are often required for proper evaluation of lesion progression to invasive disease.

5.6   Erythroplasia of Queyrat (Unifocal Intraepithelial Neoplasia)

EQ is a penile intraepithelial neoplasia that mainly affects the mucous membranes of the glans surface, inner aspect of the foreskin, or the urethral meatus of elderly men.

EQ lesions often evolve insidiously but, if untreated, the risk of progression to invasive SCC is 5–33% (Malek, 1992). Lesions occurring on keratinized areas appear less prone to progression than mucosal-located lesions.

According to Porter et al. (2002), LS is more prevalent in patients with EQ and the association with low- and high-risk HPV has been demonstrated by Wieland et al. (2000).

Wieland et al. (2000) also suggested that the presence or absence of the rare HPV type 8 may help differentiate between penile EQ and BD.

5.6.1   Clinical Manifestations

5.6.1.1   Symptoms

- Pain (uncommon)
- Pruritus
- Bleeding
- Difficulty in retracting the foreskin

5.6.1.2   Presentation

- Single, well-demarcated and slightly raised, bright red, moist plaque (Fig. 5.16a, b).
- Lesion modification to a verrucous, nodular, or ulcerated aspect is a sign of invasion (Graham and Helwig, 1973) (Fig. 5.17).

5.6.2   Differential Diagnosis

- Candidal balanitis
- Psoriasis (Fig. 5.18)
- Zoon's balanitis (Fig. 5.19)
- Erosive lichen planus
- Inflammatory granuloma
- Reiter syndrome (rare)
- Lupus erythematosus (very rare)

5.6.3   Diagnosis

- Physical examination
- Biopsy and histopathological examination

5

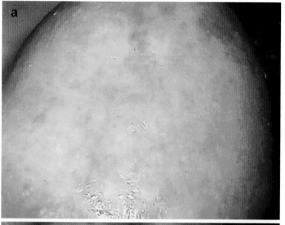

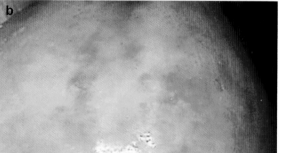

Fig. 5.16. (**a**) Erythroplasia of Queyrat (EQ)/PIN 3 located at the glans penis. (**b**) EQ – slightly raised, bright red, moist plaque

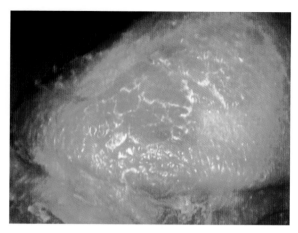

Fig. 5.18. Glans penis psoriasis

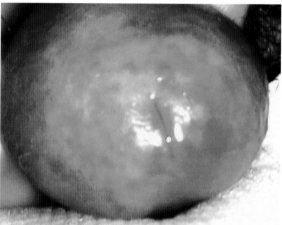

Fig. 5.19. Plasma cell balanitis (Zoon's balanitis)

Expert Advice

Early biopsy to better define diagnosis is recommended by Porter et al. (2002).

- Excisional biopsy can be performed for a small lesion located in the prepuce or in an accessible area.
- Incisional biopsy, tissue core biopsy, fine-needle aspiration, or brush biopsy can be used for larger lesions.

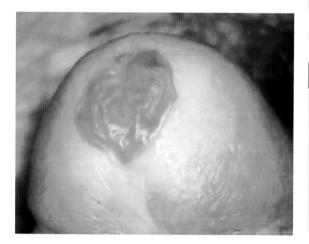

Fig. 5.17. Erythroplasia of Queyrat – discrete nodular presentation

5.6.3.1 Histological Findings

BD and EQ share histological features but, compared to the former, EQ displays more epithelial hypoplasia, fewer dyskeratotic multinucleated cells, and increased plasma cells numbers (Graham and Helwig, 1973).

5.6.4   Treatment

The recurrence rate in patients with EQ is lower than in patients with BD, reflecting the absence of hair follicles in the penile mucosa (see also BD Treatment).

Topical treatment regimens for EQ are similar to BD regimens (see above), but in a recent analysis Porter et al. (2002) reported more difficulties with the management of EQ lesions or a combination of PIN disorders.

Moreover, a penis-preserving strategy is strongly recommended when using surgical treatment approaches.

5.6.4.1   5-Fluorouracil Cream

There are only a few evidence-based reports (Tolia et al., 1976; Goette and Carson, 1976), but 5-FU cream is the preferred first-line option of Hadway et al. (2006).

5.6.4.2   Imiquimod Cream (Aldara)

Advantages

- Efficacy – complete clearance of EQ lesions associated or not with high-risk HPV (Kaspari et al., 2002; Micali et al., 2006)

Therapeutic regimen – further studies required.

5.6.4.3   Local Excision

Indications

- Small or large lesions located on the foreskin
- Not suitable for large glans penis lesions or perimeatal and urethral location, because of functional and/or cosmetic results

5.6.4.4   Circumcision

Indication

- Lesions limited to foreskin

5.6.4.5   CO$_2$ Laser

Laser CO$_2$ vaporization should extend beyond the lesion borders and an 8–10-mm safety margin is recommended by Conejo-Mir et al. (2005).

Advantages

- Excellent cosmetic and functional results
- Alternative to topical therapy in patients with penile SCC in situ (Rosemberg and Fuller, 1980)
- Effective for EQ with urethral involvement in young immunocompetent patients (Del Losada et al., 2005)

Disadvantages

- Recurrence rates following CO$_2$ laser ablation – 10–26%, according to the study performed by Porter et al. (2002)

5.6.4.6   Nd:YAG Laser

Disadvantages

- Recurrence rates – Recent data by Frimberger et al. (2002) showed that 1 of 17 patients with CIS treated with Nd:YAG laser had several recurrences and another developed nodal metastases from an apparent missed invasive disease.

5.6.4.7   Photodynamic Therapy with Methyl Aminolevulinate

Stables et al. (1999) and Lee and Ryman (2005) treated very few cases with PDT and reported good results for limited EQ lesions, but observed that extensive disease is less responsive to PDT. Further studies are recommended.

Side Effects

- Pain
- Local swelling
- Redness

5.6.4.8 Total Glans Resurfacing

Total glans resurfacing (TGR) is a novel surgical technique developed by Bracka et al. (Depasquale et al., 2000) that completely denudes the glans and subcorona of the penis down to the corpus spongiosum and Buck's fascia at the coronal sulcus, respectively. The bare surface is then covered with a healthy extragenital skin graft.

In selected cases, TGR is a promising treatment modality that offers good functional and cosmetic results without compromising oncologic control; however, additional studies and longer follow-up are needed to confirm early good results.

Indications (Hadway et al., 2006)

- Relapsing disease following topical therapy with 5-FU and imiquimod
- Extensive glans penis lesions
- Severe dysplasia
- SCC in situ lesions in young men (relapses and long treatment modalities are avoided with faster return to normal activities)

Optional Indication

- Patients who do not comply with regular follow-up

Advantages

- The specimen obtained allows for a thorough histological assessment of the disease.
- Minimal chance of recurrence.
- Normal anatomy is restored with acceptable cosmetic and functional results (Hadway et al., 2006).
- No evidence of recurrence with follow-up of 32–45 months (Palminteri et al., 2007; Hadway et al., 2006).

Disadvantages

- Surgeon experienced with the technique necessary
- Hospitalization and regional or general anesthesia required
- Immobilization for 3–4 days following the procedure

5.6.5 Follow-Up

Patients should be instructed for self-examination and self-referral if a suspicious lesion is found.

Long-term follow-up is advised by Mikhail (1980), because the risk of progression to invasive SCC is higher in EQ than in other PIN variants.

Biopsies are often required for proper evaluation of lesion progression to invasive disease, as clinical inspection can be unreliable.

5.7 Penile Lichen Sclerosus

Lichen sclerosus (LS) is a relatively common hypopigmented skin disorder, with a large incidence on genital skin.

According to new proper terminology initially proposed by Friedrich (1976) and later adopted by Ridley (1992), the term atrophic and dystrophy must be avoided when referring to LS because not all cases are histologically atrophic.

Penile LS, traditionally known as balanitis xerotica obliterans (BXO), is a chronic, progressive, and scarring dermatologic disease that may result in significant voiding complications.

It mostly affects uncircumcised middle-aged white men; however, LS has been described in 4-year-old boys (Rickwood et al., 1980) and according to Chalmers et al. (1984), it affects the young male population more often than previously assumed. In a recent long prospective study performed by Kiss et al. (2005), the peak incidence of LS occurred between the ages of 9 and 11, and nearly all affected boys had secondary phimosis.

The exact etiology of LS is unknown, but immune dysregulation is considered the factor most strongly associated with the disease (Regauer, 2005).

Recent data have shown a higher prevalence of infection with high-risk HPV types in patients with penile LS (Nasca et al., 2006; Prowse et al., 2008).

Together with low- and high-grade PIN and squamous hyperplasia, LS may be considered a precursor lesion of penile cancer (Powell et al., 2001; Cubilla et al., 2004; Velazquez and Cubilla, 2007), with a 6% risk of progression to SCC. According to Nasca et al. (2006), infection with oncogenic HPV types may enhance the risk of penile cancer development in patients with genital LS.

In a recent clinicopathologic analysis performed by Cubilla et al. (2004), LS was specifically related to well-differentiated, SCC of the penis with pseudohyperplastic features. These multicentric tumors are usually present in older patients and preferentially involve the inner mucosal surface of the foreskin.

5.7.1 Clinical Manifestations

5.7.1.1 Symptoms

- Asymptomatic at early stages
- Recurrent inflammatory symptoms (balanitis)
- Pruritus
- Glans penis hypoesthesia
- Dyspareunia
- Dysuria
- Urethritis and voiding problems because of meatal stenosis
- Difficulty or inability to retract the foreskin in uncircumcised individuals

5.7.1.2 Presentation

- Single or multiple erythematous papules or macules usually affecting the glans penis and foreskin at the early stages of the disease (Fig. 5.20a, b); in a study performed by Depasquale et al. (2000), LS was found limited to the foreskin and glans in 57% of patients. The perianal region is not affected in male individuals.
- Thin patches or plaques affecting the frenulum and foreskin (penile shaft is rarely involved).
- Presence of a typical white sclerotic ring at the tip of the foreskin.
- Mucosal fissures, petechiae, telangiectasias, and hemorrhagic lesions may occur, leading to glans penis adhesion to the prepuce at advanced stages.
- The urethral meatus and fossa navicularis may be affected resulting in urethral involvement in 20% of patients (Depasquale et al., 2000); urinary obstruction as a result of meatal stenosis was reported in 47% of the patients studied by Bainbridge et al. (1971).
- The urethra is initially affected at the level of the meatus, but with long-standing disease the mucosal

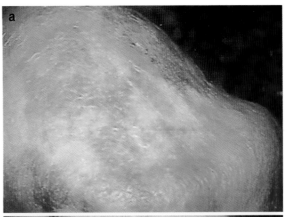
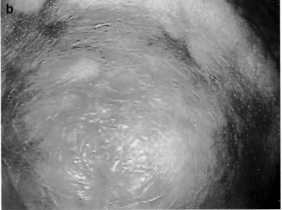

Fig. 5.20. (a) Lichen sclerosus – multiple erythematous papules or macules at the glans penis. **(b)** Lichen sclerosus – erythematous papules or macules at the glans penis

involvement and spongiofibrosis can progress proximally as far back as the posterior urethra (Fig. 5.21).

5.7.2 Diagnosis

- Physical examination.
- Biopsy and histological examination.
- Urethroscopy and retrograde urethrography are mandatory to determine the proximal extent of disease if urethral involvement is suspected.

Expert Advice

Biopsy is recommended in all patients suspected of having LS (Pugliese et al., 2007); however, the biopsy of chronically hyperplastic or ulcerated lesions of LS is mandatory to rule out SCC.

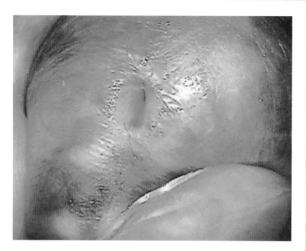

Fig. 5.21. Lichen sclerosus affecting the urethral meatus

5.7.2.1 **Histological Findings** (Fig. 5.22a, b)

- Hyperkeratosis
- Basal cells hydropic degeneration
- Sclerosis of the subepithelial collagen
- Collagen homogenization at the upper layer of the dermis
- Dermal lymphocytic infiltration
- Atrophic epidermis with loss of rete pegs

5.7.3 Treatment

5.7.3.1 **Medical**

Steroids

Indication

- Mild disease limited to the foreskin in young individuals with minimal scar formation

Advantages

- Efficacy – Steroids may improve initial symptoms and slow disease progression (Kiss et al., 2005).

Clobetasol propionate (Temovate) 0.05% cream or ointment is the topical steroid most commonly used, although it is not FDA approved for this indication; relapses may occur when treatment is discontinued.

  Therapeutic regimen – Once or twice daily for 2–3 months with gradual dose reduction.

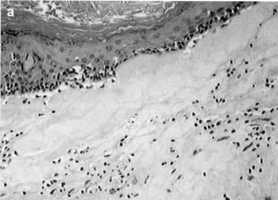
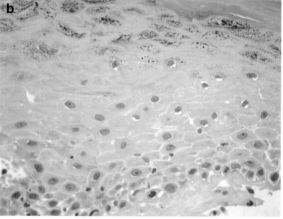

Fig. 5.22. (**a**) Lichen sclerosus. (**b**) Lichen sclerosus (LS) exhibiting marked epithelial hyperplasia (increased risk of malignant progression) (Source: Carvalho. Photograph courtesy of Filomena Marino Carvalho MD, PhD, São Paulo, Brazil)

Side Effects

- Cutaneous atrophy
- Hypopigmentation
- Contact sensitivity
- Adrenal suppression

Expert Advice

The use of potent steroids should be avoided in pediatric and in HPV-infected patients.

5.7.3.2 **Hormones**

Efficacy – There are no recent studies performed on male subjects (Pasieczny, 1977). In a recent comparative study of steroids and testosterone propionate therapy for vulvar LS, clobetasol resulted in higher remission and lower recurrence rates than hormonal therapy;

however, according to Ayhan et al. (2007) the results obtained were not statistically different.

5.7.3.3 Tacrolimus Topical (Protopic)

Tacrolimus ointment, a topical calcineurin inhibitor, is a highly selective immune modulator agent.

Advantages

● Efficacy – lower relapse rate when compared with topical betamethasone (Ebert et al., 2007)

Therapeutic regimen – A small amount of tacrolimus ointment is applied twice a day to the affected area.

Tacrolimus ointment 0.03% is prescribed to children and young boys between 2 and 15 years old.

Expert Advice

Tacrolimus use in anogenital LS may reactivate HPV infection (Bilenchi et al., 2007).

5.7.3.4 Surgical

Circumcision

Indication

● Early disease limited to the glans penis and foreskin (Depasquale et al., 2000)

Expert Advice

It is highly recommended to send all tissue removed at circumcision or meatotomy (including in the pediatric population) for pathological analysis.

CO_2 Laser

Advantages

● Efficacy – A recent study performed by Windahl (2006) showed good long-term results (80% of patients asymptomatic and without visible lesions) following CO_2 laser treatment.

Meatoplasty

● There may be recurrences when ventral meatotomy is performed for meatal stenosis correction in LS patients.
● Technique of extended meatoplasty for complex or reoperative strictures showed successful results in 87% of the patients treated by Morey et al. (2007).

Urethral Reconstruction

● Nongenital skin should preferably be used for urethroplasty because LS will likely recur using genital skin for reconstruction (Venn and Mundy, 1998).
● Despite use of buccal mucosal graft urethroplasty techniques, the recurrence rate of LS-related strictures is high in the short and long term.
● The effectiveness of one-stage buccal mucosal graft urethroplasty vs. multistage reconstruction of LS-related urethral strictures is not yet established (Levine et al., 2007).

5.7.4 Follow-Up

Long-term follow-up is advised to detect possible progression to premalignant disease or SCC.

5.8 Penile Horn

Penile horn is considered an unusual disorder as it is rarely seen in areas not exposed to sunlight.

The etiology is unclear but it usually affects individuals who had undergone adult circumcision because of a long-standing phimosis and chronic balanoposthitis.

It may also appear on the surface of preexisting penile lesions such as nevi or warts or in areas exposed to traumatic abrasions (Lowe and McCullough, 1985).

According to Solsona et al. (2004), penile horn is sporadically associated with SCC of the penis and the potential for malignant degeneration is increased in cases of recurrent disease (Cruz Guerra et al., 2005; Fields et al., 1987). A recent study performed by de la Pena Zarzuelo et al. (2001) found penile SCC arising at the base of the cutaneous horn in 37% of cases.

5

Malignant change should be suspected in a rapidly growing penile horn lesion.

5.8.1 Predisposing Factors

- Chronic preputial inflammation and phimosis
- Poor hygiene
- Traumatic abrasions
- Previous or concurrent HPV infection with oncogenic type 16 (Solivan et al., 1990)

5.8.2 Pathogenesis

Abnormal overgrowth of dry keratinized epithelium that probably occurs in response to chronic preputial inflammation and epithelial cornification.

5.8.3 Clinical Manifestations

5.8.3.1 Symptoms

- Asymptomatic
- Chronic penile discomfort

5.8.3.2 Presentation

- Single and occasionally multiple hard, exophytic, hyperkeratotic lesions of variable size (Fig. 5.23)
- Color ranges from white to yellow with an erythematous lesion base (Agarwalla et al., 2000)

5.8.4 Diagnosis

- Physical examination
- Biopsy and histopathological examination

5.8.4.1 Histological Findings

- Acanthosis
- Papillomatosis
- Intense hyperkeratosis and dyskeratosis
- Chronic inflammatory infiltrate

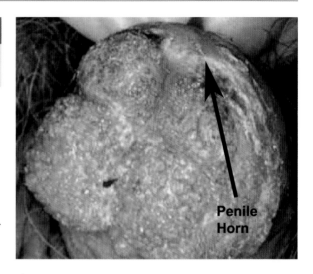

Penile Horn

Fig. 5.23. Penile horn and condylomatous lesion at the glans penis

5.8.5 Treatment

- Wide surgical excision including a margin of normal tissue at the base of the lesion
- Careful histological examination of the lesion base to exclude underlying carcinoma or a malignant transformation of the penile horn

5.8.6 Follow-Up

Close follow-up of the excision site is recommended, as these lesions have a potential to recur and become malignant.

5.9 Genital Paget's Disease

EMPD involving the penis and scrotum is exceedingly rare, with only small series or case reports described in the literature (Park et al., 2001; van Randenborgh et al., 2002; Yang et al., 2005). EMPD is a cutaneous adenocarcinoma of epidermal origin and glandular differentiation is usually involved. Chanda (1985) suggests that EMPD is a cutaneous marker of internal malignancy.

This slow-growing intraepithelial neoplasia affects elderly men (between the ages of 60 and 70), and there may be an association of penoscrotal EMPD with genitourinary cancer. The association with distant internal organ malignancy has been reported (Kim et al., 2005; Im et al., 2007), although it is a rare event with penoscrotal EMPD (Park et al., 2001). The disease may also spread to the regional lymph nodes, and lymph node metastasis is associated with a poor prognosis.

5.9.1 Clinical Manifestations

5.9.1.1 Symptoms

- Mostly asymptomatic
- Pruritus or burning pain may also occur

5.9.1.2 Presentation

- Red, moist, eroded plaque with a sharp border between normal and affected skin of the anogenital region (Fig. 5.24).

5.9.1.3 Histological Findings (Fig. 5.25)

- Presence of Paget's cells in the epidermis
- Positive immunohistochemical staining for glandular cytokeratins (Fig. 5.26), epithelial membrane antigen, and carcinoembryonic antigen (Wojnarowska and Cooper, 2003)

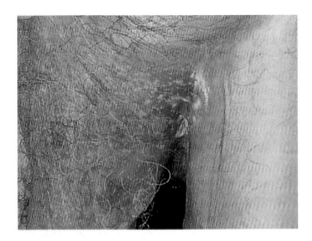

Fig. 5.24. EMPD involving the scrotum. (Source: Bolognia et al., 2003. Reproduced with permission from Elsevier)

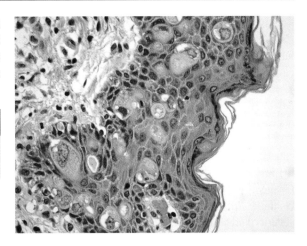

Fig. 5.25. Paget's disease. (Source: Photograph courtesy of Filomena Marino Carvalho MD, PhD, São Paulo, Brazil)

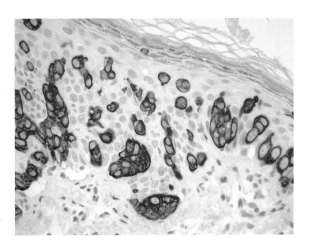

Fig. 5.26. Paget's disease – Immunohistochemical staining for glandular cytokeratins. (Source: Photograph courtesy of Filomena Marino Carvalho MD, PhD, São Paulo, Brazil)

5.9.2 Treatment

Wide local excision and immediate reconstruction with skin grafting or a local skin flap is the preferred treatment. Intraoperative frozen-section analysis is highly recommended to reduce positive margins.

5.10 Kaposi's Sarcoma

Kaposi's sarcoma (KS) is a neoplastic vascular lesion of multifocal origin occurring primarily on the extremities. KS is frequently seen in HIV-infected patients with advanced immune impairment (Tappero et al., 1993), and it is the most frequent neoplasm found in homosexual and bisexual men with AIDS. Moreover, almost 20% of patients with KS present genital lesions, but initial lesions at this region occur in only 3% of KS cases.

Primary penile KS is a relatively uncommon disorder in HIV-negative men, and histologic evaluation is necessary to establish the correct diagnosis.

The association of all types of KS with the infection caused by a virus of the Epstein-Barr family, human herpesvirus 8 (HHV-8), was recently demonstrated by Chang et al. (1994). Furthermore, according to Mendez et al. (1998), HHV-8 DNA load correlates with the severity and staging of this disease.

5.10.1 Clinical Manifestations

5.10.1.1 Symptoms

● Mostly asymptomatic

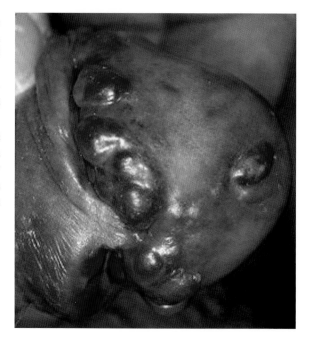

Fig. 5.27. Kaposi's sarcoma lesions at the coronal sulcus. (Source: Schwartz et al., 2008. Reproduced with permission from Elsevier)

5.10.1.2 Presentation

● Minimal glans penis or preputial lesion with nondistinctive clinical features.
● Single or multiple, red-to-purple macular lesion or skin-colored nodule (Fig. 5.27).
● Slowly growing pigmented macules are usually found in immunocompetent individuals with classical KS.
● Solitary genital lesion may be the first manifestation of KS associated with AIDS (Lowe et al., 1989).

5.10.1.3 Histological Findings

● Endothelial cell proliferation
● Fibroblastic proliferation, spindle cell bundles, and collagen dissection
● Progression from an early inflammatory or patch stage to nodular lesions of endothelialized vessels and non-endothelialized slit-like spaces (Schwartz et al., 2008)

5.10.2 Treatment

Patients should be informed that KS is a multicentric disease. Management of penile KS is usually based on the number and location of the lesions, the progression

pattern, and the immune status of the patient. Local therapies such as surgical excision, laser treatment, cryotherapy, imiquimod, or intralesional injection of chemotherapeutic agents (i.e., vinblastine) may be employed (Chun et al., 1999; Heyns and Fisher, 2005; Schwartz et al., 2008). Systemic therapies are reserved for patients with documented disseminated disease.

5.11 PIN Prevention

A recent study that evaluated the efficacy of the prophylactic quadrivalent HPV vaccine in young men reported that PIN was not detected in vaccinated individuals, but PIN 3 cases were observed in the placebo group. Moreover, penile cancer was not reported in the vaccinated or in the placebo group (Giuliano and Palefsky, 2008) (see also Sect. 11.8 in Chap. 11).

References

Agarwalla A, Agrawal CS, Thakur A, Garg VK, Joshi A, Agrawal S, Jacob M (2000) Cutaneous horn on condyloma acuminatum. Acta Derm Venereol 80: 159

Arlette JP (2003) Treatment of Bowen's disease and erythroplasia of Queyrat. Br J Dermatol 149 Suppl 66: 43–49

Axcrona K, Brennhovd B, Alfsen GC, Giercksky KE, Warloe T (2007) Photodynamic therapy with methyl aminolevulinate for atypial carcinoma in situ of the penis. Scand J Urol Nephrol 41: 507–510

Ayhan A, Guven ES, Guven S, Sakinci M, Dogan NU, Kucukali T (2007) Testosterone versus clobetasol for maintenance of vulvar lichen sclerosus associated with variable degrees of squamous cell hyperplasia. Acta Obstet Gynecol Scand 86: 715–719

Aynaud O, Bergeron C (2004) [Penile intraepithelial neoplasia]. Prog Urol 14: 100–104

Bainbridge DR, Whitaker RH, Shepheard BG (1971) Balanitis xerotica obliterans and urinary obstruction. Br J Urol 43: 487–491

Bandieramonte G, Colecchia M, Mariani L, Lo Vullo S, Pizzocaro G, Piva L, Nicolai N, Salvioni R, Lezzi V, Stefanon B, De Palo G (2008) Peniscopically controlled CO2 laser excision for conservative treatment of in situ and T1 penile carcinoma: Report on 224 patients. Eur Urol 54: 875–882

Barbagli G, Palminteri E, Mirri F, Guazzoni G, Turini D, Lazzeri M (2006) Penile carcinoma in patients with genital lichen sclerosus: A multicenter survey. J Urol 175: 1359–1363

Bergeron C (2008) [New histological terminology of vulvar intraepithelial neoplasia]. Gynecol Obstet Fertil 36: 74–78

Bilenchi R, Poggiali S, De Padova LA, Pisani C, De Paola M, Fimiani M (2007) Human papillomavirus reactivation following topical tacrolimus therapy of anogenital lichen sclerosus. Br J Dermatol 156: 405–406

Chalmers RJ, Burton PA, Bennett RF, Goring CC, Smith PJ (1984) Lichen sclerosus et atrophicus. A common and distinctive cause of phimosis in boys. Arch Dermatol 120: 1025–1027

Chanda JJ (1985) Extramammary Paget's disease: Prognosis and relationship to internal malignancy. J Am Acad Dermatol 13: 1009–1014

Chang Y, Cesarman E, Pessin MS, Lee F, Culpepper J, Knowles DM, Moore PS (1994) Identification of herpesvirus-like DNA sequences in AIDS-associated Kaposi's sarcoma. Science 266: 1865–1869

Chun YS, Chang SN, Park WH (1999) A case of classical Kaposi's sarcoma of the penis showing a good response to high-energy pulsed carbon dioxide laser therapy. J Dermatol 26: 240–243

Conejo-Mir JS, Munoz MA, Linares M, Rodriguez L, Serrano A (2005) Carbon dioxide laser treatment of erythroplasia of Queyrat: A revisited treatment to this condition. J Eur Acad Dermatol Venereol 19: 643–644

Cox NH, Eedy DJ, Morton CA (2007) Guidelines for management of Bowen's disease: 2006 update. Br J Dermatol 156: 11–21

Cruz Guerra NA, Saenz Medina J, Ursua Sarmiento I, Zamora Martinez T, Madrigal Montero R, Diego Pinto D, Tarroc Blanco A (2005) [Malignant recurrence of a penile cutaneous horn]. Arch Esp Urol 58: 61–63

Cubilla AL, Meijer CJ, Young RH (2000) Morphological features of epithelial abnormalities and precancerous lesions of the penis. Scand J Urol Nephrol Suppl 215–219

Cubilla A L, Velazquez E F, Young RH (2004) Pseudohyperplastic squamous cell carcinoma of the penis associated with lichen sclerosus. An extremely well-differentiated, nonverruciform neoplasm that preferentially affects the foreskin and is frequently misdiagnosed: A report of 10 cases of a distinctive clinicopathologic entity. Am J Surg Pathol 28: 895–900

Dawber R, Colver G (1992) Premalignant lesions. In: Dawber R, Colver G, Jackson A (eds) Cutaneous cryosurgery. Martin Dunitz, London, pp 77–93.

de Diego Rodriguez E, Villanueva Pena A, Hernandez Castrillo A, Gomez Ortega JM (2005) [Treatment of Bowen's disease of the penis with imiquimod 5% cream]. Actas Urol Esp 29: 797–800

de la Pena Zarzuelo E, Carro Rubias C, Sierra E, Delgado JA, Silmi Moyano A, Resel Estevez L (2001) [Cutaneous horn of the penis]. Arch Esp Urol 54: 367–368

Del Losada JP, Ferre A, San Roman B, Vieira V, Fonseca E (2005) Erythroplasia of Queyrat with urethral involvement: treatment with carbon dioxide laser vaporization. Dermatol Surg 31: 1454–1457

Depasquale I, Park AJ, Bracka A (2000) The treatment of balanitis xerotica obliterans. BJU Int 86: 459–465

Ebert AK, Vogt T, Rosch WH (2007) [Topical therapy of balanitis xerotica obliterans in childhood. Long-term clinical results and an overview]. Urologe A 46: 1682–1686

Feldman SB, Sexton FM, Glenn JD, Lookingbill DP (1989) Immunosuppression in men with bowenoid papulosis. Arch Dermatol 125: 651–654

Fields T, Drylie D, Wilson J (1987) Malignant evolution of penile horn. Urology 30: 65–66

Friedrich EG, Jr. (1976) Lichen sclerosus. J Reprod Med 17: 147–154

Frimberger D, Hungerhuber E, Zaak D, Waidelich R, Hofstetter A, Schneede P (2002) Penile carcinoma. Is Nd:YAG laser therapy radical enough? J Urol 168: 2418–2421; discussion 2421

Giuliano A, Palefsky J (2008) The efficacy of quadrivalent HPV (types 6/11/16/18) vaccine in reducing the incidence of HPV infection and HPV-related genital disease in young men In: European Research Organization on Genital Infection and Neoplasia – EUROGIN Nice, France

Goette DK, Carson TE (1976) Erythroplasia of Queyrat: Treatment with topical 5-fluorouracil. Cancer 38: 1498–1502

Goorney BP, Polori R (2004) A case of Bowenoid papulosis of the penis successfully treated with topical imiquimod cream 5%. Int J STD AIDS 15: 833–835

Graham JH, Helwig EB (1973) Erythroplasia of Queyrat. A clinicopathologic and histochemical study. Cancer 32: 1396–1414

Gross G, Pfister H (2004) Role of human papillomavirus in penile cancer, penile intraepithelial squamous cell neoplasias and in genital warts. Med Microbiol Immunol 193: 35–44

Guidi HGC, Stiepcich M, Andrade Z (2007) Estudo por biologia molecular de 17 neoplasias intraepiteliais penianas (Analyzis of 17 penile intraepithelial neoplasias by molecular biology techniques) [article in portuguese]. In: 31th Brazilian Congress of Urology vol 33. Braz J Urol, Salvador, Brazil

Hadway P, Corbishley CM, Watkin NA (2006) Total glans resurfacing for premalignant lesions of the penis: Initial outcome data. BJU Int 98: 532–536

Hama N, Ohtsuka T, Yamazaki S (2006) Detection of mucosal human papilloma virus DNA in bowenoid papulosis, Bowen's disease and squamous cell carcinoma of the skin. J Dermatol 33: 331–337

Heyns CF, Fisher M (2005) The urological management of the patient with acquired immunodeficiency syndrome. BJU Int 95: 709–716

Horenblas S (2008) Editorial comment on: Peniscopically controlled CO2 laser excision for conservative treatment of in situ and T1 penile carcinoma: Report on 224 patients. Eur Urol 54: 883; discussion 883–884

Ikenberg H, Gissmann L, Gross G, Grussendorf-Conen EI, zur Hausen H (1983) Human papillomavirus type-16-related DNA in genital Bowen's disease and in Bowenoid papulosis. Int J Cancer 32: 563–565

Im M, Kye KC, Kim JM, Lee JH (2007) Extramammary Paget's disease of the scrotum with adenocarcinoma of the stomach. J Am Acad Dermatol 57: S43–S45

Kaspari M, Gutzmer R, Kiehl P, Dumke P, Kapp A, Brodersen JP (2002) Imiquimod 5% cream in the treatment of human papillomavirus-16-positive erythroplasia of Queyrat. Dermatology 205: 67–69

Kim KJ, Lee DP, Lee MW, Choi JH, Moon KC, Koh JK (2005) Penoscrotal extramammary Paget's disease in a patient with rectal cancer: Double primary adenocarcinomas differentiated by immunoperoxidase staining. Am J Dermatopathol 27: 171–172

Kiss A, Kiraly L, Kutasy B, Merksz M (2005) High incidence of balanitis xerotica obliterans in boys with phimosis: Prospective 10-year study. Pediatr Dermatol 22: 305–308

Lee MR, Ryman W (2005) Erythroplasia of Queyrat treated with topical methyl aminolevulinate photodynamic therapy. Australas J Dermatol 46: 196–198

Levine LA, Strom KH, Lux MM (2007) Buccal mucosa graft urethroplasty for anterior urethral stricture repair: Evaluation of the impact of stricture location and lichen sclerosus on surgical outcome. J Urol 178: 2011–2015

Lowe FC, Lattimer DG, Metroka CE (1989) Kaposi's sarcoma of the penis in patients with acquired immunodeficiency syndrome. J Urol 142: 1475–1477

Lowe FC, McCullough AR (1985) Cutaneous horns of the penis: an approach to management. Case report and review of the literature. J Am Acad Dermatol 13: 369–373

Lucia MS, Miller GJ (1992) Histopathology of malignant lesions of the penis. Urol Clin North Am 19: 227–246

Malek RS (1992) Laser treatment of premalignant and malignant squamous cell lesions of the penis. Lasers Surg Med 12: 246–253

Mendez JC, Procop GW, Espy MJ, Paya CV, Smith TF (1998) Detection and semiquantitative analysis of human herpesvirus 8 DNA in specimens from patients with Kaposi's sarcoma. J Clin Microbiol 36: 2220–2222

Micali G, Nasca MR, De Pasquale R (2006) Erythroplasia of Queyrat treated with imiquimod 5% cream. J Am Acad Dermatol 55: 901–903

Mikhail GR (1980) Cancers, precancers, and pseudocancers on the male genitalia. A review of clinical appearances, histopathology, and management. J Dermatol Surg Oncol 6: 1027–1035

Morey AF, Lin HC, DeRosa CA, Griffith BC (2007) Fossa navicularis reconstruction: Impact of stricture length on outcomes and assessment of extended meatotomy (first stage Johanson) maneuver. J Urol 177: 184–187; discussion 187

Morton C, Horn M, Leman J, Tack B, Bedane C, Tjioe M, Ibbotson S, Khemis A, Wolf P (2006) Comparison of topical methyl aminolevulinate photodynamic therapy with cryotherapy or Fluorouracil for treatment of squamous cell carcinoma in situ: Results of a multicenter randomized trial. Arch Dermatol 142: 729–735

Nasca MR, Innocenzi D, Micali G (2006) Association of penile lichen sclerosus and oncogenic human papillomavirus infection. Int J Dermatol 45: 681–683

Nasca MR, Panetta C, Micali G, Innocenzi D (2003) Microinvasive squamous cell carcinoma arising on lichen sclerosus of the penis. J Eur Acad Dermatol Venereol 17: 337–339

Obalek S, Jablonska S, Beaudenon S, Walczak L, Orth G (1986) Bowenoid papulosis of the male and female genitalia: Risk of cervical neoplasia. J Am Acad Dermatol 14: 433–444

Ohnishi T, Kano R, Nakamura Y, Hasegawa A, Watanabe S (1999) Genital Bowen disease associated with an unusual human papillomavirus type 57b. Arch Dermatol 135: 858–859

Palminteri E, Berdondini E, Lazzeri M, Mirri F, Barbagli G (2007) Resurfacing and reconstruction of the glans penis. Eur Urol 52: 893–898

Park S, Grossfeld GD, McAninch JW, Santucci R (2001) Extramammary Paget's disease of the penis and scrotum: Excision, reconstruction, and evaluation of occult malignancy. J Urol 166: 2112–2116; discussion 2117

Pasieczny TA (1977) The treatment of balanitis xerotica obliterans with testosterone propionate ointment. Acta Derm Venereol 57: 275–277

Porter WM, Francis N, Hawkins D, Dinneen M, Bunker CB (2002) Penile intraepithelial neoplasia: clinical spectrum and treatment of 35 cases. Br J Dermatol 147: 1159–1165

Powell J, Robson A, Cranston D, Wojnarowska F, Turner R (2001) High incidence of lichen sclerosus in patients with squamous cell carcinoma of the penis. Br J Dermatol 145: 85–89

Prowse DM, Ktori EN, Chandrasekaran D, Prapa A, Baithun S (2008) Human papillomavirus-associated increase in p16INK4A expression in penile lichen sclerosus and squamous cell carcinoma. Br J Dermatol 158: 261–265

Pugliese JM, Morey AF, Peterson AC (2007) Lichen sclerosus: Review of the literature and current recommendations for management. J Urol 178: 2268–2276

Regauer S (2005) Immune dysregulation in lichen sclerosus. Eur J Cell Biol 84: 273–277

Rickwood AM, Hemalatha V, Batcup G, Spitz L (1980) Phimosis in boys. Br J Urol 52: 147–150

Ridley CM (1992) Lichen sclerosus. Dermatol Clin 10: 309–323

Rosemberg SK, Fuller TA (1980) Carbon dioxide rapid superpulsed laser treatment of erythroplasia of Queyrat. Urology 16: 181–182

Schoen EJ, Oehrli M, Colby C, Machin G (2000) The highly protective effect of newborn circumcision against invasive penile cancer. Pediatrics 105: E36

Schroeder TL, Sengelmann RD (2002) Squamous cell carcinoma in situ of the penis successfully treated with imiquimod 5% cream. J Am Acad Dermatol 46: 545–548

Schwartz RA, Janniger CK (1991) Bowenoid papulosis. 24: 261–264

Schwartz RA, Micali G, Nasca MR, Scuderi L (2008) Kaposi sarcoma: a continuing conundrum. J Am Acad Dermatol 59: 179–206; quiz 207–178

Solivan GA, Smith KJ, James WD (1990) Cutaneous horn of the penis: its association with squamous cell carcinoma and HPV-16 infection. J Am Acad Dermatol 23: 969–972

Solsona E, Algaba F, Horenblas S, Pizzocaro G, Windahl T (2004) EAU Guidelines on Penile Cancer. Eur Urol 46: 1–8

Stables GI, Stringer MR, Robinson DJ, Ash DV (1999) Erythroplasia of Queyrat treated by topical aminolaevulinic acid photodynamic therapy. Br J Dermatol 140: 514–517

Taliaferro SJ, Cohen GF (2008) Bowen's disease of the penis treated with topical imiquimod 5% cream. J Drugs Dermatol 7: 483–485

Tappero JW, Conant MA, Wolfe SF, Berger TG (1993) Kaposi's sarcoma. Epidemiology, pathogenesis, histology, clinical spectrum, staging criteria and therapy. J Am Acad Dermatol 28: 371–395

Tolia BM, Castro VL, Mouded IM, Newman HR (1976) Bowen's disease of shaft of penis. Successful treatment with 5-fluorouracil. Urology 7: 617–619

van Bezooijen BP, Horenblas S, Meinhardt W, Newling DW (2001) Laser therapy for carcinoma in situ of the penis. J Urol 166: 1670–1671

van Randenborgh H, Paul R, Nahrig J, Egelhof P, Hartung R (2002) Extramammary Paget's disease of penis and scrotum. J Urol 168: 2540–2541

Velazquez EF, Cubilla AL (2007) Penile squamous cell carcinoma: anatomic, pathologic and viral studies in Paraguay (1993–2007). Anal Quant Cytol Histol 29: 185–198

Venn SN, Mundy AR (1998) Urethroplasty for balanitis xerotica obliterans. Br J Urol 81: 735–737

von Krogh G, Horenblas S (2000) The management and prevention of premalignant penile lesions. Scand J Urol Nephrol Suppl 220–229

Wade TR, Kopf AW, Ackerman AB (1978) Bowenoid papulosis of the penis. Cancer 42: 1890–1903

Wieland U, Jurk S, Weissenborn S, Krieg T, Pfister H, Ritzkowsky A (2000) Erythroplasia of queyrat: coinfection with cutaneous carcinogenic human papillomavirus type 8 and genital papillomaviruses in a carcinoma in situ. J Invest Dermatol 115: 396–401

Wigbels B, Luger T, Metze D (2001) [Imiquimod: A new treatment possibility in bowenoid papulosis?]. Hautarzt 52: 128–131

Windahl T (2006) Is carbon dioxide laser treatment of lichen sclerosus effective in the long run? Scand J Urol Nephrol 40: 208–211

Wojnarowska F, Cooper SM (2003) Anogenital (non-venereal) disease. In: Bolognia JL, Jorizzo JL, Rapini RP (eds) Dermatology. Mosby, Edinburgh, pp 1099–1113

Yang WJ, Kim DS, Im YJ, Cho KS, Rha KH, Cho NH, Choi YD (2005) Extramammary Paget's disease of penis and scrotum. Urology 65: 972–975

Yoneta A, Yamashita T, Jin HY, Iwasawa A, Kondo S, Jimbow K (2000) Development of squamous cell carcinoma by two high-risk human papillomaviruses (HPVs), a novel HPV-67 and HPV-31 from bowenoid papulosis. Br J Dermatol 143: 604–608

Human Papillomavirus and Squamous Cell Carcinoma of the Penis

6

Simon Horenblas

Contents

6.1 Introduction

The notion that human papillomavirus (HPV) plays an important role in the etiology of cervical cancer and the sexual transmission of HPV has led to further assessment of the role of HPV in the etiology of squamous cell carcinoma of the penis. While risk factors for penile cancer, such as number of sex partners and a history of genital warts or other sexually transmitted diseases, have been known for a long time, it is becoming clear that some of these risk factors can be related to the presence of HPV (Daling et al., 2005; Bleeker et al., 2008). Several studies have shown that an infection with high-risk HPV, mainly type 16, is causally involved in the pathogenesis of penile carcinoma (Rubin et al., 2001; McCance et al., 1986; Heideman et al., 2007; Gregoire et al., 1995). The published overall prevalence of high-risk HPV DNA in penile carcinomas ranges from 30 to 100%, depending on methods of HPV detection, geographical variance, and subtype (Rubin et al., 2001; McCance et al., 1986; Maden et al., 1993). An association of a small subset of penile cancers with low-risk HPV types has also been suggested, and DNA of cutaneous HPV 8 has occasionally been detected in penile lesions (Heideman et al., 2007; Dorfman et al., 2006; Senba et al., 2006; Wieland et al., 2000).

S. Horenblas
Chief department of urology, Netherlands Cancer Institute-Anton van Leeuwenhoek Hospital, Plesmanlaan 121, 1066 CX, Amsterdam, The Netherlands
e-mail: s.horenblas@nki.nl

A. Rosenblatt, H. G. de Campos Guidi, *Human Papillomavirus*,
DOI: 10.1007/978-3-540-70974-9-6, © Springer-Verlag Berlin Heidelberg 2009

6.2   Natural History of HPV in Male Subjects

The distribution of HPV in the penis is as following, according to two studies: prepuce 28%, shaft 24%, scrotum 17%, glans 16%, and urethra 6% (Morris, 2007; Weaver et al., 2004). HPVs, most notably high-risk types, are more common in uncircumcised male subjects (Castellsague et al., 2002). A large multinational study found HPV in 19.6% of 847 uncircumcised men, but only 5.5% of 292 circumcised men; this difference was statistically significant (Castellsague et al., 2002). High-risk HPVs often produce clinically occult lesions, in contrast to low-risk HPVs that usually present as visible warts (Katelaris et al., 1988). These lesions include flat penile lesions (FPLs), which become visible only by application of dilute acetic acid to the penis (Barrasso, 1997; Hippelainen et al., 1991; Bleeker et al., 2002). FPLs are predominantly found at the mucosal site of the penis. Histological evaluation of FPLs generally shows mild changes such as squamous hyperplasia or low-grade penile intraepithelial neoplasia (PIN). High-grade PIN is uncommon, being present in about 5% of cases. FPLs are found in about 50–70% of the male sexual partners of women with cervical intraepithelial neoplasia (CIN) vs. about 10–20% in men who do not have a partner with CIN (Bleeker et al., 2006). Even higher prevalence rates (up to 36%) have been found in young male populations (Kataoka et al., 1991). Beside the association with HPV, it is important to realize that, in the case of HPV positivity, FPLs display relatively high viral load levels. The presence of high viral loads in these lesions is clinically meaningful as it indicates a potential increased risk for HPV transmission. The majority of infections are subclinical (Kohn et al., 1999).

Although the clinical course is generally benign, showing healing within 1–2 years in the majority of cases, a small percentage of FPLs remain persistently HPV-positive and do not heal. These persistent HPV-positive FPLs might progress to high-grade PIN and subsequent penile cancer.

Consistent with HPV sexual transmission, varying amounts of men whose female partner had a squamous intraepithelial lesion (SIL) had PIN (Aynaud et al., 1994). High-risk HPV was present in 75% of patients with PIN grade I, 93% with PIN grade II, and 100% of PIN grade III, which is one step removed from overt penile cancer.

6.3   Etiology of Squamous Cell Cancer of the Penis

Penile cancers are thought to arise from the progression of precursor lesions and can be subdivided into HPV-positive and HPV-negative cases. Similar to vulvar and head and neck carcinomas, squamous cell carcinomas of the basaloid and warty type display the strongest association with high-risk HPV (ranging from 70 to 100%) and their etiological relationship with high-risk HPV infection is most plausible (Cubilla et al., 1998, 2000). The remaining penile squamous cell carcinomas demonstrate about 30–50% positivity for high-risk HPV DNA. In the HPV-positive cases, HPV 16 is the predominant type found (Gregoire et al., 1995; Bezerra et al., 2001; Ferreux et al., 2003). Despite the similarities between penile and vulvar cancer, including their presence of HPV (mainly HPV 16) and their precursor lesions, a clear bimodal age distribution as is found for vulvar cancer is not clearly seen for penile cancer (Canavan and Cohen, 2002). Cubilla et al. observed a lower age of patients with basaloid or warty types (i.e., average 55 years) of cancer compared to other types of penile squamous cell carcinomas (Bleeker et al., 2002, 2006; Cubilla et al., 2004). However, in another study, including a large series of penile cancer cases, no age difference was found between HPV-positive and -negative cases (i.e., average 64 years) (Lont et al., 2006).

Cubilla et al. presented cross-sectional data of 288 invasive penile cancers and studied the presence of associated epithelial lesions (Cubilla et al., 2004). Histological evaluation showed that squamous hyperplasia, low-grade PIN, and high-grade PIN were present in 83, 59, and 44% of the cases, respectively. The observed associated lesions suggested a sequence of squamous hyperplasia to low-grade PIN to high-grade PIN. In this study a more common association was observed between squamous hyperplasia and the usual squamous, papillary, and verrucous squamous cell carcinomas than with warty or basaloid carcinomas. Conversely, high-grade PIN was present in two-thirds of the warty, basaloid, or mixed warty-basaloid tumor subtypes, in half of the usual squamous cell carcinomas, and absent in papillary and verrucous tumors. In fact, despite the lack of a clear identification of the clinical counterparts, corresponding histopathologic features between the precursor lesion and its associated tumor type were shown. Apparently, nondysplastic or mildly dysplastic lesions may directly progress into invasive cancer in at least a substantial subset of penile cancer cases. In conclusion, although there are several clear-cut differences between the types of penile squamous cell carcinoma and their precursor lesions (i.e., histomorphological features and HPV status), their clinical distinction and the underlying molecular pathogenesis for progression into invasive cancer are not clear-cut and merit further investigation. An overview of the different histopathological lesions, the presence of high-risk HPV, their clinical phenotype, and their putative transformation to penile cancer are presented in Fig. 6.1.

Multiple studies have consistently shown that there is a high prevalence of HPV in PIN (60–100%) (Barrasso et al., 1987; Porter et al., 2002). In the general population, PIN has been found in 10% of uncircumcised men compared with 6% of circumcised men.

Most cases of PIN are cleared naturally. HPV has been found in 80% of tumor specimens, 69% having the very high-risk type HPV 16. Since not all HPV types were tested for, the rate of HPV is undoubtedly higher. Condom use lowers HPV infection only slightly. The reported HPV prevalence rates of 43–100% are based on relatively small numbers (Wieland et al., 2000; Hahn et al., 1988; Ikenberg et al., 1983).

6.4 Molecular Pathogenesis

Although the etiology of penile cancers is not yet fully understood, penile carcinoma is recognized to be heterogeneous. A proportion of penile carcinomas is attributable to high-risk HPV infection, while in the remaining penile cancers molecular mechanisms independent of HPV are likely to represent the more common underlying events. An overview of the molecular pathogenesis is presented in Fig. 6.2, and will be discussed below.

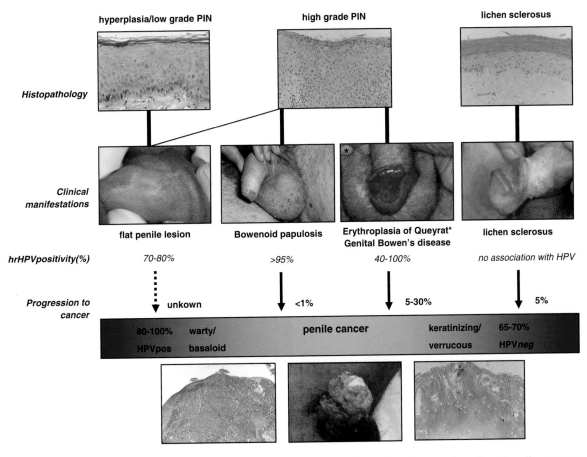

Fig. 6.1. Relationship between histology, HPV presence, clinical manifestation, and putative transformation of penile precursor lesions into penile cancer (*hrHPV* high-risk HPV) (Published with permission from Bleeker (2009))

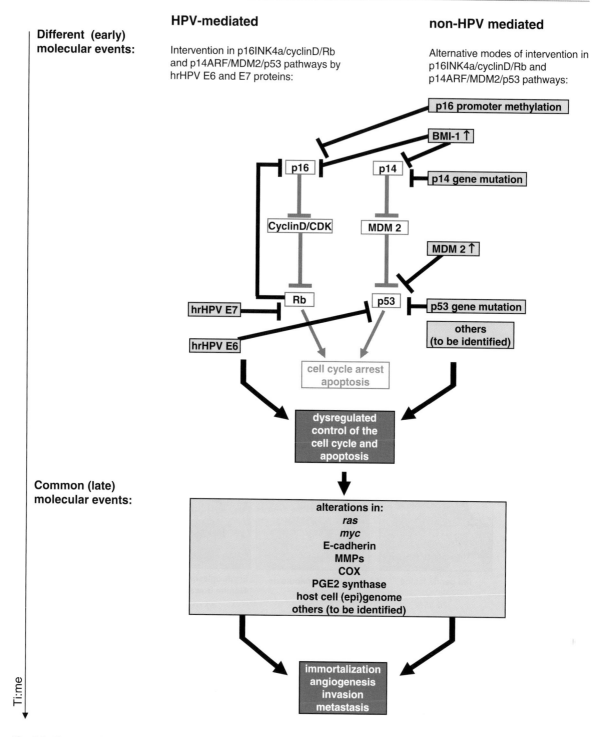

Fig. 6.2. Concept of penile molecular pathogensis. Schematic overview of modes of intervention in cellular pathways involved in early and late stages of penile carcinogenesis, and their net effect (Published with permission from Bleeker (2009))

6.4.1 HPV-Mediated Penile Carcinogenesis

High-risk HPV-associated penile cancers arise from the progression of precursor lesions caused by a high-risk HPV infection. The penile carcinogenic pathway is thought to be equivalent to high-risk HPV-mediated cervical carcinogenesis (Snijders et al., 2006). High-risk HPV-induced carcinogenesis is multistep in nature: a persistent infection with high-risk HPV is the initiating causative event, and subsequent (epi)genetic alterations are necessary for a high-risk HPV-infected cell to become fully malignant. High-risk HPVs exert their oncogenic effect by expressing the oncoproteins E6 and E7, which bind to and inactivate the p53 and Rb tumor suppressor gene products, respectively (zur Hausen, 2002; Scheffner et al., 1994). The E6 and E7 gene products of the oncogenic HPV types are required for induction and maintenance of the transformed phenotype of the infected cells. By disturbance of the $p14^{ARF}$/MDM2/p53 and $p16^{INK4a}$/cyclin D/Rb pathways, oncogenic HPV types interfere with control of the cell division cycle and apoptosis. The functional inactivation of pRb by hrHPV E7 results in the reciprocal overexpression of $p16^{INK4a}$, due to a negative feedback loop between retinoblastoma tumor suppressor protein (pRb) and $p16^{INK4a}$. Therefore, overexpression of $p16^{INK4a}$ may be used as a marker of viral involvement (Kohn et al., 1999). Subsequent host-cell (epi)genetic events involved in high-risk HPV-induced penile carcinogenesis are not well studied, but may include those identified for high-risk HPV-mediated cervical carcinogenesis, e.g., promoter methylation of CADM-1, an immunoglobulin (Ig)-like cell surface protein involved in cell–cell adhesion, and a change in the composition of the AP-1 complex, a transcription factor consisting of different proteins (e.g., c-Jun, c-Fos, or Fra-1) in homo- or heterodimer complexes (Steenbergen et al., 2001; Sastre-Garau et al., 2000). Whether the same (epi)genetic alterations are involved in high-risk HPV-mediated penile carcinogenesis as in cervical carcinogenesis warrants further research. It should be realized that despite a common causative event, differences exist between high-risk HPV-associated cervical and penile carcinoma, which are reflected by the different incidence rates and time-span of development. While penile high-risk HPV infections are as equally common as those of the cervix, the incidence of HPV-associated penile carcinoma is very rare as compared to cervical cancer (Ikenberg et al., 1983; Franceschi et al.,

2002). This may infer that penile epithelium represents a less favorable environment for virus-induced transformation compared to the epithelium of the cervical transformation zone, in which cervical cancers arise. Furthermore, the peak incidence of cervical cancer is around the age of 35–45 years, while the incidence of high-risk HPV-associated penile cancer simply increases with age. These findings suggest that there exist tissue- and/or hormonal-specific variables that influence the course of the high-risk HPV-mediated carcinogenic process that merit further attention.

6.4.2 HPV-Independent Penile Carcinogenesis

Several studies have focused on the genetic and molecular changes associated with HPV-independent penile carcinogenesis, and they have identified nonviral mechanism(s) leading to disturbance of the $p14^{ARF}$/MDM2/p53 and/or $p16^{INK4a}$/cyclin D/Rb pathways in this subset of penile carcinomas (Rubin et al., 2001; Martins et al., 2002; Leis et al., 1998; Couturier et al., 1991; Sastre-Garau et al., 2000; Campos et al., 2006; Golijanin et al., 2004; Kayes et al., 2007). Findings from Ferreux et al., revealed that there are at least two plausible mechanisms by which the $p16^{INK4a}$/cyclin D/Rb pathway can be disrupted during penile carcinogenesis in the absence of hrHPV, i.e., silencing of the $p16^{INK4a}$ gene by promoter hypermethylation in 15% of cases and overexpression of the polycomb group (PcG) gene BMI-1, which targets the INK4A/ARF locus, encoding both $p16^{INK4a}$ and $p14^{ARF}$, in 10% of cases (Kohn et al., 1999). Also, alternative high-risk HPV-independent mechanisms of $p14^{ARF}$/MDM2/p53 pathway inactivation in penile carcinogenesis have been described including somatic mutations of the p53 gene, overexpression of MDM2, and mutation of $p14^{ARF}$. An inverse correlation between high-risk HPV presence and p53 stabilization, a feature of mutated, inactive p53, has been reported in penile carcinoma (Castren et al., 1998; Pilotti et al., 1993; Ranki et al., 1995).

6.4.3 Common Molecular Events in Penile Carcinogenesis

Several other molecular events associated with penile cancer include alterations in the *ras* and *myc* genes,

E-cadherin expression, matrix metalloproteinase (MMP-2, MMP-9) expression, cyclo-oxygenase-2 (COX) pathway, and prostaglandin E2 synthase (66–70). These alterations have been described in both HPV-positive and -negative penile cancers, and are suggested to represent late events in penile carcinogenesis including disease progression, invasion, metastasis, and angiogenesis.

Evidence exists for multiple independent molecular pathways of penile carcinogenesis, with a subgroup known to be etiologically related to high-risk HPV infection. The most common disrupted pathways, both in HPV-mediated and HPV-independent penile carcinogenesis, involve the $p14^{ARF}$/MDM2/p53 and/or $p16^{INK4a}$/cyclin D/Rb pathways. To date, the etiology of penile cancers is not completely understood and additional research is necessary to fully delineate the sequence of molecular events involved in both HPV-mediated and non-HPV-associated pathways leading to penile cancer. A better understanding of the molecular mechanisms beyond the development and progression of penile cancer and its precursor lesions will aid the prevention, early detection, and development of novel therapeutic agents to reduce morbidity and mortality from penile cancer.

6.5   Prevention of HPV Infection

6.5.1   HPV Vaccination

To date, two prophylactic HPV vaccines, i.e., a bivalent HPV 16/18 vaccine Cervarix (GlaxoSmithKline Biochemicals S.A.) and a quadrivalent HPV 16/18/6/11 vaccine Gardasil (Sanofi Pasteur MSD), have been registered by the European Medicines and Evaluation Agency (EMEA) and the Federal Drug Administration (FDA). A high prophylactic efficacy of these vaccines for persistent HPV infection and incident high-grade cervical lesions has been observed in HPV-negative women in large multicentric trials (Harper et al., 2004, 2006; Villa et al., 2005). Evidence to date also suggests the safety and immunogenicity of HPV vaccines in men (10–15 years of age) and thus the vaccines have been licensed for men in some countries (Villa et al., 2005). The EMEA license for the quadrivalent vaccine includes both sexes. Although similar effects might be expected in the prevention of HPV-associated penile lesions, to date the efficacy of HPV vaccination in men is unknown and the first results are awaited in the near future. To study the efficacy of a prophylactic HPV vaccine in men, the presence of HPV-associated FPLs should not be ignored in the evaluation. This is particularly important because their existence reflects the presence of high viral load, indicating their potential increased risk for viral spread to sex partners compared to those not having FPL, being either HPV-negative or carrying very low copy numbers of HPV that are clinically irrelevant.

6.5.2   Condom Use

Although there is not 100% protection, condom use is effective in the prevention of sexually transmitted infections (STIs), including HPV (Holmes et al., 2004; Vaccarella et al., 2006; Winer et al., 2006; Nielson et al., 2007). To study whether viral shedding among sex partners might have consequences for viral persistence and the natural history of genital lesions, a randomized clinical trial was performed. In this study, sex partners were randomized for condom use, and it was shown that healing of HPV-associated genital lesions was considerably shortened in condom-using couples (Hogewoning et al., 2003; Bleeker et al., 2003). The healing time of high-risk HPV-associated FPLs was 7.4 months in male partners of the condom group compared to 13.9 months in the noncondom group.

6.6   HPV as a Prognostic Indicator in Penile Cancer

Although studies have found that HPV infection is related to the tumor subtype, the correlation with prognostic variables is still unclear.

Bezerra et al. analyzed tissue from 82 patients treated for penile carcinoma using PCR (Bezerra et al., 2001). Of these, 42 patients had lymph node metastases. HPV DNA was detected in 30.5% (25/82) samples, of which 13 were positive for HPV 16, four contained HPV 18, with the remaining samples positive for a variety of HPV DNA including HPV 45, 6/11, 31, 33, and 35. There was no correlation between HPV DNA status and 10-year survival. With a mean follow-up of 88.7 months (range, 0.1–453 months), the study concluded that HPV status was related only to lymphatic embolization and had no correlation with the prognosis. Disease-specific survival was only significantly related to the lymph node status.

In contrast, Lont et al. investigated the survival outcome in 176 patients with SCC of the penis with a mean follow-up of 95 months (Lont et al., 2006). HPV DNA detection was performed using PCR with genotyping for all the high-risk HPV subtypes. The study showed the presence of high-risk HPV DNA in 50 of the 171 patients (29%), of which 38 (76%) harbored HPV 16. Multiple logistic regression analysis found that the only factor related to the HPV status was morphea-like growth, whereby HPV-positive tumors showed less morphea-like growth. The 5-year disease-specific survival was 92% in the HPV-positive group compared to 78% in the HPV-negative group, indicating a survival advantage for patients who are HPV DNA-positive.

6.7 Conclusion

In almost half of the patients with squamous cell cancer, a clear association with high-risk HPV has been found. Based on research in cervical cancer, similar pathophysiological factors in the etiology of squamous cell cancer of the penis were found. Additionally, more insight has been gained in the non-HPV-related penile cancers. Nevertheless, for a complete understanding, even more insight is necessary, especially in the differences of natural clearance between HPV infection in men and women. However, true prevention is at hand with HPV vaccination.

References

Aynaud O, Ionesco M, Barrasso R (1994) Penile intraepithelial neoplasia – specific clinical features correlate with histologic and virologic findings. Cancer 74: 1762–1767

Barrasso R (1997) Latentand subclinical HPV external anogenital infection. Clin Dermatol 15(3): 349–353

Barrasso R, de Brux J, Croissant O, Orth G (1987) Prevalence of papillomavirus-associated penile intraepithelial neoplasia in sexual partners of women with cervical intraepithelial neoplasia. N Engl J Med 317(15): 916–923

Bezerra AL, Lopes A, Santiago GH, Ribeiro KC, Latorre MR, Villa LL (2001) Papillomavirus as a prognostic factor in carcinoma of the penis: Analysis of 82 patients treated with amputation and bilateral lymphadenectomy. Cancer 91(12): 2315–2321

Bleeker MC, Heideman DA, Snijders PJ, Horenblas S, Dillner J, Meijer CJ (2009) Penile cancer: Epidemiology, pathogenesis and prevention. World J Urol 27(2): 141–150

Bleeker MC, Hogewoning CJ, van den Brule AJ, Voorhorst FJ, Van Andel RE, Risse EK, Starink TM, Meijer CJ (2002) Lesions and human papillomavirus in male sexual partners of women with cervical intraepithelial neoplasia. J Am Acad Dermatol 47(3): 351–357

Bleeker MC, Hogewoning CJ, Voorhorst FJ, van den Brule AJ, Snijders PJ, Starink TM, Berkhof J, Meijer CJ (2003) Use promotes regression of human papillomavirus-associated penile lesions in male sexual partners of women with cervical intraepithelial neoplasia. Int J Cancer 107(5): 804–810

Bleeker MC, Snijders PF, Voorhorst FJ, Meijer CJ (2006) Penile lesions: The infectious "invisible" link in the transmission of human papillomavirus. Int J Cancer 119(11): 2505–2512

Campos RS, Lopes A, Guimaraes GC, Carvalho AL, Soares FA (2006) E-Cadherin, MMP-2, and MMP-9 as prognostic markers in penile cancer: Analysis of 125 patients. Urology 67(4): 797–802

Canavan TP, Cohen D (2002) Cancer. Am Fam Physician 66(7): 1269–1274

Castellsague X, Bosch FX, Munoz N, Meijer CJLM, Shah KV, et al. (2002)circumcision, penile human papillomavirus infection and cervical cancer in female partners. N Engl J Med 346: 1105–1112

Castren K, Vahakangas K, Heikkinen E, Ranki A (1998) Absence of P53 mutations in benign and pre-malignant male genital lesions with over-expressed P53 protein. Int J Cancer 77(5): 674–678

Couturier J, Sastre-Garau X, Schneider-Maunoury S, Labib A, Orth G (1991) Integration of papillomavirus dna near myc genes in genital carcinomas and its consequences for proto-oncogene expression. J Virol 65(8): 4534–4538

Cubilla AL, Reuter VE, Gregoire L, Ayala G, Ocampos S, Lancaster WD, Fair W (1998) Squamous cell carcinoma: A distinctive human papilloma virus- related penile neoplasm: a report of 20 cases. Am J Surg Pathol 22(6): 755–761

Cubilla AL, Velazquez EF, Young RH (2004) Lesions associated with invasive penile squamous cell carcinoma: a pathologic study of 288 Cases. Int J Surg Pathol 12(4): 351–364

Cubilla AL, Velazquez EF, Young RH (2004) Squamous cell carcinoma of the penis associated with lichen sclerosus. An extremely well-differentiated, nonverruciform neoplasm that preferentially affects the foreskin a report of 10 cases of a distinctive clinicopathologic entity. Am J Surg Pathol 28(7): 895–900

Cubilla AL, Velazques EF, Reuter VE, Oliva E, Mihm MC, Jr., Young RH (2000) Warty (Condylomatous) squamous cell carcinoma of the penis: A report of 11 cases and proposed classification of 'verruciform' penile tumors. Am J Surg Pathol 24(4): 505–512.

Daling JR, Madeleine MM, Johnson LG, Schwartz SM, Shera KA, Wurscher MA, Carter JJ, Porter PL, Galloway DA,

McDougall JK, Krieger JN (2005)Cancer: Importance of circumcision, human papillomavirus and smoking in in situ and invasive disease. Int J Cancer 116(4): 606–616

Dorfman S, Cavazza M, Cardozo J (2006) Cancer associated with so-called low-risk human papilloma virus. report of five cases from rural venezuela. Trop Doct 36(4): 232–233

Ferreux E, Lont AP, Horenblas S, Gallee MPW, Raaphorst FM, Doeberitz MV, Meijer CJLM, Snijders PJF (2003) Evidence for at least three alternative mechanisms targeting the P16(INK4A)/cyclin D/Rb pathway in penile carcinoma, one of which is mediated by high-risk human papillomavirus. J Pathol 201(1): 109–118

Franceschi S, Castellsague X, Dal Maso L, Smith JS, Plummer M, Ngelangel C, Chichareon S, Eluf-Neto J, Shah KV, Snijders PJ, Meijer CJ, Bosch FX, Munoz N (2002) Prevalence and determinants of human papillomavirus genital infection in men. Br J Cancer 86(5): 705–711

Golijanin D, Tan JY, Kazior A, Cohen EG, Russo P, Dalbagni G, Auborn KJ, Subbaramaiah K, Dannenberg AJ (2004) Cyclooxygenase-2 and microsomal prostaglandin E synthase-1 are overexpressed in squamous cell carcinoma of the penis. Clin Cancer Res. 10(3): 1024–1031

Gregoire L, Cubilla AL, Reuter VE, Haas GP, Lancaster WD (1995) Association of human papillomavirus with high-grade histologic variants of penile-invasive squamous cell carcinoma. J Natl Cancer Inst 87(22): 1705–1709

Hahn A, Loning T, Hoos A, Henke P (1988) Immunohistochemistry (S 100, KL 1) and human papillomavirus dna hybridization on morbus bowen and bowenoid papulosis. Virchows Arch A Pathol Anat Histopathol 413(2): 113–122

Harper DM, Franco EL, Wheeler C, Ferris DG, Jenkins D, Schuind A, Zahaf T, Innis B, Naud P, De Carvalho NS, Roteli-Martins CM, Teixeira J, Blatter MM, Korn AP, Quint W, Dubin G (2004) Sustained efficacy up to 4.5 yearsof a bivalent L1 virus-like particle vaccine in prevention of infection with human papillomavirus types 16 and 18 in young women: a randomised controlled trial. Lancet 364(9447): 1757–1765

Harper DM, Franco EL, Wheeler CM, Moscicki AB, Romanowski B, Roteli-Martins CM, Jenkins D, Schuind A, Costa Clemens SA, Dubin G (2006) Efficacy up to 4.5 years of a bivalent l1 virus-like particle vaccine against human papillomavirus types 16 and 18: Follow-up from a randomised control trial. Lancet 367(9518): 1247–1255

Heideman DA, Waterboer T, Pawlita M, Delis-van Diemen P, Nindl I, Leijte JA, Bonfrer JM, Horenblas S, Meijer CJ, Snijders PJ (2007) Papillomavirus-16 is the predominant type etiologically involved in penile squamous cell carcinoma. J Clin Oncol 25(29): 4550–4556

Hippelainen M, Yliskoski M, Saarikoski S, Syrjanen S, Syrjanen K (1991) Human papillomavirus lesions of the male sexual partners: The diagnostic accuracy of peniscopy [See Comments]. Genitourin Med 67(4): 291–296

Hogewoning CJ, Bleeker MC, van den Brule AJ, Voorhorst FJ, Snijders PJ, Berkhof J, Westenend PJ, Meijer CJ (2003) use promotes regression of cervical intraepithelial neoplasia and clearance of human papillomavirus: A randomized clinical trial. Int J Cancer 107(5): 811–816

Holmes KK, Levine R, Weaver M (2004) Effectiveness of condoms in preventing sexually transmitted infections. Bull World Health Organ 82(6): 454–461

Ikenberg H, Gissmann L, Gross G, Grussendorf-Conen EI, zur Hausen H (1983) Papillomavirus Type-16-related dna in genital bowen's disease and in bowenoid papulosis. Int J Cancer 32(5): 563–565

Kataoka A, Claesson U, Hansson BG, Eriksson M, Lindh E (1991) Papillomavirus infection of the male diagnosed by southern-blot hybridization and polymerase chain reaction: Comparison between urethra samples and penile biopsy samples. J Med Virol 33(3): 159–164

Katelaris PM, Cossart YE, Rose BR, Thompson CH, Sorich E, et al. (1988) Human papillomavirus: The untreated male reservoir. J Urol 140: 300–305

Kayes O, Ahmed HU, Arya M, Minhas S (2007) Molecular and genetic pathways in penile cancer. Lancet Oncol 8(5): 420–429

Kohn F-M, Pflieger-Bruss S, Schill W-B (1999) Penile skin diseases. Andrologia 31: 3–11

Leis PF, Stevens KR, Baer SC, Kadmon D, Goldberg LH, Wang XJA (1998) C-RasHa mutation in the metastasis of a human papillomavirus (HPV)-18 positive penile squamous cell carcinoma suggests a cooperative effect between HPV-18 and C-RasHa activation in malignant progression. Cancer 83(1): 122–129

Lont AP, Kroon BK, Horenblas S, Gallee MP, Berkhof J, Meijer CJ, Snijders PJ (2006) Presence of high-risk human papillomavirus dna in penile carcinoma predicts favorable outcome in survival. Int J Cancer 119(5): 1078–1081

Maden C, Sherman KJ, Beckmann AM, Hislop TG, Teh CZ, Ashley RL, Daling JR (1993) Importance of circumcision, medical conditions, and sexual activity and risk of penile cancer. J Natl Cancer Inst 85(1): 19–24

Martins AC, Faria SM, Cologna AJ, Suaid HJ, Tucci S Jr. (2002) Immunoexpression of P53 protein and proliferating cell nuclear antigen in penile carcinoma. J Urol 167(1): 89–92.

McCance DJ, Kalache A, Ashdown K, Andrade L, Menezes F, Smith P, Doll R (1986) Papillomavirus types 16 and 18 in carcinomas of the penis from Brazil. Int J Cancer 37(1): 55–59

Morris, BJ (2007) Why circumcision is a biomedical imperative for the 21st century. Bioessays. 29(11): 1147–1158.

Nielson CM, Harris RB, Dunne EF, Abrahamsen M, Papenfuss MR, Flores R, Markowitz LE, Giuliano AR (2007) Factors for anogenital human papillomavirus infection in men. J Infect Dis 196(8): 1137–1145.

Pilotti S, Donghi R, D'Amato L, Giarola M, Longoni A, Della X, Torre G, De Palo G, Pierotti MA, Rilke F (1993) Detection and P53 alteration in squamous cell verrucous malignancies of the lower genital tract. Diagn Mol Pathol 2(4): 248–256.

Porter WM, Francis N, Hawkins D, Dinneen M, Bunker CB (2002) Intraepithelial neoplasia: Clinical spectrum and treatment of 35 cases. Br J Dermatol 147(6): 1159–1165

Ranki A, Lassus J, Niemi KM (1995) Relation of P53 tumor suppressor protein expression to human papillomavirus (HPV) DNA and to cellular atypia in male genital warts and in premalignant lesions. Acta Derm Venereol. 75(3): 180–186

Rubin MA, Kleter B, Zhou M, Ayala G, Cubilla AL, Quint WG, Pirog EC (2001) Detection and typing of human papillomavirus dna in penile carcinoma: evidence for multiple independent pathways of penile carcinogenesis. Am J Pathol 159(4): 1211–1218

Sastre-Garau X, Favre M, Couturier J, Orth G (2000) patterns of alteration of Myc genes associated with integration of human papillomavirus type 16 or type 45 DNA in two genital tumours. J Gen Virol 81(Pt 8): 1983–1993

Scheffner M, Romanczuk H, Munger K, Huibregtse JM, Mietz JA, Howley PM (1994) Functions of human papillomavirus proteins. Curr Top Microbiol Immunol 186: 83–99

Senba M, Kumatori A, Fujita S, Jutavijittum P, Yousukh A, Moriuchi T, Nakamura T, Toriyama K (2006) Prevalence of human papillomavirus genotypes in penile cancers from Northern Thailand. J Med Virol 78(10): 1341–1346

Snijders PJ, Steenbergen RD, Heideman DA, Meijer CJ (2006) HPV-mediated cervical carcinogenesis: concepts and clinical implications. J Pathol 208(2): 152–164

Steenbergen RD, Kramer D, Meijer CJ, Walboomers JM, Trott DA, Cuthbert AP, Newbold RF, Overkamp WJ, Zdzienicka MZ, Snijders PJ (2001) Suppression by chromosome 6 in a human papillomavirus type 16-immortalized keratinocyte cell line and in a cervical cancer cell line. J Natl Cancer Inst 93(11): 865–872

Vaccarella S, Franceschi S, Herrero R, Munoz N, Snijders PJ, Clifford GM, Smith JS, Lazcano-Ponce E, Sukvirach S, Shin HR, de Sanjose S, Molano M, Matos E, Ferreccio C, Anh PT, Thomas JO, Meijer CJ (2006) Behavior, condom use, and human papillomavirus: pooled analysis of the iarc human papillomavirus prevalence surveys. Cancer Epidemiol Biomarkers Prev 15(2): 326–333

Villa LL, Costa RL, Petta CA, Andrade RP, Ault KA, Giuliano AR, Wheeler CM, Koutsky LA, Malm C, Lehtinen M, Skjeldestad FE, Olsson SE, Steinwall M, Brown DR, Kurman RJ, Ronnett BM, Stoler MH, Ferenczy A, Harper DM, Tamms GM, Yu J, Lupinacci L, Railkar R, Taddeo FJ, Jansen KU, Esser MT, Sings HL, Saah AJ, Barr E (2005)Quadrivalent human papillomavirus (Types 6, 11, 16, and 18) L1 virus-like particle vaccine in young women: A randomised double-blind placebo-controlled multicentre phase ii efficacy trial. Lancet Oncol 6(5): 271–278

Weaver BA, Feng Q, Holmes KK, Kiviat N, Lee SK et al. (2004) Evaluation of genital sites and sampling techniques for detection of human papillomavirus DNA in men. J Infect Dis 189: 677–685

Wieland U, Jurk S, Weissenborn S, Krieg T, Pfister H, Ritzkowsky A (2000) Erythroplasia of Queyrat: coinfection with cutaneous carcinogenic human papillomavirus type 8 and genital papillomaviruses in a carcinoma in situ. J Invest Dermatol 115(3): 396–401

Winer RL, Hughes JP, Feng Q, O'Reilly S, Kiviat NB, Holmes KK, Koutsky LA (2006) Use and the risk of genital human papillomavirus infection in young women. N Engl J Med 354(25): 2645–2654

zur Hausen H (2002) Papillomaviruses and cancer: From basic studies to clinical application. Nat Rev Cancer 2(5): 342–350

Part III

Human Papillomavirus and Other Anogenital Premalignant Diseases

Human Papillomavirus and Anal Intraepithelial Neoplasia

7

Alberto Rosenblatt and Homero Gustavo de Campos Guidi

Contents

A. Rosenblatt (✉)
Albert Einstein Jewish Hospital, Sao Paulo, Brasil
e-mail: albrose1@gmail.com

7.1   Introduction

Human papillomavirus (HPV)-associated malignancies other than cervical cancer have increased in recent decades and one of the most challenging is squamous cell carcinoma of the anus (SCCA).

This chapter reviews and discusses the recent findings related to anal intraepithelial neoplasia (AIN), the precursor lesion of anal SCC, including grading, terminology, and management of anal dysplastic lesions. A complete discussion of anal carcinoma is beyond the scope of this book, and readers interested in the subject should refer to the specialized literature (Abbasakoor and Boulos, 2005; Shepherd, 2007).

7.2   Overview

Squamous cell carcinoma of the anus (SCCA) and perianal skin is relatively uncommon, accounting for about 4% of all lower gastrointestinal cancers in the United States. However, evidence shows that the incidence of both anal SCC and AIN is increasing in both genders, particularly in high-risk groups such as individuals infected with the human immunodeficiency virus (HIV) and immunosuppressed patients.

The prevalence of AIN in surgically removed perianal/anal warts is higher than previously reported. In a recent retrospective analysis, McCloskey et al. (2007) found an overall AIN rate of 33% (with 20% high-grade AIN) in men without HIV infection and 78%

A. Rosenblatt, H. G. de Campos Guidi, *Human Papillomavirus*,
DOI: 10.1007/978-3-540-70974-9-7, © Springer-Verlag Berlin Heidelberg 2009

(52% high-grade AIN) in HIV-infected men. In HIV-negative female subjects, the overall rate of AIN in perianal/anal warts was 8.3%, with high-grade AIN present in 2.8% of specimens. According to the investigators, the presented data support the judicious pathological analysis of all HPV-related lesions removed from the anogenital region.

The anal squamocolumnar junction is anatomically very similar to the squamocolumnar junction of the cervix. This active transformation zone is particularly vulnerable to HPV infection and its related oncogenic effects, particularly in women where the anal squamocolumnar junction is more exteriorized than in men. It is currently believed that basal cell invasion by the virus occurs in a period of approximately 24 h, and the HPV life cycle and infection are initiated when viruses reach this cell layer.

AIN shares many disease characteristics with cervical intraepithelial neoplasia (CIN) and is considered a precursor lesion of anal invasive disease.

However, as opposed to CIN lesions, the natural history of AIN is still not completely understood. The regression rate is questionable in low-grade AIN, as it could simply reflect inconsistent pathologic reporting or poor clinical follow-up. Concerning high-grade AIN, Shepherd (2007) showed that these lesions may remain in a quiescent state for long periods of time in immunocompetent subjects, but have a tendency to rapidly progress in HIV/AIDS patients.

Anal cancer is highly associated with HPV infection, particularly with oncogenic type 16, although several other high-risk HPV types are also involved in the pathogenesis of this disease (Palmer et al., 1987; Youk et al., 2001; Shroyer et al., 1995).

7.2.1   Anal HPV Infection and Associated Diseases in Men

HIV-positive men, and particularly infected men who have sex with men (MSM), are at increased risk of anal HPV infection (Fig. 7.1), AIN, and anal cancer (Melbye et al., 1994; Carter et al., 1995; Chin-Hong and Palefsky, 2005; Chin-Hong et al., 2005; Kreuter et al., 2005) (Table 7.1). The exact mechanism is still unknown, but it is likely related to an immunosuppressive status.

However, the risk of acquiring anal HPV infection is also high in heterosexual men and in HIV-negative sexually active MSM (Chin-Hong et al., 2004) (Table 7.1).

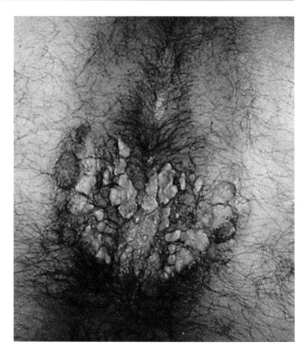

Fig. 7.1. Anal condyloma. (Source: Photograph courtesy of Carlos Walter Sobrado Jr MD, PhD, São Paulo, Brazil)

Nyitray et al. (2008) reported that the overall prevalence of anal HPV infection (at the anal canal and/or perianal region) in men who acknowledged having had no prior sexual intercourse with men was 24.8%, suggesting the possibility of distinct routes of HPV transmission (such as spread from the penis or from sexual partners via fingers or other objects). In the HIV-negative MSM group, Ching-Hong detected HPV DNA in the anal canal in 57% of 1,218 individuals aged 18–89 years, and the prevalence of low-grade squamous intraepithelial lesions (LSILs) and high-grade squamous intraepithelial lesions (HSILs) was 15% and 5%, respectively (Chin-Hong et al., 2005).

In addition, Palefsky et al. (1998c) showed that the relative risk of HIV-positive men developing incident HSILs is 3.7 higher than HIV-negative men.

7.2.2   Anal HPV Infection and Associated Diseases in Women

The prevalence of anal HPV infection in cytologically (cervical) normal and abnormal women has recently been analyzed. Goodman et al. (2008) detected anal HPV infection in 42% of women without cervical abnormalities at the time of study enrollment, and more

Table 7.1 Risk factors for anal HPV infection, AIN, and anal neoplasia

---

Risk factors associated with anal HPV infection in heterosexual male subjects (Nyitray et al., 2008)

- Lifetime number of female sex partners
- Frequency of sex with females during the preceding month

Risk factors associated with anal HPV infection in HIV-negative MSM (Chin-Hong et al., 2004)

- Receptive anal intercourse during the preceding 6 months
- >Five sex partners during the preceding 6 months

Most significant risk factors for anal HPV detection (Palefsky et al., 1998b)

- Presence of anal HPV infection
- History of receptive anal intercourse
- HIV infection
- Low CD4+ levels

Risk factors for developing low-grade SIL (LSIL) in HIV-negative MSM (Chin-Hong et al., 2005)

- >Five male receptive anal sex partners
- Use of poppers (alkyl nitrites) or injection drugs two or more times per month in the previous 6 months
- Older age at first receptive anal intercourse
- Infection with multiple HPV types

Risk factors for developing high-grade SIL (HSIL) (Palefsky et al., 1998a)

- HIV infection
- Low CD4 cell counts
- Persistent anal HPV infection
- Multifocal genital intraepithelial neoplasia in female subjects (Scholefield et al., 1992)

Risk factors associated with carcinoma of the anus (Ryan et al., 2000; Welton et al., 2004; Fagan et al., 2005)

- AIN 3 (HSIL)
- HPV infection
- HIV infection and immunosuppression
- Anoreceptive intercourse/multiple sexual partners
- History of cervical intraepithelial neoplasia (CIN)/cervical cancer
- Host genetic changes
- Other sexually acquired diseases
- Cigarette smoking

HPV human papillomavirus; *HIV* human immunodeficiency virus; *MSM* men who have sex with men; *AIN* anal intraepithelial neoplasia; *CIN* cervical intraepithelial neoplasia; *LSIL* low-grade squamous intraepithelial lesion; *HSIL* high-grade squamous intraepithelial lesion

than half of these were oncogenic types. But the risk of acquisition of an incident high-risk anal HPV infection was increased significantly (91% greater risk) in women with a cervical HPV infection at baseline. Moreover, a significant inverse relationship was found for incident oncogenic anal HPV infection and the women's age. Anal intercourse and spread of HPV from the cervix/vagina/vulva or even from sexual partners via fingers/toys may play a causative role in viral transmission to the anal region of women.

According to Scholefield et al. (1992), the incidence of AIN is also high (16-fold increase) in women with multifocal genital intraepithelial neoplasia and the increased association of AIN, CIN, and vulvar intraepithelial neoplasia (VIN) is probably related to the shared exposure to oncogenic HPV infections (Rabkin et al., 1992; Frisch et al., 1997; Frisch et al., 1999; Fox, 2006) (Fig. 7.2a, b). Furthermore, Holly et al. (2001) demonstrated that the risk of abnormal anal cytology is also higher in HIV-positive women than in HIV-negative women presenting high-risk behavior.

Nevertheless, anal carcinoma rates are not as high as the reported rates of anal dysplastic lesions.

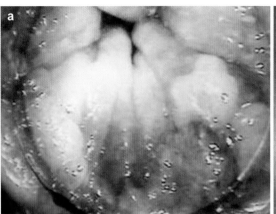

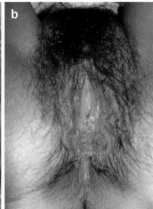

Fig. 7.2. (**a**) Anal condyloma. (**b**) Vulvar and perianal condyloma. (Source: Photograph courtesy of Nadir Oyakawa, MD, PhD, São Paulo, Brazil)

7.3 Clinical Manifestations

The majority of patients have no visible lesions, but nonspecific macroscopic changes may occur in the anal mucosa and/or perianal region:

- Raised hyperemia or white desquamative lesions
- Pigmentation (Fig. 7.3)
- Ulceration or verrucous lesions (according to Kreuter et al. (2005), the presence of the latter has been usually associated with increased risk of progression to invasive disease)

7.3.1 Symptoms

- Asymptomatic
- Local symptoms such as, pruritus, irritation, pain, tenesmus, and bleeding discharge

7.4 Differential Diagnosis

For further details (on the differential diagnosis), the reader is referred to reports by Buechner and by Wacker and Hartschuh (Buechner, (2002); Wacker and Hartschuh, (2004)).

7.4.1 Benign Conditions

- Essential pruritus
- Chronic perianal dermatitis, contact urticaria, and allergic contact dermatitis
- Parasites and fungal infections
- Seborrheic keratoses and hidradenitis suppurativa

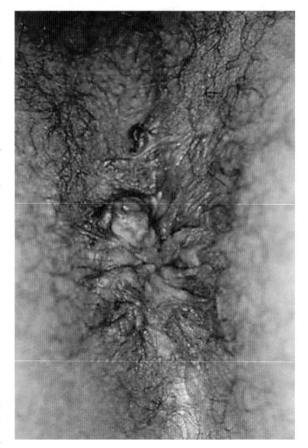

Fig. 7.3. Anal intraepithelial neoplasia. (Source: Photograph courtesy of Carlos Walter Sobrado Jr MD, PhD, São Paulo, Brazil)

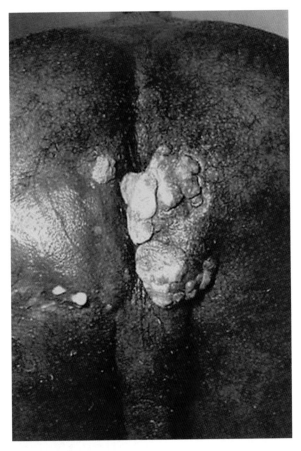

Fig. 7.4. Perianal Buschke-Löwenstein tumor. (Source: Photograph courtesy of Carlos Walter Sobrado Jr MD, PhD, São Paulo, Brazil)

7.4.2 Malignant Conditions

- Giant verrucous carcinoma of the perianal region (Buschke-Löwenstein tumor) (Fig. 7.4)
- Extramammary Paget's disease
- Cutaneous T cell lymphoma
- Basal cell carcinoma
- Langerhans cell histiocytosis
- Anorectal melanoma (rare)

7.5 Diagnosis

7.5.1 Anal Cytology and Histology

Chin-Hong et al. (2008) analyzed patient- and clinician-collected anal cytology samples to screen for HPV-associated AIN in HIV-positive and -negative MSM. The investigators reported a higher sensitivity of cytology in detecting AIN for clinician-collected than for patient-collected specimens and for HIV-positive vs. HIV-negative men. The specificity of cytology in detecting AIN was higher in HIV-negative than HIV-positive men.

However, given the high probability of AIN in a patient with a negative cytology result (23% for HIV-negative men and 45% for HIV-positive men with self-collected specimen), anoscopy should still be considered in those individuals with a single negative Pap test result.

> Anal cytology is a useful screening method for detecting premalignant anal lesions associated with HPV, and the detection rate is increased with repeated cytology screening (Jay et al., 1997; Nadal et al., 2007).

7.5.2 AIN Grading and Terminology

> AIN grading is based on anal cytology and histopathologic confirmation (Jay et al., 1997).

AIN grading remains controversial. As for the cervix, the grading of AIN is based on morphologic criteria and tissue architecture, where the level of epithelial involvement by disorderly growth and cytologic atypia are analyzed. In addition, the histological features of AIN are usually combined with those associated with HPV infection (i.e., presence of koilocytosis and dyskeratosis) (Shepherd, 2007):

AIN 1 – dysplasia involves less than one-third of the squamous mucosa thickness.

AIN 2 – dysplasia involves more than one-third, but less than two-thirds of the mucosa.

AIN 3 – dysplasia involves more than two-thirds of the mucosa thickness.

Carcinoma in situ is now categorized as grade AIN 3.

Because of reported interobserver variations using the "three-tiered" grading system, particularly for AIN grade 1 and 2, the utilization of a Bethesda-type categorization is recommended (i.e., low- and high-grade AIN), where:

- Low-grade AIN encompasses AIN 1 and AIN 2.
- High-grade AIN corresponds to AIN 3 (Scholefield, 1999).

AIN can also be referred to as anal squamous intraepithelial lesion (SIL); hence, low-grade anal squamous intraepithelial lesion (LSIL) is equivalent to histologic grade AIN 1 (Martin and Bower, 2001), whereas high-grade anal squamous intraepithelial lesion (HSIL) corresponds to AIN 2 or 3.

Specimens exhibiting insufficient abnormalities to be interpreted as SIL, and those with rare atypical squamous cells but without definitive cellular evidence for SIL, should be classified as atypical squamous cells of undetermined significance (ASCUS) (see also Chap. 8).

7.5.3   Anal and Perianal Brush Samples for Molecular Tests

Perianal and anal canal specimens can be obtained by brushing and then be analyzed for HPV DNA using polymerase chain reaction (PCR) and genotyping.

Goldstone (2008) recently evaluated the use of the Hybrid Capture 2 test in HIV-positive and -negative MSM exhibiting ASCUS. The investigators reported that referring only patients with high-risk HPV types for high-resolution anoscopy (HRA) can reduce the number of procedures by more than 50%.

Studies show that HIV patients harbor different types of HPV DNA, including intermediate-risk and high-risk HPV types other than 16–18. Furthermore, regional differences in type prevalence have been also reported in these patients (Nyitray et al., 2008; Goodman et al., 2008; Tsai et al., 2008).

7.5.4   High-Resolution Anoscopy and Targeted Biopsies

High-resolution anoscopy (HRA) is a minimally invasive procedure (equivalent to cervical colposcopy) that enables visualization and biopsy of abnormal lesions (Fig. 7.5).

HRA should be performed if ASCUS, LSIL, or HSIL is found on the anal Pap smear (Chin-Hong and Palefsky, 2002).

Moreover, since subclinical anal HPV infection should be considered in the differential diagnoses of idiopathic anal pruritus, HRA can also be recommended in individuals presenting this common disorder (Magi et al., 2003; Magi et al., 2006).

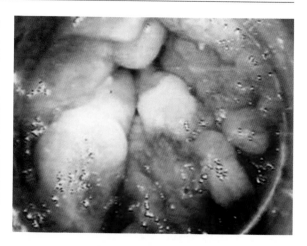

Fig. 7.5. High-resolution anoscopy showing acetowhitening of the anal mucosa. (Source: Photograph courtesy of Nadir Oyakawa, MD, PhD, São Paulo, Brazil)

How to Perform HRA

HRA is an office procedure and anesthesia is not required. A digital rectal examination (DRE) is also performed at the time of the procedure.

Initially, the perianal skin and perineum are examined under magnification following application of acetic acid 5% (Fig. 7.6a, b). After introduction of a disposable anoscope (Fig. 7.7), gauze wrapped around a cotton-tipped swab soaked in 3% acetic acid solution is generously applied to the anal canal and perianal area. The solution is allowed to saturate the epithelium for a couple of minutes and the swab is then removed. The whitening of the mucosa (Fig. 7.8a, b) produced by the vinegar solution in areas of abnormal transitional epithelium facilitates examination with a magnifying instrument (colposcope/ microscope). Lugol's iodine solution is then applied after the acetic acid, and the anus is examined once again with the magnifying instrument.

- HSILs do not take up the iodine solution and the suspected areas appear yellow-to-tan, whereas normal tissue or LSILs become dark brown or black.

High-resolution anoscopy and targeted surgical destruction:

Suspected HSIL areas (Fig. 7.9) are then selectively destroyed under direct visualization (see below - Anoscopic changes associated with HSIL (Sect. 7.5.5) and Sect 7.6).

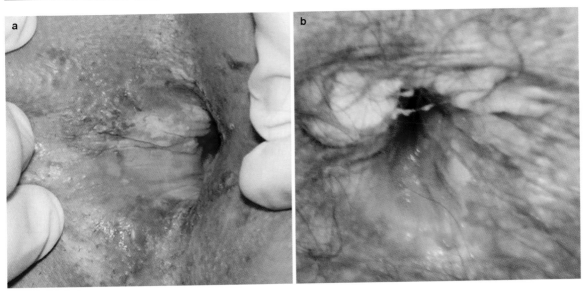

Fig. 7.6. (a.b) Acetowhitening and condylomatous lesions in the anal/perianal area. (Source: Photograph courtesy of Sidney Roberto Nadal MD, PhD, São Paulo, Brazil)

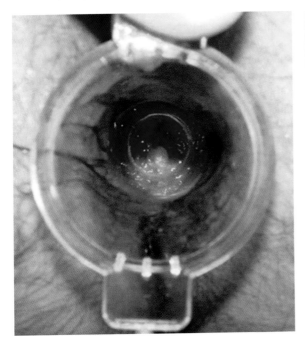

Fig. 7.7. HPV-related anal lesion identified after introduction of a disposable anoscope. (Source: Photograph courtesy of Sidney Roberto Nadal MD, PhD, São Paulo, Brazil)

Important

● Normal mucosa in between treated areas should be preserved, with an effort to prevent anal stenosis.

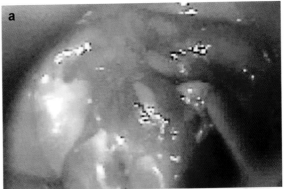
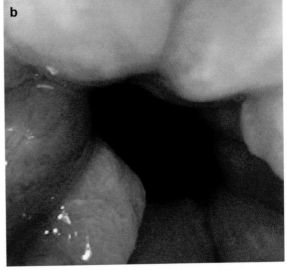

Fig. 7.8. (a) High-resolution anoscopy showing acetowhite lesions (Source: Nadal. Photograph courtesy of Sidney Roberto Nadal MD, PhD, São Paulo, Brazil). (b) Acetowhite lesions of the anal canal (Source: Photograph courtesy of Toshiro Tomishige MD, PhD, São Paulo, Brazil)

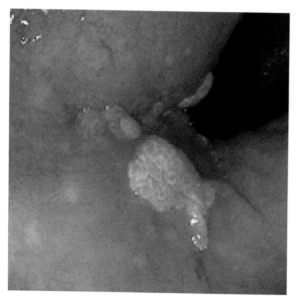

Fig. 7.9 HPV-related lesion in the rectal ampulla (Source: Photograph courtesy of Toshiro Tomishige MD, PhD, São Paulo, Brazil)

7.5.5 Anoscopic Changes Associated with HSIL

Anoscopic changes most often associated with HSIL are similar to those seen in cervical colposcopy and peniscopy:

- Acetowhite lesions exhibiting specific vascular characteristics such as punctuate vessels, mosaicism, or honeycomb patterns (Pineda et al., 2006).
- Papillation and ulceration.
- HSIL involved areas not displaying the characteristic vascular changes associated with acetic acid can also be identified by their lack of Lugol's iodine uptake.
- High-grade lesions tend to be flat, although a warty or exophytic appearance can also occur. Furthermore, HSIL can also be present in the deeper portions of typical condylomata and LSIL lesions (Goldstone et al., 2001).

Expert Advice

HRA in conjunction with anal cytology is an effective way to detect AIN. Moreover, HRA associated with anal cytology and DRE is an effective method to prevent anal cancer and/or facilitate the early diagnosis of anal neoplasia. However, even when the infrastructure for the screening and treatment of AIN is lacking, every individual at risk of anal HPV infection should be screened for anal cancer by DRE.

7.5.6 Cellular Markers

Walts et al. (2006) and Bean et al. (2007) demonstrated that the immunohistochemical expression of p16 and Ki67 is a useful method to refine the diagnosis and grading of AIN, particularly for high-grade disease.

Moreover, Kreuter et al. (2007) recently showed that p16 may be a useful adjunct marker for the evaluation of treatment response in HPV-associated AIN.

7.6 Treatment for Anogenital Warts and AIN

Treatment of anal and perianal warts is similar to HPV-related genital lesions (see Chap. 3).

However, reliable treatment modalities for the management of AIN are still lacking and good treatment results are probably best achieved in centers with a special interest in this disease.

Recurrence rates are high, particularly in HIV-positive patients, and likely reflect the multifocal nature of the disease. Some authors recommend close surveillance with HRA every 6 months as a treatment option for extensive and multifocal high-grade AIN in the anal canal (Chin-Hong and Palefsky, 2002; Devaraj and Cosman, 2006; Scholefield et al., 2005).

However, (Pineda et al., 2008) recently reviewed their 10-year experience with high-grade SIL treated with HRA-targeted surgical destruction. There was high-grade SIL persistence in 18.7% of patients and a planned staged therapy was performed. Recurrences were reported in 57% of cases at an average of 19 months and surgery was required in 23% of these patients. Progression to invasive anal neoplasia occurred in 1.2% of cases despite adequate treatment, and no evidence of disease was reported in 78% of patients at the last follow-up visit. The authors concluded that HRA-targeted destruction combined with office-based surveillance and therapy is superior to close observation or traditional mapping procedures. The study even suggested that circumferential or near-circumferential high-grade SIL (reflecting a "field defect") can still be managed by this treatment modality.

Moreover, contrary to previous findings by the same investigators, the high recurrence rates reported in previous studies (Chang et al., 2002) represented patients who had persistent disease after their initial operation. With the aim of preserving normal mucosa and skin,

Table 7.2 Recommended treatment modalities for anal warts and AIN

Topical treatments

- Podophyllotoxin solution or gel
- Trichloroacetic acid (TCA)
- Imiquimod 5% cream
- Cidofovir gel
- Photodynamic therapy (ALA-PDT)

Ablative treatments

- Infrared coagulation (IRC)
- Cryotherapy
- Surgical excision
- Electrocautery
- Carbon dioxide (CO_2) laser

HSIL was intentionally left behind, but lesion persistence was mistakenly reported as recurrence.

Therapeutic strategies can be divided into topical (podophyllotoxin, trichloroacetic acid, imiquimod, cidofovir, photodynamic therapy) and ablative (infrared coagulation, cryotherapy, surgical excision, electrocautery, or CO_2 laser vaporization) (Table 7.2).

> **Expert Advice**
>
> Patients with large-volume, circumferential, or near-circumferential HSIL disease should be offered a staged procedure (usually performed 3 months after the previous surgery), to prevent excessive tissue destruction and anal stenosis (Pineda et al., 2008).

7.6.1 Topical Treatments

7.6.1.1 Podophyllotoxin (see Chap. 3).

Disadvantages

- High recurrence rates have been observed by de Gois et al. (2005) in HIV-infected patients.

7.6.1.2 Trichloroacetic Acid

Trichloroacetic acid (TCA) can be used for individual, small to medium-sized high-grade lesions (Fox, 2006). However, controlled studies evaluating TCA for anal dysplasia are limited.

Advantages

- Efficacy – In a preliminary study, Tinmouth and Lytwyn (2005) showed that short-term clearance results using TCA for high-grade AIN were similar to infrared coagulation results.

Disadvantages

- Physician-applied therapy

Adverse Effects

- Burning sensation following TCA application that lasts for up to 10 min
- Pain
- Ulceration

7.6.1.3 Imiquimod 5% Cream (Aldara)

Topical 5% imiquimod use has been shown to be safe and effective (including in reducing recurrences) for the treatment of HPV-related anogenital lesions (Fig. 7.10a–d). Herrera et al. (2007) reported imiquimod cream efficacy in treating related lesions in HIV-infected patients, especially when used for longer periods (up to 20 weeks).

In a recent study evaluating the use of self-applied suppositories containing 5% imiquimod following surgical ablation of intra-anal warts in a small group of HIV-infected patients, Kreuter et al. (2006) reported efficacy in reducing the viral load of low- and high-risk HPV DNA. In addition, the same study showed regression of high-grade AIN lesions in three of seven patients after the use of 5% imiquimod suppositories, suggesting a beneficial role of the decrease in oncogenic HPV DNA load.

Advantages

- Patient-applied cream

Disadvantages

- Not FDA approved for use at the anal canal

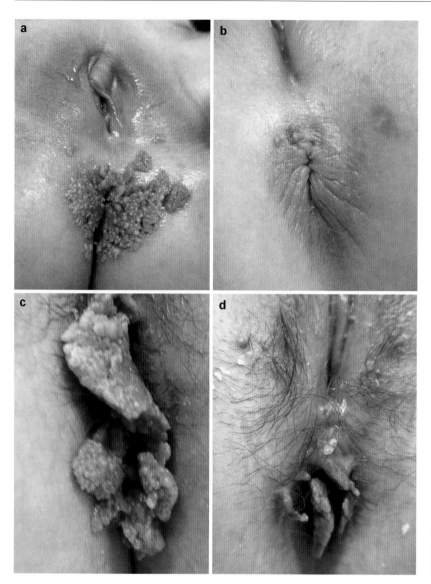

Fig. 7.10. (**a**) Anal and perianal condyloma in a 2-year-old girl. (**b**) Anal and perianal region after topical imiquimod use (Source: Oyakawa). (**c**) Anal and perianal condyloma in a 13-year-old girl. (**d**) Anal and perianal region after topical Imiquimod use (Source: Photograph courtesy of Nadir Oyakawa, MD, PhD, São Paulo, Brazil)

Side Effects

Local

- Hyperemia, swelling, pruritus, bleeding
- Blisters, flaking, scaling, dryness, or thickening of the skin
- Burning, stinging, pain in the treated area

Systemic

- Headache
- Diarrhea
- Back pain
- Fatigue
- Fever

7.6.1.4   Cidofovir 1% Gel

Cidofovir 1% gel has been used for relapsing and multifocal HPV-related anogenital lesions in HIV-positive patients (Orlando et al., 2002). However, controlled studies evaluating cidofovir for anal dysplasia have not been performed.

How to Use

Cidofovir gel is applied topically 5 days a week for up to 6 weeks.

Advantages

- Patient-applied gel.
- Efficacy – In a recent study that evaluated surgery and topical cidofovir in HIV-infected patients with anogenital warts, Orlando et al. (2002) showed a complete response in 76.2% of patients treated with cidofovir 1% gel and in 100% of subjects treated by a combination of electrocautery–cidofovir.

Disadvantages

- Expensive.
- Not FDA approved for this indication.
- Unstandardized preparation.
- Recurrence was observed in 35.29% of patients using cidofovir 1% gel and 73.68% of patients treated by surgical excision using electrocautery (Orlando et al., 2002).

Adverse Effects

- Local mucosal erosion is a common and sometimes severe event.
- Pain.
- No systemic side effects.

7.6.1.5 Photodynamic Therapy

Aminolevulinic acid (ALA) is the photosensitizer agent most commonly used in photodynamic therapy (PDT). Early results show that PDT can be used as a successful alternative to surgical excision for anal carcinoma in situ, but further prospective studies are still needed.

How to Use (Webber and Fromm, 2004)

Photosensitizer delta-ALA is given orally. Approximately 4 h later, the entire anal circumference is submitted to photodynamic therapy.

Advantages

- Efficacy – In a recent study evaluating PDT in HIV-positive patients with anal carcinoma in situ, Webber and Fromm (2004) showed consistent downgrading of cytologic findings during the 5 months of follow-up.

Adverse Effects

- Mild burning and/or stinging sensation during irradiation
- Liver function test abnormalities (usually return to baseline values within 2 weeks)

7.6.2 Ablative Treatments

7.6.2.1 Infrared Coagulation

Pulsed irradiation in the infrared range is applied to the dysplastic anal mucosa resulting in controlled tissue destruction. Targeted procedures using HRA to identify and infrared coagulation (IRC) to destroy HSIL can be performed in the office with patients under local anesthesia (Goldstone et al., 2005). Both low-volume HSILs and large-volume disease in a staged approach are amenable to IRC therapy (Pineda et al., 2008).

Advantages

- FDA approved for the treatment of anal warts and hemorrhoids.
- Response rate – 64% for biopsy-proven HSIL, in a recent retrospective study performed by Cranston et al. (2008) that evaluated infrared coagulation treatment of high-grade anal dysplasia in a cohort of HIV-positive MSM. Goldstone et al. (2007) reported cure rates of 72% for individual lesions in HIV-positive MSM and 81% after the first treatment in HIV-negative MSM patients.

Disadvantages

- Not approved for the treatment of ASIL.
- Recurrence rate is high in HIV-infected patients, according to Goldstone et al. (2005).

Adverse Effects

● Immediate or delayed bleeding
● Infection

7.6.2.2 Surgical Excision

Excision of the affected skin and mucosa using Metzenbaum scissors and a scalpel is performed in the operating room with the patient under anesthesia.

Indication

● Lesions greater than 1 cm^2
● Noncircumferential lesions

Disadvantages

● Incomplete excision
● Possible need for skin grafting
● Permanent or temporary fecal diversion

Adverse Effects

● Postoperative pain
● Bleeding
● Anal stenosis
● Fecal incontinence

Expert Advice

Targeted destruction of lesions guided by HRA is safe and effective, avoiding the risk of anal incontinence or stenosis (Pineda et al., 2006).

7.6.2.3 Electrocautery

Targeted procedures using HRA to identify HSIL and destruction of involved lesions using needle-tip electrocautery are usually performed in the operating room.

In a prospective study that evaluated HRA-targeted destruction of HSIL with needle-tip electrocautery in 29 HIV-positive and 8 HIV-negative MSM patients, Chang et al. (2002) reported recurrence rates of 79% in the former group and 0% in the HIV-negative subjects.

Adverse Effects

● Postoperative pain

7.6.2.4 CO$_2$ Laser

Carbon dioxide (CO$_2$) laser can be used for anal and perianal warts, but studies evaluating targeted procedures using HRA and CO$_2$ laser treatment for anal dysplasia are limited.

Disadvantages

● CO$_2$ laser is usually performed in the operating room with the patient under anesthesia.

Adverse Effects

● Postoperative pain

Expert Advice

Despite available ablative therapies, giant perianal condyloma (Buschke-Löwenstein tumor) (Fig. 7.11) is a highly recurrent disease. Sobrado et al. (2000) reported that radiation therapy is an optional treatment, and it can be used in selected cases as an initial cytoreductive approach before other ablative modalities (laser or surgical excision) are used.

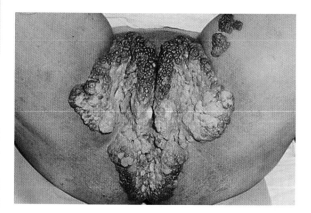

Fig. 7.11. Buschke-Löwenstein tumor involving the anogenital area. (Source: Photograph courtesy of Carlos Walter Sobrado Jr. MD, PhD, São Paulo, Brazil)

7.7 Surveillance

Surveillance for anal dysplastic lesions is performed with cytology, HRA, and DRE (Pineda et al., 2008).

In individuals exhibiting atypical squamous cells of unknown significance (ASCUS) or low-grade squamous intraepithelial lesions (LSILs) and no HRA evidence of HSIL:

- Cytology and HRA should be repeated every 6 months.

In patients exhibiting cytological findings of atypical squamous cells "cannot rule out high-grade squamous intraepithelial lesion" (ASC-H), or HSIL cytology:

- HRA is performed in less than 4 months, coupled with biopsies to confirm recurrent disease or when induration or a mass is found during DRE.

7.8 Anal Disease Screening

Who should be screened for AIN? (For further details, the reader is referred to reports by Chin-Hong and Palefsky (2002), de Sanjose and Palefsky (2002) and Benson et al (2004)).

High-risk groups such as:

- Men who have sex with men
- HIV-infected individuals (regardless of the means of HIV acquisition)

Other groups who should be considered:

- Women with cervical cancer, high-grade vulvar disease, or vulvar cancer
- Individuals presenting with HPV-related perianal lesions
- Transplant recipients

7.9 Prevention of HPV-Related Anal Warts and AIN

A recent study that evaluated the efficacy of the prophylactic quadrivalent HPV vaccine in a large group of HPV-naïve sexually active *young* men (3,400 hetero-sexuals and 600 MSM) aged 16–26 years reported that AIN was not detected in vaccinated individuals. Moreover, Gardasil was 89.4% effective in preventing HPV-related anogenital warts (Giuliano et al., 2008) (see also Sect.11.8 in Chap. 11)

References

Abbasakoor F, Boulos PB (2005) Anal intraepithelial neoplasia. Br J Surg 92: 277–290

Bean SM, Eltoum I, Horton DK, Whitlow L, Chhieng DC (2007) Immunohistochemical expression of p16 and Ki-67 correlates with degree of anal intraepithelial neoplasia. Am J Surg Pathol 31: 555–561

Benson CA, Kaplan JE, Masur H, Pau A, Holmes KK (2004) Treating opportunistic infections among HIV-infected adults and adolescents: recommendations from CDC, the National Institutes of Health, and the HIV Medicine Association/ Infectious Diseases Society of America. MMWR Recomm Rep 53: 1–112

Buechner SA (2002) Common skin disorders of the penis. BJU Int 90: 498–506

Carter PS, de Ruiter A, Whatrup C, Katz DR, Ewings P, Mindel A, Northover JM (1995) Human immunodeficiency virus infection and genital warts as risk factors for anal intraepithelial neoplasia in homosexual men. Br J Surg 82: 473–474

Chang GJ, Berry JM, Jay N, Palefsky JM, Welton ML (2002) Surgical treatment of high-grade anal squamous intraepithelial lesions: A prospective study. Dis Colon Rectum 45: 453–458

Chin-Hong PV, Berry JM, Cheng SC, Catania JA, Da Costa M, Darragh TM, Fishman F, Jay N, Pollack LM, Palefsky JM (2008) Comparison of patient- and clinician-collected anal cytology samples to screen for human papillomavirus-associated anal intraepithelial neoplasia in men who have sex with men. Ann Intern Med 149: 300–306

Chin-Hong PV, Palefsky JM (2002) Natural history and clinical management of anal human papillomavirus disease in men and women infected with human immunodeficiency virus. Clin Infect Dis 35: 1127–1134

Chin-Hong PV, Palefsky JM (2005) Human papillomavirus anogenital disease in HIV-infected individuals. Dermatol Ther 18: 67–76

Chin-Hong PV, Vittinghoff E, Cranston RD, Browne L, Buchbinder S, Colfax G, Da Costa M, Darragh T, Benet DJ, Judson F, Koblin B, Mayer KH, Palefsky JM (2005) Age-related prevalence of anal cancer precursors in homosexual men: The EXPLORE study. J Natl Cancer Inst 97: 896–905

Chin-Hong PV, Vittinghoff E, Cranston RD, Buchbinder S, Cohen D, Colfax G, Da Costa M, Darragh T, Hess E, Judson F, Koblin B, Madison M, Palefsky JM (2004) Age-specific prevalence of anal human papillomavirus infection in HIV-negative sexually active men who have sex with men: The EXPLORE study. J Infect Dis 190: 2070–2076

Cranston RD, Hirschowitz SL, Cortina G, Moe AA (2008) A retrospective clinical study of the treatment of high-grade anal dysplasia by infrared coagulation in a population of HIV-positive men who have sex with men. Int J STD AIDS 19: 118–120

de Gois NM, Costa RR, Kesselring F, de Freitas VG, Ribalta JC, Kobata MP, Taha NS (2005) Grade 3 vulvar and anal intra-epithelial neoplasia in a HIV seropositive child–therapeutic result: Case report. Clin Exp Obstet Gynecol 32: 138–140

de Sanjose S, Palefsky J (2002) Cervical and anal HPV infections in HIV positive women and men. Virus Res 89: 201–211

Devaraj B, Cosman BC (2006) Expectant management of anal squamous dysplasia in patients with HIV. Dis Colon Rectum 49: 36–40

Fagan SP, Bellows CF, 3rd, Albo D, Rodriquez-Barradas M, Feanny M, Awad SS, Berger DH (2005) Length of human immunodeficiency virus disease and not immune status is a risk factor for development of anal carcinoma. Am J Surg 190: 732–735

Fox PA (2006) Human papillomavirus and anal intraepithelial neoplasia. Curr Opin Infect Dis 19: 62–66

Frisch M, Fenger C, van den Brule AJ, Sorensen P, Meijer CJ, Walboomers JM, Adami HO, Melbye M, Glimelius B (1999) Variants of squamous cell carcinoma of the anal canal and perianal skin and their relation to human papillomaviruses. Cancer Res 59: 753–757

Frisch M, Glimelius B, van den Brule AJ, Wohlfahrt J, Meijer CJ, Walboomers JM, Goldman S, Svensson C, Adami HO, Melbye M (1997) Sexually transmitted infection as a cause of anal cancer. N Engl J Med 337: 1350–1358

Giuliano A, Palefsky J, Coutlee F (2008) The efficay of quadrivalent HPV (types 6/11/16/18) vaccine in reducing the incidence of HPV infection and HPV-related genital disease in young men. In: European Research Organization on Genital Infection and Neoplasia – EUROGIN, Nice, France

Goldstone SE, Hundert JS, Huyett JW (2007) Infrared coagulator ablation of high-grade anal squamous intraepithelial lesions in HIV-negative males who have sex with males. Dis Colon Rectum 50: 565–575

Goldstone SE, Kawalek AZ, Goldstone RN, Goldstone AB (2008) Hybrid Capture II detection of oncogenic human papillomavirus: A useful tool when evaluating men who have sex with men with atypical squamous cells of undetermined significance on anal cytology. Dis Colon Rectum 51: 1130–1136

Goldstone SE, Kawalek AZ, Huyett JW (2005) Infrared coagulator: a useful tool for treating anal squamous intraepithelial lesions. Dis Colon Rectum 48: 1042–1054

Goldstone SE, Winkler B, Ufford LJ, Alt E, Palefsky JM (2001) High prevalence of anal squamous intraepithelial lesions and squamous-cell carcinoma in men who have sex with men as seen in a surgical practice. Dis Colon Rectum 44: 690–698

Goodman MT, Shvetsov YB, McDuffie K, Wilkens LR, Zhu X, Ning L, Killeen J, Kamemoto L, Hernandez BY (2008) Acquisition of anal human papillomavirus (HPV) infection in women: The Hawaii HPV Cohort study. J Infect Dis 197: 957–966

Herrera S, Correa LA, Wolff JC, Gaviria A, Tyring SK, Sanclemente G (2007) Effect of imiquimod in anogenital warts from HIV-positive men. J Clin Virol 39: 210–214

Holly EA, Ralston ML, Darragh TM, Greenblatt RM, Jay N, Palefsky JM (2001) Prevalence and risk factors for anal squamous intraepithelial lesions in women. J Natl Cancer Inst 93: 843–849

Jay N, Berry JM, Hogeboom CJ, Holly EA, Darragh TM, Palefsky JM (1997) Colposcopic appearance of anal squamous intraepithelial lesions: Relationship to histopathology. Dis Colon Rectum 40: 919–928

Kreuter A, Brockmeyer NH, Hochdorfer B, Weissenborn SJ, Stucker M, Swoboda J, Altmeyer P, Pfister H, Wieland U (2005) Clinical spectrum and virologic characteristics of anal intraepithelial neoplasia in HIV infection. J Am Acad Dermatol 52: 603–608

Kreuter A, Brockmeyer NH, Weissenborn SJ, Wafaisade A, Pfister H, Altmeyer P, Wieland U (2006) 5% imiquimod suppositories decrease the DNA load of intra-anal HPV types 6 and 11 in HIV-infected men after surgical ablation of condylomata acuminata. Arch Dermatol 142: 243–244

Kreuter A, Wieland U, Gambichler T, Altmeyer P, Pfister H, Tenner-Racz K, Racz P, Potthoff A, Brockmeyer NH (2007) p16ink4a expression decreases during imiquimod treatment of anal intraepithelial neoplasia in human immunodeficiency virus-infected men and correlates with the decline of lesional high-risk human papillomavirus DNA load. Br J Dermatol 157: 523–530

Magi JC, Rodrigues MRS, Guerra GMLSR, Costa ACL, Formiga GJS (2003) Subclinical human papillomavirus in the differential diagnosis of the etiology of anal pruritus [O Papilomavirus humano (HPV) na forma subclínica como diagnóstico diferencial da etiologia do prurido anal] [article in portuguese]. Rev bras Coloproct 23: 273–277

Magi JC, Rodrigues MRS, Guerra GMLSR, Costa MC, Costa ACL, Villa LL, Formiga GJS (2006) Histopathological and PCR results for clinical and subclinical forms of HPV anal infection – Study of four groups of patients In: Rev bras Coloproct, vol 26, Rio de Janeiro, pp 406–413

Martin F, Bower M (2001) Anal intraepithelial neoplasia in HIV positive people. Sex Transm Infect 77: 327–331

McCloskey JC, Metcalf C, French MA, Flexman JP, Burke V, Beilin LJ (2007) The frequency of high-grade intraepithelial neoplasia in anal/perianal warts is higher than previously recognized. Int J STD AIDS 18: 538–542

Melbye M, Cote TR, Kessler L, Gail M, Biggar RJ (1994) High incidence of anal cancer among AIDS patients. The AIDS/Cancer Working Group. Lancet 343: 636–639

Nadal SR, Calore EE, Nadal LR, Horta SH, Manzione CR (2007) [Anal cytology for screening of pre-neoplasic lesions]. Rev Assoc Med Bras 53: 147–151

Nyitray A, Nielson CM, Harris RB, Flores R, Abrahamsen M, Dunne EF, Giuliano AR (2008) Prevalence of and risk factors for anal human papillomavirus infection in heterosexual men. J Infect Dis 197: 1676–1684

Orlando G, Fasolo MM, Beretta R, Merli S, Cargnel A (2002) Combined surgery and cidofovir is an effective treatment for genital warts in HIV-infected patients. AIDS 16: 447–450

Palefsky JM, Holly EA, Ralston ML, Jay N (1998b) Prevalence and risk factors for human papillomavirus infection of the anal canal in human immunodeficiency virus (HIV)-positive and HIV-negative homosexual men. J Infect Dis 177: 361–367

Palefsky JM, Holly EA, Ralston ML, Jay N, Berry JM, Darragh TM (1998c) High incidence of anal high-grade squamous intra-epithelial lesions among HIV-positive and HIV-negative homosexual and bisexual men. AIDS 12: 495–503

Palmer JG, Shepherd NA, Jass JR, Crawford LV, Northover JM (1987) Human papillomavirus type 16 DNA in anal squamous cell carcinoma. Lancet 2: 42

Pineda CE, Berry JM, Jay N, Palefsky JM, Welton ML (2008) High-resolution anoscopy targeted surgical destruction of anal high-grade squamous intraepithelial lesions: A ten-year experience. Dis Colon Rectum 51: 829–835; discussion 835–827

Pineda CE, Berry JM, Welton ML (2006) High resolution anoscopy and targeted treatment of high-grade squamous intraepithelial lesions. Dis Colon Rectum 49: 126

Rabkin CS, Biggar RJ, Melbye M, Curtis RE (1992) Second primary cancers following anal and cervical carcinoma: Evidence of shared etiologic factors. Am J Epidemiol 136: 54–58

Ryan DP, Compton CC, Mayer RJ (2000) Carcinoma of the anal canal. N Engl J Med 342: 792–800

Scholefield JH (1999) Anal intraepithelial neoplasia. Br J Surg 86: 1363–1364

Scholefield JH, Castle MT, Watson NF (2005) Malignant transformation of high-grade anal intraepithelial neoplasia. Br J Surg 92: 1133–1136

Scholefield JH, Hickson WG, Smith JH, Rogers K, Sharp F (1992) Anal intraepithelial neoplasia: Part of a multifocal disease process. Lancet 340: 1271–1273

Shepherd NA (2007) Anal intraepithelial neoplasia and other neoplastic precursor lesions of the anal canal and perianal region. Gastroenterol Clin North Am 36: 969–987, ix

Shroyer KR, Brookes CG, Markham NE, Shroyer AL (1995) Detection of human papillomavirus in anorectal squamous cell carcinoma. Correlation with basaloid pattern of differentiation. Am J Clin Pathol 104: 299–305

Sobrado CW, Mester M, Nadalin W, Nahas SC, Bocchini SF, Habr-Gama A (2000) Radiation-induced total regression of a highly recurrent giant perianal condyloma: report of case. Dis Colon Rectum 43: 257–260

Tinmouth J, Lytwyn A (2005) Treatment of high grade anal dysplasia with trichloroacetic acid and infra red coagulation [PosterP033]. In: 22nd International Papillomavirus Conference, Vancouver, Canada

Tsai TF, Kuo GT, Kuo LT, Hsiao CH (2008) Prevalence status and association with human papilloma virus of anal squamous proliferative lesions in a patient sample in Taiwan. Sex Transm Dis 35: 721–724

Wacker J, Hartschuh W (2004) [Differential diagnosis of chronic perianal dermatitis. Premalignant and malignant disorders]. Hautarzt 55: 266–272

Walts AE, Lechago J, Bose S (2006) P16 and Ki67 immunostaining is a useful adjunct in the assessment of biopsies for HPV-associated anal intraepithelial neoplasia. Am J Surg Pathol 30: 795–801

Webber J, Fromm D (2004) Photodynamic therapy for carcinoma in situ of the anus. Arch Surg 139: 259–261

Welton ML, Sharkey FE, Kahlenberg MS (2004) The etiology and epidemiology of anal cancer. Surg Oncol Clin N Am 13: 263–275

Youk EG, Ku JL, Park JG (2001) Detection and typing of human papillomavirus in anal epidermoid carcinomas: Sequence variation in the E7 gene of human papillomavirus Type 16. Dis Colon Rectum 44: 236–242

Human Papillomavirus and Cervical Intraepithelial Neoplasia

8

Alberto Rosenblatt and Homero Gustavo de Campos Guidi

Contents

8.1 Introduction

This chapter reviews gynecological diseases associated with human papillomavirus (HPV) infection, particularly the terminology and grading of premalignant cervical lesions as well as general guidelines for the treatment of these disorders. The aim is to provide updated information that will help urologists and medical practitioners understand the diagnosis (including the different grading systems currently in use) and management of cervical intraepithelial neoplasia in the female partner. A full discussion of gynecological malignancies is beyond the scope of this book, and the interested reader should refer to specific literature.

8.2 Overview

Cervical cancer is the second most common cancer among women worldwide and one of the leading causes of women's death in developing countries (Parkin et al., 2005).

Nevertheless, cervical premalignant conditions (also known as cervical intraepithelial neoplasia (CIN)) evolve slowly and these precancerous lesions can be discovered and treated before progression to invasive cervical carcinoma (ICC) occurs.

Furthermore, in countries where organized cervical cancer surveillance has been implemented with a routine Papanicolaou (Pap) smear screening program, the ICC incidence and mortality have seen a dramatic reduction.

A. Rosenblatt (✉)
Albert Einstein Jewish Hospital, Sao Paulo, Brasil
e-mail: albrose1@gmail.com

A. Rosenblatt, H. G. de Campos Guidi, *Human Papillomavirus*,
DOI: 10.1007/978-3-540-70974-9-8, © Springer-Verlag Berlin Heidelberg 2009

Sexually active young women are more susceptible to HPV infection and the peak age of infection is in the 20- to 24-year-old group. According to Moscicki (2008), abnormal cytology is frequently observed in these young women, but most of these findings are related to the HPV infection and are transient. In addition, clearance of HPV infection is higher in young female individuals.

However, in a small number of adolescents and in older female groups, viral infection tends to persist. There is enough evidence to support the fact that the presence and persistence of high-risk HPV infection are necessary for the development of high-grade squamous intraepithelial lesions (HSILs) and invasive cervical cancer (Wallin et al., 1999; Walboomers et al., 1999; Munoz et al., 2003).

Eventually, only a small percentage of all HPV-associated lesions will ultimately progress to ICC if no intervention occurs.

8.3 Terminology and Grading of Cervical Dysplastic Lesions

Different terminology systems can be used to report a cytology (Pap smear) test (Table 8.1), but it is important to differentiate between:

Table 8.1 Cervical diagnostic terminology. (Source: Safaeian et al. (2007a). Reprinted with permission from Elsevier)

Dysplasia	CIN	Bethesda
Atypia	Atypia	ASCUS (Fig. 8.1)
HPV	HPV	
Mild dysplasia	CIN 1 (Fig. 8.3)	
Moderate dysplasia	CIN 2	LSIL
Severe dysplasia	CIN 3	HSIL (Fig. 8.2)
CIS		

ASCUS atypical squamous cells of undetermined significance; *CIN* cervical intraepithelial neoplasia; *HPV* human papillomavirus; *LSIL* low-grade squamous intraepithelial lesion; *HSIL* high-grade squamous intraepithelial lesion; *CIS* carcinoma in situ

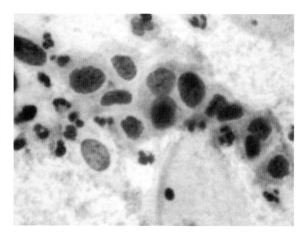

Fig. 8.2. High-grade squamous intraepithelial lesion (HSIL). (Source: Photograph courtesy of Filomena Marino Carvalho MD, PhD, São Paulo, Brazil)

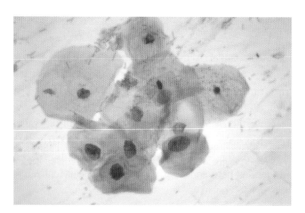

Fig. 8.1. Atypical squamous cells of undetermined significance (ASCUS). (Source: Photograph courtesy of Filomena Marino Carvalho MD, PhD, São Paulo, Brazil)

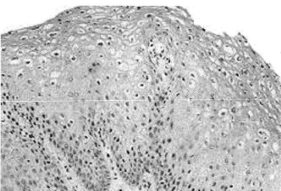

Fig. 8.3. CIN 1. (Source: Photograph courtesy of Filomena Marino Carvalho MD, PhD, São Paulo, Brazil)

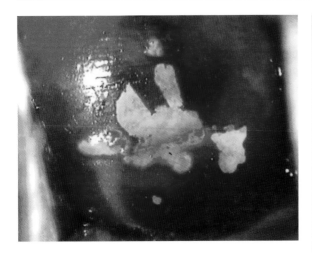

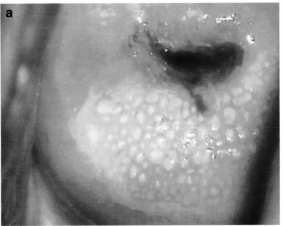

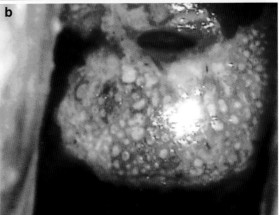

Fig. 8.4. CIN 2 (histology report) after Lugol's solution application. (Source: Photograph courtesy of Nadir Oyakawa, MD, PhD, São Paulo, Brazil)

- Cytologic abnormalities
  - Low-grade intraepithelial squamous lesions (LSILs)
  - High-grade intraepithelial squamous lesions (HSILs)
- Histologic abnormalities (CIN)

The CIN classification is based on morphologic criteria and is widely used in cervical histopathology, but Pap test results are commonly reported using the Bethesda system.

CIN 2 can be regarded as a combination of lesions that may potentially regress or become premalignant (Fig. 8.4)

Carcinoma in situ (CIS) is now encompassed under the same category as severe dysplasia (CIN 3), and histologic CIN 3 (Fig. 8.5a–c) is considered to be the "true cancer precursor."

In the Bethesda system, HPV-related cellular changes are categorized under "squamous intraepithelial lesion."LSIL corresponds to acute HPV infection, irrespective of type, resulting in mild and usually transient cytological abnormalities. HSIL is highly associated with persistent HPV infection, mostly caused by oncogenic types.

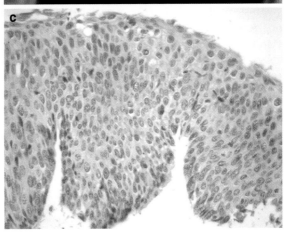

Fig. 8.5. (**a**) CIN 3/CIS (histology report). (**b**) CIN 3/CIS (histology report) after Lugol's solution application (Source: Photograph courtesy of Nadir Oyakawa, MD, PhD, São Paulo, Brazil). (**c**) CIN 3 (Source: Photograph courtesy of Filomena Marino Carvalho MD, PhD, São Paulo, Brazil)

Important

Treatment decisions are based on histology and not on cytology grade.

8.4 Risk Factors for Cervical Cancer Development

- Early age at onset of sexual activity and multiple sexual partners
- High-risk sexual partner
- Multiparity
- History of sexually transmitted diseases (STDs)
- Immunosuppression
- Cigarette smoking

8.5 Natural History of Cervical Dysplastic Lesions

The natural history of CIN is linked to the presence of high-risk HPV and, in a recent meta-analysis performed by Koshiol et al. (2008), HPV persistence was validated as a marker for cervical cancer risk.

Accordingly, the risk of cervical cancer is extremely low in women not infected with oncogenic HPV types.

Only 15% of women with a negative Pap smear and a positive HPV test result will develop abnormal cytology results within 5 years, and HPV infection is required for CIN 3 promotion and maintenance.

Most LSILs are usually associated with HPV infection and have a tendency to regress spontaneously (Moscicki et al., 2004) (Fig. 8.6).

Nobbenhuis et al. (2001) reported that high-risk HPV clearance preceded regression of cervical lesions by an average of 3 months.

Furthermore, Safaeian et al. (2007a) reported that high-grade morphological abnormalities can appear de novo from persistent HPV infection without progressing from low-grade changes.

8.5.1 CIN 2 and 3

CIN 2 is associated with significant spontaneous regression (approximately 40% over 2 years). However:

- High-grade dysplasia (HSIL or grade 2–3 CIN) is likely to progress to ICC, particularly in the group of HIV-positive women where ICC behavior is likely to be more aggressive (Maiman et al., 1997).
- Persistent high-risk HPV infection is necessary for the development of almost all invasive cervical cancers (Fig. 8.7).

8.6 Clinical Manifestations

8.6.1 Symptoms

- Premalignant intraepithelial dysplasia is generally asymptomatic, but local symptoms such as, pruritus, irritation, dyspareunia, and abnormal vaginal discharge may occur.

8.7 Diagnosis

According to Goodman et al. (2008), the risk of acquisition of an incident high-risk anal HPV infection is increased significantly (91% greater risk) in women with cervical HPV infection. Moreover, the incidence of anal intraepithelial neoplasia (AIN) is also high (16-fold increase) in women with multifocal genital intraepithelial neoplasia (Scholefield et al., 1992), and the increased association of AIN, CIN, and vulvar intraepithelial neoplasia (VIN) (Fig. 8.8a–d) is probably related to the shared exposure to high-risk HPV types. Therefore, a thorough investigation of the anogenital region for HPV infection and associated premalignant diseases is recommended by some investigators.

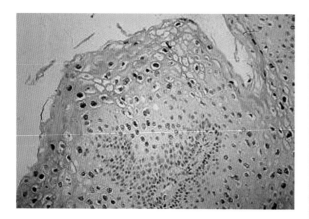

Fig. 8.6. CIN 1 associated with HPV 16/18 detection by in situ hybridization (ISH). (Source: Photograph courtesy of Monica Stiepcich MD, PhD, São Paulo, Brazil)

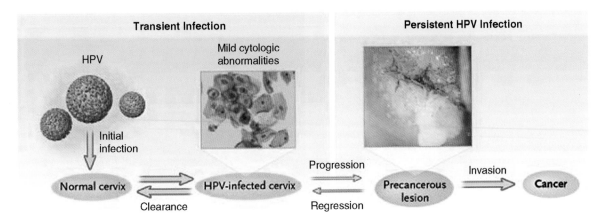

Fig. 8.7. Steps in cervical carcinogenesis (Source: From Wright and Schiffman (2003). Reproduced with permission from Massachusetts Medical Society)

8.7.1 Colposcopy with Acetowhite Test

Colposcopy with acetic acid 5% application (Fig. 8.9) is performed when frank dysplasia (i.e., LSILs in premenopausal women and HSIL in all female subjects) is found on cytology. Colposcopic-directed biopsy of suspicious lesions is done to assess histology.

Women with persistent LSIL or presenting with high-risk HPV infection should undergo multiple colposcopic examinations over time.

> Atrophic changes in postmenopausal women may result in the cytologic diagnosis of LSIL. Therefore, these women can be managed similarly to those with a diagnosis of atypical squamous cells of undetermined significance (ASCUS) (i.e., cytologic evaluation repeated at 6 and 12 months and HPV DNA testing).

8.7.2 Biomarkers

8.7.2.1 HPV DNA Testing

See also Chap. 2.

Molecular HPV testing can now further refine most cytologic findings of ASCUS.

- Negative cytological results associated with positive high-risk HPV DNA test results (the risk of having an undetected CIN 2 or greater is quite low, ranging from 2.4 to 5.1%):

  - Colposcopy is not routinely performed.
  - HPV DNA testing in combination with a Pap test is repeated at 1 year, according to the 2006 consensus guidelines for the management of women with abnormal cervical cancer screening test results (Wright et al., 2007a).

- ASCUS associated with a positive high-risk HPV DNA testing (the risk of developing CIN 3 is 15.2% at 12-month follow-up, according to Safaeian et al. (2007b)):

  - Colposcopy with directed biopsy as needed is recommended.

> LSIL should be managed as ASCUS associated with a positive high-risk HPV DNA test result (studies show that the prevalence of CIN 2 or greater identified at initial colposcopy among women with LSIL is 12–16%).

- ASCUS associated with a negative high-risk HPV DNA test result (low risk of developing CIN 2/3):
  - Cytology is repeated after 1 year or longer depending on age and screening history (Safaeian et al., 2007b).

8

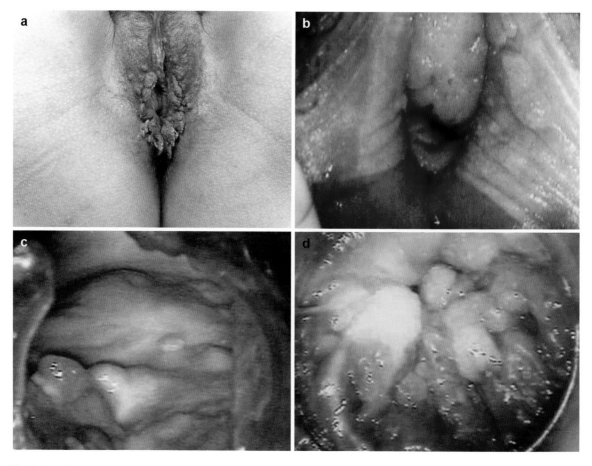

Fig. 8.8. (a) Vulvar and perianal condyloma. **(b)** HPV-associated vulvar intraepithelial neoplasia 1 (VIN 1) (histology). **(c)** Vaginal carcinoma in situ (CIS) (histology) post-hysterectomy. **(d)** High-resolution anoscopy (HRA) showing acetowhitening of the anal mucosa (Source: Photograph courtesy of Nadir Oyakawa, MD, PhD, São Paulo, Brazil)

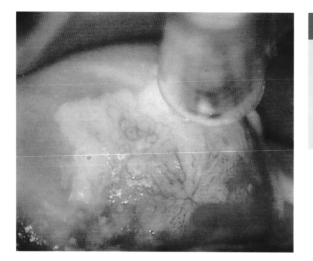

Fig. 8.9. Colposcopic findings after acetic acid 5% application (Source: Photograph courtesy of Maricy Tacla MD, PhD, São Paulo, Brazil)

Expert Advice

HPV DNA testing is not useful in adolescents and *should not be used*. In addition, Spitzer (2007) recommended that colposcopic evaluation in this age-group should be delayed in most cases, and should be performed only if cytological abnormalities persist or are of high grade (HSIL)

8.8 Treatment for HSIL and CIN

8.8.1 High-Grade Squamous Intraepithelial Lesions

Findings of HSIL on cytology carry a high risk of significant cervical disease. Therefore, according to the 2006 consensus guidelines for the management of women with abnormal cervical cancer screening test (Wright et al., 2007a):

- Colposcopy and directed biopsy of visible lesions are recommended, including endocervical assessment in nonpregnant women and thorough vaginal visualization, particularly when a Pap scan-related lesion is not found.

In cases where a lesion consistent with CIN 2 or 3 is found in nonpregnant women who may be at risk to be lost to follow-up, a loop electrosurgical excision procedure (LEEP) (see Sect 8.9.1.1) at the same visit as the colposcopy is recommended. In this "see and treat" modality, cervical biopsy is not performed and an endocervical assessment can be done after the LEEP (Wright et al., 2007b).

However, HSIL in adolescents should be managed with colposcopy and observation for up to 24 months, using both colposcopy and cytology at 6-month intervals. Immediate LEEP (i.e., "see and treat") is not indicated in this age-group.

8.8.2 CIN 1

Surveillance with Pap smear is recommended, particularly in young women as most cases of CIN 1 spontaneously regress without the need for treatment (Wright et al., 2007b). In a recent study, Moscicki (2008) suggested that adolescents should be followed up with yearly cytology indefinitely or until HSIL or CIN 2/3 develops.

Women with CIN 1 preceded by ASCUS, ASC-H, or LSIL should be followed up with Pap tests repeated at 6 and 12 months, or preferably HPV testing at 12 months (Wright et al., 2007b).

Persistent CIN 1 should not be treated before 2 years and a longer surveillance is also preferred in women who are planning a pregnancy.

Pregnant women with a histological diagnosis of CIN 1 should not be treated and surveillance only is the recommended management option.

8.8.3 CIN 2 and 3

Excision or ablation is recommended for nonpregnant women presenting with CIN 2 and 3. However, CIN 2 in adolescents should be managed as CIN 1, since there is a high rate of spontaneous lesion regression and clearance in this group (Wright et al., 2007b). Treatment is recommended for adolescents presenting with CIN 3 or CIN 2/3 that persists for 24 months.

8.9 Treatment Modalities

8.9.1 Excisional Procedures

8.9.1.1 Loop Electrosurgical Excision /Large Loop Excision of the Transformation Zone

LEEP and large loop excision of the transformation zone (LLETZ) are safe and effective treatment options for CIN, with high cure rates reported at 1 year (Spitzer, 2007).

Advantages

- Outpatient procedure under local anesthesia.
- More effective than cryotherapy for CIN 2 and 3 (Kleinberg et al., 2003).
- Efficacy – Kjellberg and Tavelin (2007) reported that LEEP conization is a safe and timesaving "see and treat" modality after an HSIL Pap smear result.

Adverse Effects

Subsequent risk of pregnancy complications

In a recent study that evaluated data from the ASCUS-LSIL Triage Study, Kreimer et al. (2007) reported that HPV types that are likely to persist or reappear after LEEP treatment for CIN 2 or 3 are mostly HPV types in the alpha3 species, which are all noncarcinogenic and therefore unlikely to cause disease.

8.9.1.2 Cold-Knife Conization

Indications

Cold-knife conization is usually performed in cases where a more accurate pathologic interpretation of the specimen is required, such as a suspected microinvasion or adenocarcinoma of the cervix.

Disadvantages

- General/peridural anesthesia required

Adverse Effects

- Risk of hemorrhage
- Subsequent risk of pregnancy complications

8.9.2 Ablative Procedures

> **Expert Advice**
>
> Application of Lugol's solution to the cervix may help define the area to be treated (Fig. 8.10a-d). Because of the lack of glycogen in the dysplastic cells, high-grade cervical lesions do not take up the iodine solution (Lugol's negative). Therefore, HSILs appear yellow-to-tan, whereas normal tissue or LSILs appear dark brown or black.

8.9.2.1 Cryotherapy

A vaginal probe is used and the 3–5–3 freeze technique is usually employed (freeze for 3 min twice, with a 5-min thaw interval between cycles).

Advantages

- Considered the least expensive strategy for CIN 2 and 3 (Kleinberg et al., 2003).
- Office-based procedure.

- Efficacy – In a recent large-series analysis, Luciani et al. (2008) showed that 1 year after cryotherapy 70% of CIN 3 lesions were cured.

Disadvantages

- Considered the least effective strategy for CIN 2 and 3 (Kleinberg et al., 2003)

Adverse Effects

- Colic pain and occasionally a vasovagal reflex during the procedure
- Watery discharge that may last for several weeks after cryotherapy

8.9.2.2 CO_2 Laser or Nd:YAG Laser

Advantages

- Efficacy – In a long follow-up study using Nd:YAG laser conization, Ueda et al. (2006) showed that incomplete CIN excision occurred in 12.3% of cases, although a failure rate (persistence or recurrence) was found in only 1.2% of cases.

Disadvantages

- Laser expertise is needed.
- General/peridural anesthesia is required.
- Hospital-based procedure.

8.10 Post-treatment Follow-Up

Treatment of precancerous lesions of the cervix usually results in clearance of HPV infection. However, the risk of lesion recurrence after the treatment of CIN 2/3 with LEEP is 2–3% when specimen margins are negative and 5–15% when margins are positive. In a recent study, Xi et al. (2007) showed that 10% of women with CIN 3 and baseline infection with HPV 16 who were treated with LEEP developed CIN 2/3 in 2 years.

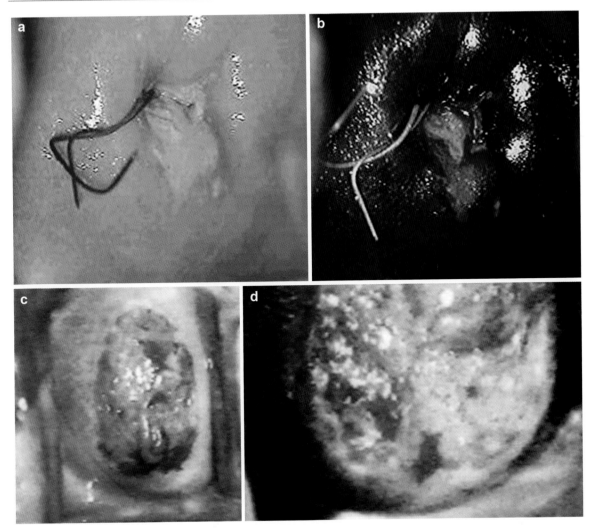

Fig. 8.10. (**a**) Cervical acetowhite lesion. (**b**) Cervical lesion after Lugol's solution application (Source: Photograph courtesy of Maricy Tacla MD, PhD, São Paulo, Brazil). (**c**) CIN 3 (histology report). (**d**) CIN 3 (histology report) after Lugol's solution application (Source: Photograph courtesy of Nadir Oyakawa, MD, PhD, São Paulo, Brazil)

HPV DNA testing can be a helpful diagnostic tool in the follow-up of patients after treatment of precancerous cervical lesions (Aerssens et al., 2008), and Cuzick et al. (2006) recently supported its use as the sole primary screening test.

In addition, Houfflin Debarge et al. (2003) suggested that the frequency of follow-up could be reduced in patients presenting free margins and negative post-treatment HPV test results.

Women should undergo cytology tests at 6 and 12 months after treatment of CIN (Wright et al., 2007b). HPV DNA testing at 6 and 12 months after treatment is also recommended for women with CIN 2 and 3, and colposcopy should be performed on those presenting with high-risk HPV type infection (Wright, 2007b).

UK guidelines recommend annual Pap tests for 9 years and colposcopy in cases of positive cytology. However, based on consistent observations that most recurrences of CIN are in the first 2–3 years after treatment, Kitchener et al. (2008) recommended a shorter follow-up before these women return to routine screening.

8.11 Prevention

Sexual behavior changes such as initiating sexual life at a later age, use of condoms, limiting the number of sexual partners, as well as avoiding high-risk partners

8

are important measures aimed at reducing the risk of HPV infection and other STDs.

Avoidance of cigarette smoking is also recommended, because tobacco is a known cofactor for the development of cervical cancer.

Prophylactic HPV vaccination should be offered to girls before onset of sexual activity; however, the universal vaccination of men and women may become necessary to adequately control HPV infection and related cervical diseases, therefore complementing secondary screening programs (i.e., Pap smears) (see also Chap. 11).

8.12   Screening

The first Pap smear should be performed 3 years from initiation of sexual activity or at age 21 years (whichever comes first), and repeated subsequently at least every 3 years (US Preventive Services Task Force. Screening for cervical cancer: recommendations and rationale).

Women up to the age of 30 years should undergo either annual cytologic screening or biennial screening if a liquid-based Pap test is used, according to the American Cancer Society guidelines (Smith et al., 2002); thereafter, the screening interval may be increased to every 2–3 years based on previous cytology test results and risk factors.

HPV testing or newer Pap test technologies for screening are not currently recommended (US Preventive Services Task Force. Screening for cervical cancer: recommendations and rationale). However, in a recent analysis, Goldhaber-Fiebert et al. (2008) concluded that the use of HPV DNA testing as a triage test for equivocal results in younger vaccinated and unvaccinated women may be more cost-effective than current screening recommendations.

Women older than 65 years should not be routinely screened for cervical cancer if recent Pap smears were normal and are not otherwise at high risk for cervical cancer (i.e., recent unprotected intercourse with new sexual partner).

> Screening must be performed even in vaccinated populations, since HPV infection and related diseases may also occur with other high-risk HPV strains not covered by currently available vaccines.

References

Aerssens A, Claeys P, Garcia A, Sturtewagen Y, Velasquez R, Vanden Broeck D, Vansteelandt S, Temmerman M, Cuvelier CA (2008) Natural history and clearance of HPV after treatment of precancerous cervical lesions. Histopathology 52: 381–386

Cuzick J, Clavel C, Petry KU, Meijer CJ, Hoyer H, Ratnam S, Szarewski A, Birembaut P, Kulasingam S, Sasieni P, Iftner T (2006) Overview of the European and North American studies on HPV testing in primary cervical cancer screening. Int J Cancer 119: 1095–1101

Goldhaber-Fiebert JD, Stout NK, Salomon JA, Kuntz KM, Goldie SJ (2008) Cost-effectiveness of cervical cancer screening with human papillomavirus DNA testing and HPV-16,18 vaccination. J Natl Cancer Inst 100: 308–320

Goodman MT, Shvetsov YB, McDuffie K, Wilkens LR, Zhu X, Ning L, Killeen J, Kamemoto L, Hernandez BY (2008) Acquisition of anal human papillomavirus (HPV) infection in women: The Hawaii HPV Cohort study. J Infect Dis 197: 957–966

Houfflin Debarge V, Collinet P, Vinatier D, Ego A, Dewilde A, Boman F, Leroy JL (2003) Value of human papillomavirus testing after conization by loop electrosurgical excision for high-grade squamous intraepithelial lesions. Gynecol Oncol 90: 587–592

Kitchener HC, Walker PG, Nelson L, Hadwin R, Patnick J, Anthony GB, Sargent A, Wood J, Moore C, Cruickshank ME (2008) HPV testing as an adjunct to cytology in the follow up of women treated for cervical intraepithelial neoplasia. BJOG 115: 1001–1007

Kjellberg L, Tavelin B (2007) 'See and treat' regime by LEEP conisation is a safe and time saving procedure among women with cytological high-grade squamous intraepithelial lesion. Acta Obstet Gynecol Scand 86: 1140–1144

Kleinberg MJ, Straughn JM, Jr., Stringer JS, Partridge EE (2003) A cost-effectiveness analysis of management strategies for cervical intraepithelial neoplasia grades 2 and 3. Am J Obstet Gynecol 188: 1186–1188

Koshiol J, Lindsay L, Pimenta JM, Poole C, Jenkins D, Smith JS (2008) Persistent human papillomavirus infection and cervical neoplasia: A systematic review and meta-analysis. Am J Epidemiol 168: 123–137

Kreimer AR, Katki HA, Schiffman M, Wheeler CM, Castle PE (2007) Viral determinants of human papillomavirus persistence following loop electrical excision procedure treatment for cervical intraepithelial neoplasia grade 2 or 3. Cancer Epidemiol Biomarkers Prev 16: 11–16

Luciani S, Gonzales M, Munoz S, Jeronimo J, Robles S (2008) Effectiveness of cryotherapy treatment for cervical intraepithelial neoplasia. Int J Gynaecol Obstet 101: 172–177

Maiman M, Fruchter RG, Clark M, Arrastia CD, Matthews R, Gates EJ (1997) Cervical cancer as an AIDS-defining illness. Obstet Gynecol 89: 76–80

Moscicki AB (2008) Conservative management of adolescents with abnormal cytology and histology. J Natl Compr Canc Netw 6: 101–106

Moscicki AB, Shiboski S, Hills NK, Powell KJ, Jay N, Hanson EN, Miller S, Canjura-Clayton KL, Farhat S, Broering JM, Darragh TM (2004) Regression of low-grade squamous intraepithelial lesions in young women. Lancet 364: 1678–1683

Munoz N, Bosch FX, de Sanjose S, Herrero R, Castellsague X, Shah KV, Snijders PJ, Meijer CJ (2003) Epidemiologic classification of human papillomavirus types associated with cervical cancer. N Engl J Med 348: 518–527

Nobbenhuis MA, Helmerhorst TJ, van den Brule AJ, Rozendaal L, Voorhorst FJ, Bezemer PD, Verheijen RH, Meijer CJ (2001) Cytological regression and clearance of high-risk human papillomavirus in women with an abnormal cervical smear. Lancet 358: 1782–1783

Parkin DM, Bray F, Ferlay J, Pisani P (2005) Global cancer statistics, 2002. CA Cancer J Clin 55: 74–108

Safaeian M, Solomon D, Castle PE (2007a) Cervical cancer prevention–cervical screening: Science in evolution. Obstet Gynecol Clin North Am 34: 739–760, ix

Safaeian M, Solomon D, Wacholder S, Schiffman M, Castle P (2007b) Risk of precancer and follow-up management strategies for women with human papillomavirus-negative atypical squamous cells of undetermined significance. Obstet Gynecol 109: 1325–1331

Scholefield JH, Hickson WG, Smith JH, Rogers K, Sharp F (1992) Anal intraepithelial neoplasia: Part of a multifocal disease process. Lancet 340: 1271–1273

Smith RA, Cokkinides V, von Eschenbach AC, Levin B, Cohen C, Runowicz CD, Sener S, Saslow D, Eyre HJ (2002) American Cancer Society guidelines for the early detection of cancer. CA Cancer J Clin 52: 8–22

Spitzer M (2007) Screening and management of women and girls with human papillomavirus infection. Gynecol Oncol 107: S14–S18

Ueda M, Ueki K, Kanemura M, Izuma S, Yamaguchi H, Nishiyama K, Tanaka Y, Terai Y, Ueki M (2006) Diagnostic and therapeutic laser conization for cervical intraepithelial neoplasia. Gynecol Oncol 101: 143–146

U.S. Preventive Services Task Force. Screening for cervical cancer: Recommendations and rationale [available at: http://www.ahrq.gov/clinic/3rduspstf/cervcan/cervcanrr.htm] (viewed on 14/09/2008)

U.S. Preventive Services Task Force. Screening for cervical cancer: Recommendations and rationale In: Agency for Healthcare R, and Quality, (ed). U.S. Department of Health and Human Services

Walboomers JM, Jacobs MV, Manos MM, Bosch FX, Kummer JA, Shah KV, Snijders PJ, Peto J, Meijer CJ, Munoz N (1999) Human papillomavirus is a necessary cause of invasive cervical cancer worldwide. J Pathol 189: 12–19

Wallin KL, Wiklund F, Angstrom T, Bergman F, Stendahl U, Wadell G, Hallmans G, Dillner J (1999) Type-specific persistence of human papillomavirus DNA before the development of invasive cervical cancer. N Engl J Med 341: 1633–1638

Wright TC, Jr., Massad LS, Dunton CJ, Spitzer M, Wilkinson EJ, Solomon D (2007a) 2006 consensus guidelines for the management of women with abnormal cervical cancer screening tests. Am J Obstet Gynecol 197: 346–355

Wright TC, Jr., Massad LS, Dunton CJ, Spitzer M, Wilkinson EJ, Solomon D (2007b) 2006 consensus guidelines for the management of women with cervical intraepithelial neoplasia or adenocarcinoma in situ. Am J Obstet Gynecol 197: 340–345

Wright TC, Jr., Schiffman M (2003) Adding a test for human papillomavirus DNA to cervical-cancer screening. N Engl J Med 348: 489–490

Xi LF, Kiviat NB, Wheeler CM, Kreimer A, Ho J, Koutsky LA (2007) Risk of cervical intraepithelial neoplasia grade 2 or 3 after loop electrosurgical excision procedure associated with human papillomavirus type 16 variants. J Infect Dis 195: 1340–1344

Part IV

Human Papillomavirus Infection and Immunosuppression

Human Papillomavirus Infection in HIV-Infected Individuals

9

Alberto Rosenblatt and Homero Gustavo de Campos Guidi

Contents

9.1 Introduction

The body's natural defenses are able to spontaneously clear more than 90% of all human papillomavirus (HPV) infections in healthy, immunocompetent individuals, but in human immunodeficiency virus (HIV)-positive individuals the burden of the HPV infection and related anogenital diseases is higher.

In addition to the indirect effects of HIV-associated immune suppression, HPV has evolved to directly subvert and evade immune responses, allowing the virus to replicate undetected by the host.

Failure of virus clearance with subsequent HPV infection persistence is associated with poor immunological response and an increased risk of HPV-related diseases, including cancer.

This chapter reviews the most recent data related to the effects of HIV infection and immune suppression on HPV infection, with particular emphasis on anogenital neoplasia. It briefly discusses the HPV

A. Rosenblatt (✉)
Albert Einstein Jewish Hospital, Sao Paulo, Brasil
e-mail: albrose1@gmail.com

A. Rosenblatt, H. G. de Campos Guidi, *Human Papillomavirus*,
DOI: 10.1007/978-3-540-70974-9-9, © Springer-Verlag Berlin Heidelberg 2009

infectious cycle and its immune evasion methods, and it also addresses anogenital screening, treatment considerations, and surveillance (anal intraepithelial neoplasia (AIN) is detailed in Chap. 7).

The chapter ends with a short update on HPV vaccines in HIV-infected individuals, although a complete discussion of HPV vaccines can be found in Chap. 11.

9.2   Overview

9.2.1   HPV-HIV Coinfection in Women

The seroprevalence of oncogenic HPV type 16 among HIV-positive women has been estimated at approximately 50%, according to a recent study that evaluated immunoglobulin G response to HPV 16 capsids (Viscidi et al., 2003a).

HPV DNA of multiple and concurrent HPV types is more prevalent in cervicovaginal specimens of HIV-positive women than in noninfected subjects (Sun et al., 1995; Kreiss et al., 1992), and infection with multiple HPV types has been associated with cervical carcinogenesis.

The prevalence of squamous intraepithelial lesions (SILs) among HIV-infected women ranges between 12 and 76% (Clark et al., 1993; Massad et al., 1999; Parham et al., 2006), and Trottier et al. (2006) reported that coinfection with oncogenic HPV types 16 and 58 increased the risk of developing SIL.

HPV infection, particularly with high-risk HPV 16 and 18, is associated with the majority of vulvar and vaginal cancers (Hampl et al., 2006). Furthermore, the risk of developing anogenital neoplasias is increased in HIV-positive women (Fig. 9.1a, b) compared to HIV-negative subjects (Frisch et al., 2000; Jamieson et al., 2006).

9.2.2   HPV-HIV Coinfection in Men

HPV infection is common in HIV-infected male subjects and, in a large study performed by Palefsky et al. (1998c), HPV infection was found in 95% of HIV-positive men who have sex with men (MSM). Moreover, according to a recent report (CDR, 2006), the number of cases of anogenital warts occurring in MSM in the United Kingdom increased by 76% between 1996 and 2005.

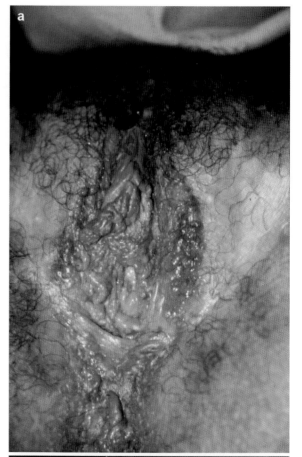

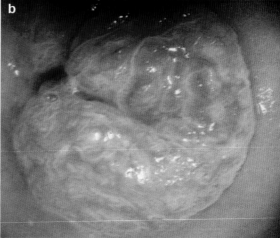

Fig. 9.1. (**a**) Vulvar Bowen's disease in an HIV-positive woman. (**b**) Invasive cervical cancer (Source: Photograph courtesy of Nadir Oyakawa, MD, PhD, São Paulo, Brazil)

HPV DNA has been detected at different anatomic locations in 50% of HIV-positive men, with a high prevalence of simultaneous HPV infection at different

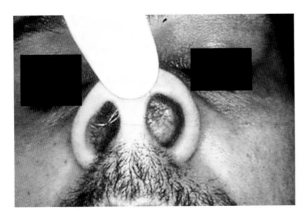

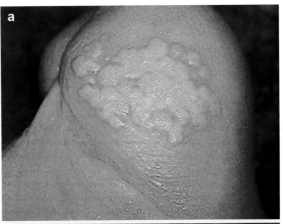

Fig. 9.2. HPV-related lesion in the left nasal cavity of an HIV-positive patient with anal intraepithelial neoplasia (Source: Photograph courtesy of Carlos Walter Sobrado Jr., MD, PhD, São Paulo, Brazil)

sites (penis, mouth, and anus) (Fig. 9.2) in the same individual (Sirera et al., 2006).

According to a recent analysis performed by Hagensee et al. (2004), HPV DNA detection in HIV-infected subjects was highest in the anal and perianal regions.

In a retrospective study evaluating carbon dioxide (CO_2) laser treatment efficacy for HPV-associated anogenital lesions in immunocompetent and immunosuppressed patients (HIV-infected and therapeutically immunosuppressed), Aynaud et al. (2008) found that anogenital intraepithelial lesions were significantly more common in HIV-positive patients (47.4%) than in immunocompetent individuals (20.2%). The dysplastic lesions exhibited a higher grade in 25% of cases and also covered a larger surface area (see also Chaps. 5 and 7).

The risk of anal neoplasia in HIV-positive men is reported to be two to six times higher than in HIV-negative subjects (Ryan et al., 2000; Goedert et al., 1998), and the reported prevalence of the putative anal cancer precursor high-grade squamous intraepithelial lesion (HSIL) is 52% in HIV-positive MSM (Palefsky et al., 2005) and 5% in immunosuppressed patients (Ogunbiyi et al., 1994).

The prevalence of penile (Fig. 9.3a, b) and oral HPV infection in HIV-infected men is 36 and 30%, respectively. Moreover, Heideman et al. (2007) recently reported that HPV 16 was the main type etiologically involved in the development of penile squamous cell carcinoma (SCC). Incidentally, the reported frequency of penile cancers in HIV-positive men is two to three times higher than the occurrence rate in their noninfected counterparts.

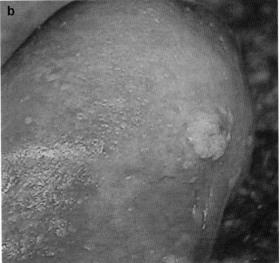

Fig. 9.3. (**a**) Glans lesions in an HIV-positive patient; virology HPV 18. (**b**) Glans papular lesion in an HIV-positive patient; virology HPV 16

HPV infection in immunocompromised individuals may also affect atypical sites (Fig. 9.2) (Handisurya et al., 2007), with a high prevalence of oncogenic types (Kojic and Cu-Uvin, 2007).

9.3   HPV Infectious Cycle

See also Chap. 11.

HPV infects basal keratinocytes and the viral life cycle follows the differentiation stages of the host epithelial cell. Expression of early gene products (E1, E2, E5, E6, and E7) is activated in the basal and suprabasal layers of the epithelium. However, late gene expression of

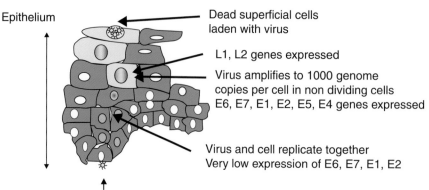

Replication cycle of genital hr HPV

Fig. 9.4. Replication cycle of high-risk (*hr*) HVP (see also text for further explanation) (Source: Stanley, 2006. Reproduced with permission from Elsevier)

high levels of capsid viral proteins (L1 and L2), the expression of protein responsible for HPV DNA replication and encapsidation (E4), along with final viral assembly will only occur in the upper layers of the squamous epithelia (Sterling et al., 1993; Stanley, 1994; Middleton et al., 2003). As virus-laden superficial cells desquamate, HPVs are released into the environment (Fig. 9.4).

9.4   Effects of Host Immune Status on the Risk of HPV Infection

The cell-mediated immunity is the main component involved in clearing HPV infections. However, Shrestha et al. (2007) recently evaluated the effects of interleukin-10 (IL-10) gene polymorphisms on the clearance of high-risk HPV infection in a cohort of HIV-infected young female subjects. The results of this study support the hypothesis that HPV clearance may be under host genetic influence.

In immunocompetent individuals, DNA from oncogenic HPV types is no longer observed (i.e., clearance of infection) after 8–14 months, and low-risk types are usually cleared in 5–6 months (Giuliano et al., 2002; Brown et al., 2005; Franco et al., 1999).

However, observing the long interval between HPV infection and lesion manifestation, it appears that efficient virus immune evasion methods seem to delay or prevent the host immune response mechanism from clearing or controlling the infection, resulting in a chronic and persistent viral presence.

Long-lasting infection with high-risk HPV types may increase the risk of progression to high-grade SILs and invasive carcinoma (Remmink et al., 1995; Liaw et al., 1999).

9.5   Host Immune Evasion Methods of HPV

The exclusively intraepithelial viral infectious cycle is itself an efficient immune evasion mechanism, exposing minimal amounts of replicating virus particles in a noninflammatory milieu to the host immune surveillance cells.

Viral gene expression is confined to cells with squamous maturation potential, and the mature infectious virus is released with the differentiating keratinocyte, a cell already programmed to die and desquamate.

As the virus is not involved in the cell death, the host immune system becomes unaware of the infection and, as a result, there is little or no release of proinflammatory cytokines that are important for squamous epithelial immune responses (Kupper and Fuhlbrigge, 2004).

In addition, oncogenic HPV types encode proteins (E6 and E7) that inhibit p53 and Rb1, important tumor suppression proteins (Munger et al., 1989; Heck et al., 1992; Werness et al., 1990).

HPV E6 and E7 proteins also downregulate interferon (IFN)-a gene expression (Chang and Laimins, 2000; Nees et al., 2001) and directly interact with IFN signaling pathways (Barnard and McMillan, 1999),

Fig. 9.5. Schematic representation of HPV-associated lesions and malignant transformation (see also text)

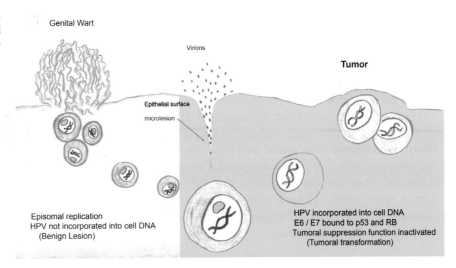

inhibiting an important antiviral defense system. According to Stern (2005), these oncoproteins are implicated in the mechanisms that promote viral persistence and cancer progression (Fig. 9.5).

> In addition to its potent antiviral features, type-1 IFNs (INF-a and INF-b) display immunostimulatory, antiproliferative, and antiangiogenic properties.

Studies have shown that high-risk HPV 16 may more efficiently evade host immune surveillance than other HPV types; consequently, progression to high-grade intraepithelial lesions and invasive carcinoma is likely if a cell-mediated immune response is not generated during persistent HPV 16 infection.

9.6   HPV Infection in Immunosuppressed Individuals

HPV infection flourishes, persists, and recurs in HIV-positive patients as their local immune responses are usually unpredictable.

van Benthem et al. (2000) reported that HIV-infected women have a significantly increased risk for HPV infection occurrence. In addition, HIV-infected individuals usually harbor multiple HPV types and additional ones can be detected over time, particularly among those with lower CD4+ levels. They are more prone to long-lasting infection or latent HPV infection reactivation rather than acquisition of new infection through recent sexual contact, presumably as a result of immunosuppression

(Breese et al., 1995; van der Snoek et al., 2003; Strickler et al., 2005; Palefsky and Holly, 2003).

> Silverberg et al. (2006) recently demonstrated that measurement of serial HPV 16 serum antibodies is a useful diagnostic tool for identifying HPV 16 replication.

> According to these investigators, rising antibody levels among HIV-positive female patients may reflect reactivation of a latent HPV infection, whereas among their HIV-negative counterparts, it may result from HPV reinfection.

HIV-positive female patients have a greater tendency to develop cervical SILs than HIV-negative individuals.

A high quantitative HPV load has been associated with both histological severity and lesion size, and the potential use of HPV load measurement as a risk marker for cervical disease was lately suggested by Lillo and Uberti-Foppa (2006).

Furthermore, female subjects with high HIV viral load are at increased risk of developing cervical HPV infection with oncogenic types and cervical dysplasias (Massad et al., 1999).

Minkoff et al. (2008) found an increased risk of detection of both prevalent and incident high-risk HPV types and an increased risk of SIL in HIV-positive cocaine users, which may be related to the potential immunosuppressive effect of the drug on HIV-infected patients. However, recent data by Syrjanen (2008) showed that drug abuse itself is not a risk factor for high-risk HPV infection, but rather it seems to be associated with risky sexual behavior.

HIV-infected male patients have an increased incidence of anal HPV infection with oncogenic risk types (Critchlow et al., 1998), although infection with multiple HPV genotypes is very common.

In a histological assessment of anogenital HPV infection in HIV-infected male patients, Aynaud et al. (1998) demonstrated that penile exophytic lesions were associated with low-grade intraepithelial neoplasia and high-grade dysplastic lesions in 36% and 22% of cases, respectively. The same study suggested that development of high-risk HPV-associated lesions is facilitated by immune suppression.

Recent analysis evaluating the effectiveness of using urine samples as a noninvasive alternative for HPV testing showed that molecular biological methods that detect HPV DNA in urine can be reliably used for screening genital HPV infection in both HIV-infected men and women (Smits et al., 2005; Jong et al., 2008).

9.7   Relationship Between Declining CD4+ Levels, HPV Infection, and Anogenital Cancers

HPV anogenital infections have been associated with a declining CD4 cell count (Clark et al., 1993), and Fennema et al. (1995) reported that the risk for recurrent genital warts was strongly associated with decreased $CD4^+$ levels.

In a recent study in Africa, Yamada et al. (2008) showed that cervical HPV infection was present in 49% of HIV-positive women compared to 17% of HIV-negative counterparts. Moreover, the investigators found that high-risk HPV infection and low $CD4^+$ T cell counts are risk factors for cervical cancer.

However, data suggest that lower $CD4^+$ levels (i.e., immunosuppression) may play a more important role in the earlier stages of HPV-related disease (up to and including high-grade cervical intraepithelial neoplasia (CIN) and AIN), rather than in the progression from high-grade anogenital lesions to invasive disease (Palefsky and Holly, 2003).

A recent study performed by Strickler et al. (2003) evaluated HPV DNA detection in cervicovaginal lavage specimens of HIV-infected patients with cervical cancer.

The results showed that HPV 16 detection levels were not greatly affected by diminished CD4+ T cells. This could suggest that HPV 16 may evade host immune surveillance more efficiently than other HPV types, contributing to its strong association with cervical neoplasia

A low CD4 cell count is a known risk factor for anal high-grade SIL (HSIL) development (Palefsky et al., 1998c), but Fagan et al. (2005) reported that the incidence of anal cancer in HIV-positive individuals is not related to low $CD4^+$ levels or HIV viral load. This finding suggests that host genetic changes may play a more influential role in the progression from high-grade AIN to invasive neoplasia (Gagne et al., 2005).

9.8   Relationship between HIV/HPV Coinfection and CIN/Cervical Cancer

See also Chap. 8.

A better understanding of the contribution of HIV to the increased risk of HPV infection and CIN is still required. However, diminished HPV-specific immune responses resulting from HIV infection may allow for viral and high-grade CIN persistence with the subsequent accumulation of genetic changes that are influential in lesion progression to invasive disease.

Invasive cervical carcinoma (ICC) became an acquired immunodeficiency syndrome (AIDS)-defining illness in the early 1990s, and it is likely the most common AIDS-related malignancy among HIV-positive women in countries with a high HPV prevalence (Maiman et al., 1997). Fortunately, the incidence and associated mortality rate of ICC is low in places with adequate cervical cytological screening.

However, Massad et al. (1999) reported that the prevalence and incidence of CIN was increased among HIV-positive individuals, with abnormal cervical cytological results found in 38% of HIV-positive women compared with 16% of the HIV-negative subjects.

9.8.1   Natural History of CIN in the HIV-Infected Patient

In the HIV-infected group, SILs have been shown to be more aggressive, multifocal, and extensive (Fruchter et al., 1996).

Table 9.1 Known risk factors for cervical intraepithelial neoplasia among HIV-infected women

• Decreased CD4 cell count
• High human immunodeficiency viral load (HIVL)
• Human papillomavirus (HPV) infection

Furthermore, Maiman et al. (1997) demonstrated that high-grade dysplasia (HSIL or grade 2–3 CIN) is likely to progress to ICC, particularly in HIV-positive women where ICC behavior is more aggressive.

Risk factors for CIN among HIV-positive women are listed in Table 9.1.

However, Lehtovirta et al. (2008) recently demonstrated that the risk of developing CIN was not associated with decreased levels of CD4 lymphocytes, HIV infection duration, antiretroviral treatment, or plasma HIVL (high human immunodeficiency viral load). According to these investigators, HIV-positive women have a higher risk of CIN in association with bacterial vaginosis (BV), whereas parity lowered the risk.

9.8.2 Cervical Disease Screening for HIV-Infected Women

A Pap smear should be performed at the time of diagnosis of HIV infection, and repeated in 6 months if results are normal.

Women with a previous history of normal cytological findings and at least two normal Pap smears can then undergo an annual screening.

The Pap smear should be repeated in 3 months if inflammation or atypia is demonstrated.

Colposcopic examination is recommended when Pap smear results exhibit persistent atypia, SIL, or HPV findings.

9.8.3 Treatment Considerations for Anogenital Warts and CIN in HIV-Infected Women

See also Chap. 8.

HIV-positive female patients with cervical SIL (regardless of grade) require more aggressive therapy than HIV-negative subjects.

Excisional procedures are recommended by Nappi et al. (2005), and sometimes multiple treatment modalities are needed. However, recurrence rates after treatment are high in this group of patients.

9.9 Relationship Between HIV/HPV Coinfection and AIN/Anal Cancer

See also Chap. 7.

AIN is considered a precursor lesion of anal SCC, and the progression of AIN lesions to anal neoplasia in immunosuppressed individuals was recently demonstrated by Scholefield et al. (2005).

There is an increased incidence of anal HPV infection in HIV-infected male patients (Kreuter et al., 2005) and high-risk types are commonly detected (Critchlow et al., 1998).

In a study evaluating prevalence of AIN lesions in HIV-positive and -negative homosexual and bisexual men, Palefsky et al. (1998b) showed that the incidence rate of AIN in HIV-positive homosexual men was 52%, compared to 17% in HIV-negative individuals. Furthermore, HIV-positive men have a higher risk of anal neoplasia than HIV-negative subjects (Ryan et al., 2000; Goedert et al., 1998).

Pineda et al. recently reviewed 246 patients (among those 182 HIV-positive and 12 immunocompromised) with both HSIL and LSIL, who were managed with high-resolution anoscopy (HRA)-targeted surgical destruction. Recurrences were documented in 57% of the 200 patients treated in a single-stage procedure, and the authors reported that lesion recurrence correlated with extent of disease but not with HIV status (Pineda et al., 2008).

> Fagan et al. (2005) showed that HIV disease duration was the most significant factor for the development of invasive anal carcinoma in HIV-infected individuals with HPV.

9.9.1 Natural History of AIN in the HIV-Infected Patient

The natural history of AIN is poorly understood, being the subject of current active investigation.

Low-grade AIN (AIN 1 and 2) lesions may regress in up to 30% of cases (Scholefield et al., 1992; Scholefield et al., 1994), but Palefsky et al. (1998a) reported progression of LSIL to HSIL in more than 50% of HIV-positive homosexual men during a 2-year follow-up. The same authors showed that high-grade lesions rarely regress in these patients.

Immunosuppressed patients seem to have multifocal disease and show an increased rate of progression to invasive anal carcinoma (Scholefield et al., 2005; Watson et al., 2006).

9.9.2 Anal Disease Screening for HIV-Infected Individuals

HIV-positive MSM should have a Pap smear annually and patients with cytological results exhibiting atypical squamous cells of undetermined significance (ASCUS), high-grade change (ASC-H), LSIL, and HSIL should be referred to HRA and biopsy.

Cranston et al. (2007) recently reported that abnormal anal cytology was highly predicative of anal dysplasia on biopsy specimens.

In addition to the increased risk of developing AIN and anal cancer, the risk of penile cancer is also moderately increased in HIV-positive MSM. However, data concerning the precursor lesion penile intraepithelial neoplasia (PIN) in this group of patients are limited. Kreuter et al. (2008) studied a large group of HIV-positive MSM patients and detected PIN in 4.2% and AIN in 59.3% of these patients. Furthermore, nearly all patients diagnosed with PIN had a concurrent AIN lesion, and all PIN lesions showed immunohistochemical staining for p16(INK4a) that correlated both with the histological grade and with high-risk HPV DNA load. These findings suggest that HIV-positive MSM should be screened for both PIN and AIN.

9.9.3 Treatment Considerations for Anogenital Warts and AIN in HIV-Infected Individuals

See also Chap. 7.

9.9.3.1 Imiquimod 5%

Although topical 5% imiquimod is not licensed for use in the anal canal, Herrera et al. (2007) recently demonstrated that it is safe and effective for the treatment of HPV-related anogenital lesions in HIV-infected patients.

9.9.3.2 Cidofovir 1% Gel

Cidofovir 1% gel has been found more effective than surgery for HPV-related anogenital lesions in HIV-positive patients (Orlando et al., 2002).

9.9.3.3 Infrared Coagulation

Cranston et al. (2008) reported efficacy rates of 64% for biopsy-proven HSIL in HIV-positive MSM. Goldstone et al. (2007) using HRA and targeted surgical destruction with infrared coagulation (IRC) in the office reported cure rates of 72% for individual lesions in HIV-positive MSM.

9.9.3.4 Excisional Surgery and Electrocautery

Mapping of the lesions with punch biopsies associated with intraoperative frozen section analysis and wide local excision of involved areas is a nontargeted therapy that is associated with high recurrence rates and increased morbidity (Margenthaler et al., 2004; Brown et al., 1999).

However, targeted procedures using HRA to identify HSIL are safer and can be performed in the operating room using needle-tip electrocautery to destroy the lesions (Pineda et al., 2008). In their recent 10-year retrospective analysis of 246 patients (among them, 79% HIV-positive or immunocompromised), Pineda et al. showed that HRA and targeted surgical destruction of anal HSIL offer excellent disease-free status and less progression to invasive anal disease than expectant management (see below, *Observation ("Watch and Wait" Approach)*).

9.9.3.5 CO_2 Laser

CO_2 laser treatment can be an effective choice, even in cases of repeated laser sessions if lesions recur or persist. Aynaud et al. (2008) evaluated remission and relapse rates in immunocompetent and immunosuppressed individuals with condyloma and high-grade intraepithelial neoplasms (IENs 3) treated with CO_2 laser. The study showed clinical absence of lesions in 81.2% of cases at 1 month, irrespective of immune status. IEN 3 lesions in remission at 1 month maintained the remission status at 6 months. There was recurrence in 12.6% of cases and persistence in 6.6% of cases. The investigators reported that lesion persistence was more frequently observed in HIV-positive patients, while recurrences were found mainly in immunocompetent and therapeutically immunosuppressed patients.

9.9.3.6 Observation ("Watch and Wait" Approach)

HIV-infected patients presenting with extensive and multifocal anal squamous dysplasia can be followed up with physical examination surveillance only, since morbidity and recurrences are high using any of the current treatment modalities.

Patients should be instructed for self-referral if new anal symptoms or worsening of presenting symptoms develop, and close follow-up is recommended with HRA and repeated biopsies for new or suspicious lesions (Chin-Hong and Palefsky, 2002; Devaraj and Cosman, 2006).

Further studies regarding AIN treatment for HIV-positive individuals are required.

> **Expert Advice**
>
> Visible lesions of the anal and perianal region in HIV-infected individuals should be carefully evaluated, including with pathological studies, because of the increased occurrence of low- and high-grade anal disease in this group of patients (Sanclemente et al., 2007).

9.10 HAART in HPV-Associated Neoplasias

Treatment of HIV has evolved from monotherapy to a combination of three or more antiretroviral drugs (HAART or highly active antiretroviral therapy).

More than 20 single anti-HIV drugs have been approved by the U.S. Food and Drug Administration and new drugs are under active development or are already in clinical trials (FDA Approved Drugs and Investigational Drugs, AIDSinfo).

The introduction of current HAART regimens has contributed to the many advances seen in the management of HIV-infected patients. HAART has decreased the incidence of opportunistic infections, resulting in fewer hospital admissions and fewer HIV-related deaths (Murphy et al., 2001; Vandamme et al., 1998).

9.11 HAART in HPV-Associated Cervical Disease

There are conflicting results in the literature regarding the impact of HAART on the persistence of both HPV infection and cervical abnormalities (Heard et al., 1998; Lillo et al., 2001).

Luque et al. (2001) reported a diminished detection of HPV DNA in cervical specimens of HIV-infected women on antiretroviral therapy compared to subjects without antiretroviral treatment.

In the long follow-up study performed by Soncini et al. (2007), HAART significantly reduced the risk of developing CIN, while Minkoff et al. (2001) reported that women on HAART were less likely to have cervical disease progression.

Sirera et al. (2008), in a recent retrospective analysis, showed that when CD4 cell count was high, the incidence of cervical SIL in HIV-positive women treated with HAART was similar to infected women not on HAART. In addition, Moore et al. (2002) reported that higher CD4$^+$ levels at or following the initiation of HAART appeared to have a positive effect on CIN regression.

> HIV-positive women, whether or not on HAART, should continue to be actively screened and treated for CIN (Heard et al., 2006).

9.12 HAART in HPV-Associated Anal Disease

According to Palefsky et al. (2005), the detection of high-grade AIN has not been reduced since HAART introduction.

Hoffman et al. (1999) showed that CD4 count levels previous to anal cancer treatment may determine the response of HIV-positive patients to chemoradiation and their ability to tolerate potential therapy-related toxicity. Furthermore, HIV-infected patients with CD4 counts of more than 200 cells/ml should usually be treated with combined chemoradiation, similarly to non-HIV-infected individuals (Berry et al., 2004).

HIV-positive patients with anal cancer on HAART demonstrated an improved ability to sustain cancer treatment using full chemoradiation and an improved local tumor control (Cleator et al., 2000; Place et al., 2001).

In summary, studies failed to demonstrate a clear relationship between HPV-associated anal and cervical neoplasia and diminished immunity as measured by low $CD4^+$ T cell levels. Therapy with highly active antiretroviral drugs is not effective for anal and cervical neoplasia in HIV-positive individuals, and the incidence of these cancers has not changed since HAART introduction (Chiao et al., 2005; Bower et al., 2006).

9.13 HAART in HPV-Associated Oral Disease

An increase in oral HPV infection has been reported in white HIV-infected men on HAART (72%) as compared with those not on HAART (29%) (Cameron et al., 2005).

9.14 Surveillance

HIV and HPV coinfected individuals require a close surveillance in order to detect early squamous cell cancer transformation and progression in the penis, anus, cervix, vagina, vulva, and mouth.

Current data available reinforce a policy of continued screening and aggressive treatment of CIN in HIV-infected women, and assessment of $CD4^+$ levels and HPV DNA testing may be useful risk indicators (Nappi et al., 2005).

Surveillance of AIN in HIV patients is best achieved by HRA with multiple targeted biopsies every 4–6 months, as long as dysplasia persists (Chang and Welton, 2003; Chin-Hong et al., 2005) (see also Chap. 7).

Further studies of anal cytology screening methods are required.

9.15 Considerations Regarding HPV Prophylactic and Therapeutic Vaccines in HIV-Infected Individuals

9.15.1 Prophylactic Vaccines

Newly developed HPV prophylactic vaccines will likely influence HPV-related diseases in immunocompetent individuals, including the prevention of cervical lesions caused by the high-risk HPV types 16 and 18 (see Chap. 11).

However, the influence that prophylactic vaccines will have in immunosuppressed individuals is still unknown.

Natural immunity against HPV involves a strong localized cell-mediated response and the subsequent generation of serum-neutralizing antibodies (Stanley, 2006).

Viscidi et al. (2003b) recently evaluated serum immunoglobulin A (IgA) response to HPV 16 capsids in a large group of HIV-positive and high-risk HIV-negative women. IgA seropositivity was higher in HIV-positive female subjects and was associated with progression of high-grade cytological abnormalities, suggesting that IgA response to HPV 16 may be a marker of viral persistence.

HPV prophylactic vaccine induces the production of neutralizing antibodies. Thus, since the immune response in HIV-infected individuals with well-preserved CD4 count levels is still effective, HPV vaccines could also benefit this particular group of individuals. In addition, it has been demonstrated that HIV-positive women are able to generate HPV antibodies (particularly against oncogenic HPV 16) even with a low $CD4^+$ level (Strickler et al., 2003).

In a recent study, Goncalves et al. (2008) reported that infection with HPV 18 was commonly found in both the anal and genital region of HIV-positive women, suggesting that current HPV vaccines may prevent anal HPV infection in immunocompromised individuals.

Limited information is now available about the safety and immune response of the quadrivalent HPV vaccine in young male subjects (Block et al., 2006; Reisinger et al., 2007). In addition, a recent study showed that the quadrivalent HPV vaccine was 100% effective in preventing AIN, PIN and penile cancer in young immunocompetent male individuals (Giuliano and Palefsky, 2008) (see also Sect. 11.8 in Chap. 11).

Further clinical studies in both immunocompetent and immunosuppressed subjects are required.

9.15.2 Therapeutic Vaccines

Therapeutic vaccines directed against HPV-infected cells are likely to improve local immune responses, resulting in potential regression of associated anogenital dysplastic lesions.

Therapeutic vaccines could particularly benefit HIV-infected individuals, because of the increased risk of HPV infection occurrence in these patients and the associated high rates of recurrence found after the treatment of anal squamous intraepithelial lesions (ASILs).

There are no commercially available licensed vaccines intended for therapeutic use against ASILs, but clinical studies are being performed on HIV-positive and HIV-negative high-risk subjects.

Two vaccines have been evaluated and only data from phase-I/II clinical trials for ASILs are available (Berry and Palefsky, 2003).

A phase-I safety study of SGN-00101 (HspE7), designed to treat high-grade AIN in HIV-positive individuals, showed regression of HSIL in about one-third of participants (Palefsky et al., 2006) and clearance of HPV infection in 60% of patients in whom anal lesions regressed.

Therapeutic vaccination may be useful at the early stages of cervical and anal disease, but further evidence for clinical efficacy is still needed.

References

Aynaud O, Buffet M, Roman P, Plantier F, Dupin N (2008) Study of persistence and recurrence rates in 106 patients with con-dyloma and intraepithelial neoplasia after CO_2 laser treatment. Eur J Dermatol 18: 153–158

Aynaud O, Piron D, Barrasso R, Poveda JD (1998) Comparison of clinical, histological, and virological symptoms of HPV in HIV-1 infected men and immunocompetent subjects. Sex Transm Infect 74: 32–34

Barnard P, McMillan NA (1999) The human papillomavirus E7 oncoprotein abrogates signaling mediated by interferon-alpha. Virology 259: 305–313

Berry JM, Palefsky JM (2003) A review of human papillomavirus vaccines: From basic science to clinical trials. Front Biosci 8: s333–s345

Berry JM, Palefsky JM, Welton ML (2004) Anal cancer and its precursors in HIV-positive patients: Perspectives and management. Surg Oncol Clin N Am 13: 355–373

Block SL, Nolan T, Sattler C, Barr E, Giacoletti KE, Marchant CD, Castellsague X, Rusche SA, Lukac S, Bryan JT, Cavanaugh PF, Jr., Reisinger KS (2006) Comparison of the immunogenicity and reactogenicity of a prophylactic quadrivalent human papillomavirus (types 6, 11, 16, and 18) L1 virus-like particle vaccine in male and female adolescents and young adult women. Pediatrics 118: 2135–2145

Bower M, Palmieri C, Dhillon T (2006) AIDS-related malignancies: Changing epidemiology and the impact of highly active antiretroviral therapy. Curr Opin Infect Dis 19: 14–19

Breese PL, Judson FN, Penley KA, Douglas JM, Jr. (1995) Anal human papillomavirus infection among homosexual and bisexual men: Prevalence of type-specific infection and association with human immunodeficiency virus. Sex Transm Dis 22: 7–14

Brown DR, Shew ML, Qadadri B, Neptune N, Vargas M, Tu W, Juliar BE, Breen TE, Fortenberry JD (2005) A longitudinal study of genital human papillomavirus infection in a cohort of closely followed adolescent women. J Infect Dis 191: 182–192

Brown SR, Skinner P, Tidy J, Smith JH, Sharp F, Hosie KB (1999) Outcome after surgical resection for high-grade anal intraepithelial neoplasia (Bowen's disease). Br J Surg 86: 1063–1066

Cameron JE, Mercante D, O'Brien M, Gaffga AM, Leigh JE, Fidel PL, Jr., Hagensee ME (2005) The impact of highly active antiretroviral therapy and immunodeficiency on human papillomavirus infection of the oral cavity of human immunodeficiency virus-seropositive adults. Sex Transm Dis 32: 703–709

CDR W (2006) Trends in anogenital warts and anogenital herpes simplex virus infection in the United Kingdom: 1996 to 2005. In: Communicable Disease Report Weekly (CDR Weekly), vol 16. Health Protection Agency

Chang GJ, Welton ML (2003) Anal neoplasia. Sem Colon Rectal Surg 14: 111–118

Chang YE, Laimins LA (2000) Microarray analysis identifies interferon-inducible genes and Stat-1 as major transcriptional targets of human papillomavirus type 31. J Virol 74: 4174–4182

Chiao EY, Krown SE, Stier EA, Schrag D (2005) A population-based analysis of temporal trends in the incidence of squamous anal canal cancer in relation to the HIV epidemic. J Acquir Immune Defic Syndr 40: 451–455

Chin-Hong PV, Palefsky JM (2002) Natural history and clinical management of anal human papillomavirus disease in men and women infected with human immunodeficiency virus. Clin Infect Dis 35: 1127–1134

Chin-Hong PV, Vittinghoff E, Cranston RD, Browne L, Buchbinder S, Colfax G, Da Costa M, Darragh T, Benet DJ, Judson F, Koblin B, Mayer KH, Palefsky JM (2005) Age-related prevalence of anal cancer precursors in homosexual men: The EXPLORE study. J Natl Cancer Inst 97: 896–905

Clark RA, Brandon W, Dumestre J, Pindaro C (1993) Clinical manifestations of infection with the human immunodeficiency virus in women in Louisiana. Clin Infect Dis 17: 165–172

Cleator S, Fife K, Nelson M, Gazzard B, Phillips R, Bower M (2000) Treatment of HIV-associated invasive anal cancer with combined chemoradiation. Eur J Cancer 36: 754–758

Cranston RD, Hart SD, Gornbein JA, Hirschowitz SL, Cortina G, Moe AA (2007) The prevalence, and predictive value, of abnormal anal cytology to diagnose anal dysplasia in a population of HIV-positive men who have sex with men. Int J STD AIDS 18: 77–80

Cranston RD, Hirschowitz SL, Cortina G, Moe AA (2008) A retrospective clinical study of the treatment of high-grade anal dysplasia by infrared coagulation in a population of HIV-positive men who have sex with men. Int J STD AIDS 19: 118–120

Critchlow CW, Hawes SE, Kuypers JM, Goldbaum GM, Holmes KK, Surawicz CM, Kiviat NB (1998) Effect of HIV infection on the natural history of anal human papillomavirus infection. AIDS 12: 1177–1184

Devaraj B, Cosman BC (2006) Expectant management of anal squamous dysplasia in patients with HIV. Dis Colon Rectum 49: 36–40

Fagan SP, Bellows CF, 3rd, Albo D, Rodriquez-Barradas M, Feanny M, Awad SS, Berger DH (2005) Length of human immunodeficiency virus disease and not immune status is a risk factor for development of anal carcinoma. Am J Surg 190: 732–735

Fennema JS, van Ameijden EJ, Coutinho RA, van den Hoek AA (1995) HIV, sexually transmitted diseases and gynaecologic disorders in women: Increased risk for genital herpes and warts among HIV-infected prostitutes in Amsterdam. AIDS 9: 1071–1078

Franco EL, Villa LL, Sobrinho JP, Prado JM, Rousseau MC, Desy M, Rohan TE (1999) Epidemiology of acquisition and clearance of cervical human papillomavirus infection in women from a high-risk area for cervical cancer. J Infect Dis 180: 1415–1423

Frisch M, Biggar RJ, Goedert JJ (2000) Human papillomavirus-associated cancers in patients with human immunodeficiency virus infection and acquired immunodeficiency syndrome. J Natl Cancer Inst 92: 1500–1510

Fruchter RG, Maiman M, Sedlis A, Bartley L, Camilien L, Arrastia CD (1996) Multiple recurrences of cervical intraepithelial neoplasia in women with the human immunodeficiency virus. Obstet Gynecol 87: 338–344

Gagne SE, Jensen R, Polvi A, Da Costa M, Ginzinger D, Efird JT, Holly EA, Darragh T, Palefsky JM (2005) High-resolution analysis of genomic alterations and human papillomavirus integration in anal intraepithelial neoplasia. J Acquir Immune Defic Syndr 40: 182–189

Giuliano AR, Papenfuss M, Abrahamsen M, Inserra P (2002) Differences in factors associated with oncogenic and nonon-cogenic human papillomavirus infection at the United States-Mexico border. Cancer Epidemiol Biomarkers Prev 11: 930–934

Goedert JJ, Cote TR, Virgo P, Scoppa SM, Kingma DW, Gail MH, Jaffe ES, Biggar RJ (1998) Spectrum of AIDS-associated malignant disorders. Lancet 351: 1833–1839

Goldstone SE, Hundert JS, Huyett JW (2007) Infrared coagulator ablation of high-grade anal squamous intraepithelial lesions in HIV-negative males who have sex with males. Dis Colon Rectum 50: 565–575

Goncalves MA, Randi G, Arslan A, Villa LL, Burattini MN, Franceschi S, Donadi EA, Massad E (2008) HPV type infection in different anogenital sites among HIV-positive Brazilian women. Infect Agent Cancer 3: 5

Giuliano A, Palefsky J (2008) The efficacy of quadrivalent HPV (types 6/11/16/18) vaccine in reducing the incidence of HPV infection and HPV-related genital disease in young men In: European Research Organization on Genital Infection and Neoplasia – EUROGIN Nice , France

Hagensee ME, Cameron JE, Leigh JE, Clark RA (2004) Human papillomavirus infection and disease in HIV-infected individuals. Am J Med Sci 328: 57–63

Hampl M, Sarajuuri H, Wentzensen N, Bender HG, Kueppers V (2006) Effect of human papillomavirus vaccines on vulvar, vaginal, and anal intraepithelial lesions and vulvar cancer. Obstet Gynecol 108: 1361–1368

Handisurya A, Rieger A, Bankier A, Koller A, Salat A, Stingl G, Kirnbauer R (2007) Human papillomavirus type 26 infection causing multiple invasive squamous cell carcinomas of the fingernails in an AIDS patient under highly active antiretroviral therapy. Br J Dermatol 157: 788–794

Heard I, Potard V, Costagliola D (2006) Limited impact of immunosuppression and HAART on the incidence of cervical squamous intraepithelial lesions in HIV-positive women. Antivir Ther 11: 1091–1096

Heard I, Schmitz V, Costagliola D, Orth G, Kazatchkine MD (1998) Early regression of cervical lesions in HIV-seropositive women receiving highly active antiretroviral therapy. AIDS 12: 1459–1464

Heck DV, Yee CL, Howley PM, Munger K (1992) Efficiency of binding the retinoblastoma protein correlates with the transforming capacity of the E7 oncoproteins of the human papillomaviruses. Proc Natl Acad Sci U S A 89: 4442–4446

Heideman DA, Waterboer T, Pawlita M, Delis-van Diemen P, Nindl I, Leijte JA, Bonfrer JM, Horenblas S, Meijer CJ, Snijders PJ (2007) Human papillomavirus-16 is the predominant type etiologically involved in penile squamous cell carcinoma. J Clin Oncol 25: 4550–4556

Herrera S, Correa LA, Wolff JC, Gaviria A, Tyring SK, Sanclemente G (2007) Effect of imiquimod in anogenital warts from HIV-positive men. J Clin Virol 39: 210–214

Hoffman R, Welton ML, Klencke B, Weinberg V, Krieg R (1999) The significance of pretreatment CD4 count on the outcome and treatment tolerance of HIV-positive patients with anal cancer. Int J Radiat Oncol Biol Phys 44: 127–131

Jamieson DJ, Paramsothy P, Cu-Uvin S, Duerr A, Group HIVERS (2006) Vulvar, vaginal, and perianal intraepithelial neoplasia in women with or at risk for human immunodeficiency virus. Obstet Gynecol 107: 1023–1028

Jong E, Mulder JW, van Gorp EC, Wagenaar JK, Derksen J, Westerga J, Tol A, Smits PH (2008) The prevalence of human papillomavirus (HPV) infection in paired urine and cervical smear samples of HIV-infected women. J Clin Virol 41: 111–115

Kojic EM, Cu-Uvin S (2007) Update: Human papillomavirus infection remains highly prevalent and persistent among HIV-infected individuals. Curr Opin Oncol 19: 464–469

Kreiss JK, Kiviat NB, Plummer FA, Roberts PL, Waiyaki P, Ngugi E, Holmes KK (1992) Human immunodeficiency virus, human papillomavirus, and cervical intraepithelial neoplasia in Nairobi prostitutes. Sex Transm Dis 19: 54–59

Kreuter A, Brockmeyer NH, Hochdorfer B, Weissenborn SJ, Stucker M, Swoboda J, Altmeyer P, Pfister H, Wieland U (2005) Clinical spectrum and virologic characteristics of anal intraepithelial neoplasia in HIV infection. J Am Acad Dermatol 52: 603–608

Kreuter A, Brockmeyer NH, Weissenborn SJ, Gambichler T, Stucker M, Altmeyer P, Pfister H, Wieland U (2008) Penile intraepithelial neoplasia is frequent in HIV-positive men with anal dysplasia. J Invest Dermatol 128: 2316–2324

Kupper TS, Fuhlbrigge RC (2004) Immune surveillance in the skin: Mechanisms and clinical consequences. Nat Rev Immunol 4: 211–222

Lehtovirta P, Paavonen J, Heikinheimo O (2008) Risk factors, diagnosis and prognosis of cervical intraepithelial neoplasia among HIV-infected women. Int J STD AIDS 19: 37–41

Liaw KL, Glass AG, Manos MM, Greer CE, Scott DR, Sherman M, Burk RD, Kurman RJ, Wacholder S, Rush BB, Cadell DM, Lawler P, Tabor D, Schiffman M (1999) Detection of human papillomavirus DNA in cytologically normal women and subsequent cervical squamous intraepithelial lesions. J Natl Cancer Inst 91: 954–960

Lillo FB, Ferrari D, Veglia F, Origoni M, Grasso MA, Lodini S, Mastrorilli E, Taccagni G, Lazzarin A, Uberti-Foppa C (2001) Human papillomavirus infection and associated cervical disease in human immunodeficiency virus-infected women: Effect of highly active antiretroviral therapy. J Infect Dis 184: 547–551

Lillo FB, Uberti-Foppa C (2006) Human papillomavirus viral load: A possible marker for cervical disease in HIV-infected women. J Antimicrob Chemother 57: 810–814

Luque AE, Li H, Demeter LM, Reichman RC (2001) Effect of highly active antiretroviral therapy (HAART) on human papillomavirus (HPV) infection and disease among HIV-infected women. In: 8th Conference on retroviruses and opportunistic infections, Chicago

Maiman M, Fruchter RG, Clark M, Arrastia CD, Matthews R, Gates EJ (1997) Cervical cancer as an AIDS-defining illness. Obstet Gynecol 89: 76–80

Margenthaler JA, Dietz DW, Mutch MG, Birnbaum EH, Kodner IJ, Fleshman JW (2004) Outcomes, risk of other malignancies, and need for formal mapping procedures in patients with perianal Bowen's disease. Dis Colon Rectum 47: 1655–1660; discussion 1660–1651

Massad LS, Riester KA, Anastos KM, Fruchter RG, Palefsky JM, Burk RD, Burns D, Greenblatt RM, Muderspach LI, Miotti P (1999) Prevalence and predictors of squamous cell abnormalities in Papanicolaou smears from women infected with HIV-1. Women's Interagency HIV Study Group. J Acquir Immune Defic Syndr 21: 33–41

Middleton K, Peh W, Southern S, Griffin H, Sotlar K, Nakahara T, El-Sherif A, Morris L, Seth R, Hibma M, Jenkins D,

Lambert P, Coleman N, Doorbar J (2003) Organization of human papillomavirus productive cycle during neoplastic progression provides a basis for selection of diagnostic markers. J Virol 77: 10186–10201

Minkoff H, Ahdieh L, Massad LS, Anastos K, Watts DH, Melnick S, Muderspach L, Burk R, Palefsky J (2001) The effect of highly active antiretroviral therapy on cervical cytologic changes associated with oncogenic HPV among HIV-infected women. AIDS 15: 2157–2164

Minkoff H, Zhong Y, Strickler HD, Watts DH, Palefsky JM, Levine AM, D'Souza G, Howard AA, Plankey M, Massad LS, Burk R (2008) The relationship between cocaine use and human papillomavirus infections in HIV-seropositive and HIV-seronegative women. Infect Dis Obstet Gynecol 2008: 587082

Moore AL, Sabin CA, Madge S, Mocroft A, Reid W, Johnson MA (2002) Highly active antiretroviral therapy and cervical intraepithelial neoplasia. AIDS 16: 927–929

Munger K, Werness BA, Dyson N, Phelps WC, Harlow E, Howley PM (1989) Complex formation of human papillomavirus E7 proteins with the retinoblastoma tumor suppressor gene product. EMBO J 8: 4099–4105

Murphy EL, Collier AC, Kalish LA, Assmann SF, Para MF, Flanigan TP, Kumar PN, Mintz L, Wallach FR, Nemo GJ (2001) Highly active antiretroviral therapy decreases mortality and morbidity in patients with advanced HIV disease. Ann Intern Med 135: 17–26

Nappi L, Carriero C, Bettocchi S, Herrero J, Vimercati A, Putignano G (2005) Cervical squamous intraepithelial lesions of low-grade in HIV-infected women: recurrence, persistence, and progression, in treated and untreated women. Eur J Obstet Gynecol Reprod Biol 121: 226–232

Nees M, Geoghegan JM, Hyman T, Frank S, Miller L, Woodworth CD (2001) Papillomavirus type 16 oncogenes downregulate expression of interferon-responsive genes and upregulate proliferation-associated and NF-kappaB-responsive genes in cervical keratinocytes. J Virol 75: 4283–4296

Ogunbiyi OA, Scholefield JH, Raftery AT, Smith JH, Duffy S, Sharp F, Rogers K (1994) Prevalence of anal human papillomavirus infection and intraepithelial neoplasia in renal allograft recipients. Br J Surg 81: 365–367

Orlando G, Fasolo MM, Beretta R, Merli S, Cargnel A (2002) Combined surgery and cidofovir is an effective treatment for genital warts in HIV-infected patients. AIDS 16: 447–450

Palefsky JM, Berry JM, Jay N, Krogstad M, Da Costa M, Darragh TM, Lee JY (2006) A trial of SGN-00101 (HspE7) to treat high-grade anal intraepithelial neoplasia in HIV-positive individuals. AIDS 20: 1151–1155

Palefsky JM, Holly EA (2003) Chapter 6: Immunosuppression and co-infection with HIV. J Natl Cancer Inst Monogr: 41–46

Palefsky JM, Holly EA, Efirdc JT, Da Costa M, Jay N, Berry JM, Darragh TM (2005) Anal intraepithelial neoplasia in the highly active antiretroviral therapy era among HIV-positive men who have sex with men. AIDS 19: 1407–1414

Palefsky JM, Holly EA, Hogeboom CJ, Ralston ML, DaCosta MM, Botts R, Berry JM, Jay N, Darragh TM (1998a) Virologic, immunologic, and clinical parameters in the incidence and progression of anal squamous intraepithelial lesions in HIV-positive and HIV-negative homosexual men. J Acquir Immune Defic Syndr Hum Retrovirol 17: 314–319

Palefsky JM, Holly EA, Ralston ML, Arthur SP, Jay N, Berry JM, DaCosta MM, Botts R, Darragh TM (1998b) Anal squamous intraepithelial lesions in HIV-positive and HIV-negative homosexual and bisexual men: prevalence and risk factors. J Acquir Immune Defic Syndr Hum Retrovirol 17: 320–326

Palefsky JM, Holly EA, Ralston ML, Jay N (1998c) Prevalence and risk factors for human papillomavirus infection of the anal canal in human immunodeficiency virus (HIV)-positive and HIV-negative homosexual men. J Infect Dis 177: 361–367

Parham GP, Sahasrabuddhe VV, Mwanahamuntu MH, Shepherd BE, Hicks ML, Stringer EM, Vermund SH (2006) Prevalence and predictors of squamous intraepithelial lesions of the cervix in HIV-infected women in Lusaka, Zambia. Gynecol Oncol 103: 1017–1022

Pineda CE, Berry JM, Jay N, Palefsky JM, Welton ML (2008) High-resolution anoscopy targeted surgical destruction of anal high-grade squamous intraepithelial lesions: a ten-year experience. Dis Colon Rectum 51: 829–835; discussion 835–827

Place RJ, Gregorcyk SG, Huber PJ, Simmang CL (2001) Outcome analysis of HIV-positive patients with anal squamous cell carcinoma. Dis Colon Rectum 44: 506–512

Reisinger KS, Block SL, Lazcano-Ponce E, Samakoses R, Esser MT, Erick J, Puchalski D, Giacoletti KE, Sings HL, Lukac S, Alvarez FB, Barr E (2007) Safety and persistent immunogenicity of a quadrivalent human papillomavirus types 6, 11, 16, 18 L1 virus-like particle vaccine in preadolescents and adolescents: A randomized controlled trial. Pediatr Infect Dis J 26: 201–209

Remmink AJ, Walboomers JM, Helmerhorst TJ, Voorhorst FJ, Rozendaal L, Risse EK, Meijer CJ, Kenemans P (1995) The presence of persistent high-risk HPV genotypes in dysplastic cervical lesions is associated with progressive disease: Natural history up to 36 months. Int J Cancer 61: 306–311

Ryan DP, Compton CC, Mayer RJ (2000) Carcinoma of the anal canal. N Engl J Med 342: 792–800

Sanclemente G, Herrera S, Tyring SK, Rady PL, Zuleta JJ, Correa LA, He Q, Wolff JC (2007) Human papillomavirus (HPV) viral load and HPV type in the clinical outcome of HIV-positive patients treated with imiquimod for anogenital warts and anal intraepithelial neoplasia. J Eur Acad Dermatol Venereol 21: 1054–1060

Scholefield JH, Castle MT, Watson NF (2005) Malignant transformation of high-grade anal intraepithelial neoplasia. Br J Surg 92: 1133–1136

Scholefield JH, Hickson WG, Smith JH, Rogers K, Sharp F (1992) Anal intraepithelial neoplasia: Part of a multifocal disease process. Lancet 340: 1271–1273

Scholefield JH, Ogunbiyi OA, Smith JH, Rogers K, Sharp F (1994) Treatment of anal intraepithelial neoplasia. Br J Surg 81: 1238–1240

Shrestha S, Wang C, Aissani B, Wilson CM, Tang J, Kaslow RA (2007) Interleukin-10 gene (IL10) polymorphisms and human papillomavirus clearance among immunosuppressed adolescents. Cancer Epidemiol Biomarkers Prev 16: 1626–1632

Silverberg MJ, Schneider MF, Silver B, Anastos KM, Burk RD, Minkoff H, Palefsky J, Levine AM, Viscidi RP (2006) Serological detection of human papillomavirus type 16 infection in human immunodeficiency virus (HIV)-positive

and high-risk HIV-negative women. Clin Vaccine Immunol 13: 511–519

Sirera G, Videla S, Lopez-Blazquez R, Llatjos M, Tarrats A, Castella E, Grane N, Tural C, Rey-Joly C, Clotet B (2008) Highly active antiretroviral therapy and incidence of cervical squamous intraepithelial lesions among HIV-infected women with normal cytology and CD4 counts above 350 cells/mm3. J Antimicrob Chemother 61: 191–194

Sirera G, Videla S, Pinol M, Canadas MP, Llatjos M, Ballesteros AL, Garcia-Cuyas F, Castella E, Guerola R, Tural C, Rey-Joly C, Clotet B (2006) High prevalence of human papillomavirus infection in the anus, penis and mouth in HIV-positive men. AIDS 20: 1201–1204

Smits PH, Bakker R, Jong E, Mulder JW, Meenhorst PL, Kleter B, van Doorn LJ, Quint WG (2005) High prevalence of human papillomavirus infections in urine samples from human immunodeficiency virus-infected men. J Clin Microbiol 43: 5936–5939

Soncini E, Zoncada A, Condemi V, Antoni AD, Bocchialini E, Soregotti P (2007) Reduction of the risk of cervical intraepithelial neoplasia in HIV-infected women treated with highly active antiretroviral therapy. Acta Biomed 78: 36–40

Stanley M (2006) Immune responses to human papillomavirus. Vaccine 24 Suppl 1: S16–22

Stanley MA (1994) Replication of human papillomaviruses in cell culture. Antiviral Res 24: 1–15

Sterling JC, Skepper JN, Stanley MA (1993) Immunoelectron microscopical localization of human papillomavirus type 16 L1 and E4 proteins in cervical keratinocytes cultured in vivo. J Invest Dermatol 100: 154–158

Stern PL (2005) Immune control of human papillomavirus (HPV) associated anogenital disease and potential for vaccination. J Clin Virol 32 Suppl 1: S72–S81

Strickler HD, Burk RD, Fazzari M, Anastos K, Minkoff H, Massad LS, Hall C, Bacon M, Levine AM, Watts DH, Silverberg MJ, Xue X, Schlecht NF, Melnick S, Palefsky JM (2005) Natural history and possible reactivation of human papillomavirus in human immunodeficiency virus-positive women. J Natl Cancer Inst 97: 577–586

Strickler HD, Palefsky JM, Shah KV, Anastos K, Klein RS, Minkoff H, Duerr A, Massad LS, Celentano DD, Hall C, Fazzari M, Cu-Uvin S, Bacon M, Schuman P, Levine AM, Durante AJ, Gange S, Melnick S, Burk RD (2003) Human papillomavirus type 16 and immune status in human immunodeficiency virus-seropositive women. J Natl Cancer Inst 95: 1062–1071

Sun XW, Ellerbrock TV, Lungu O, Chiasson MA, Bush TJ, Wright TC, Jr. (1995) Human papillomavirus infection in human immunodeficiency virus-seropositive women. Obstet Gynecol 85: 680–686

Syrjanen K (2008) New concepts on risk factors of HPV and novel screening strategies for cervical cancer precursors. Eur J Gynaecol Oncol 29: 205–221

Trottier H, Mahmud S, Costa MC, Sobrinho JP, Duarte-Franco E, Rohan TE, Ferenczy A, Villa LL, Franco EL (2006) Human papillomavirus infections with multiple types and risk of cervical neoplasia. Cancer Epidemiol Biomarkers Prev 15: 1274–1280

van Benthem BH, Prins M, Larsen C, Delmas MC, Brunet JB, van den Hoek A (2000) Sexually transmitted infections in European HIV-infected women: incidence in relation to time from infection. European Study on the Natural History of HIV Infection in Women. AIDS 14: 595–603

van der Snoek EM, Niesters HG, Mulder PG, van Doornum GJ, Osterhaus AD, van der Meijden WI (2003) Human papillomavirus infection in men who have sex with men participating in a Dutch gay-cohort study. Sex Transm Dis 30: 639–644

Vandamme AM, Van Vaerenbergh K, De Clercq E (1998) Anti-human immunodeficiency virus drug combination strategies. Antivir Chem Chemother 9: 187–203

Viscidi RP, Ahdieh-Grant L, Clayman B, Fox K, Massad LS, Cu-Uvin S, Shah KV, Anastos KM, Squires KE, Duerr A, Jamieson DJ, Burk RD, Klein RS, Minkoff H, Palefsky J, Strickler H, Schuman P, Piessens E, Miotti P (2003a) Serum immunoglobulin G response to human papillomavirus type 16 virus-like particles in human immunodeficiency virus (HIV)-positive and risk-matched HIV-negative women. J Infect Dis 187: 194–205

Viscidi RP, Ahdieh-Grant L, Schneider MF, Clayman B, Massad LS, Anastos KM, Burk RD, Minkoff H, Palefsky J, Levine A, Strickler H (2003b) Serum immunoglobulin A response to human papillomavirus type 16 virus-like particles in human immunodeficiency virus (HIV)-positive and high-risk HIV-negative women. J Infect Dis 188: 1834–1844

Watson AJ, Smith BB, Whitehead MR, Sykes PH, Frizelle FA (2006) Malignant progression of anal intra-epithelial neoplasia. ANZ J Surg 76: 715–717

Werness BA, Levine AJ, Howley PM (1990) Association of human papillomavirus types 16 and 18 E6 proteins with p53. Science 248: 76–79

Yamada R, Sasagawa T, Kirumbi LW, Kingoro A, Karanja DK, Kiptoo M, Nakitare GW, Ichimura H, Inoue M (2008) Human papillomavirus infection and cervical abnormalities in Nairobi, Kenya, an area with a high prevalence of human immunodeficiency virus infection. J Med Virol 80: 847–855

Human Papillomavirus and CO$_2$ Laser Treatment

10

Alberto Rosenblatt and Homero Gustavo de Campos Guidi

Contents

10.1 Introduction

The acronym LASER stands for "light amplification by the stimulated emission of radiation" and it was coined by the American physicist Gordon Gould, considered by some as the "inventor of the laser."

Medical lasers deliver the exact amount of energy to the target tissue, thus sparing contiguous structures, a principle called selective photothermolysis.

A. Rosenblatt (✉)
Albert Einstein Jewish Hospital, Sao Paulo, Brasil
e-mail: albrose1@gmail.com

Lasers containing carbon dioxide (CO$_2$) gas are called CO$_2$ lasers (Fig. 10.1a–c). These devices emit an invisible infrared light at a wavelength of 10,600 nm, which is absorbed by intracellular and extracellular water, the main constituent of human tissue. Heat is then produced, which results in tissue vaporization and coagulative necrosis of superficial epidermal layers.

This chapter briefly reviews CO$_2$ lasers, with particular focus on the use of CO$_2$ lasers in the treatment of HPV-related genital lesions.

10.2 Historic Background

In the treatise *On the Quantum Mechanics of Radiation*, published in 1917 by Albert Einstein (Einstein, 1917), the fundamentals of light emission by an atom were initially proposed. The basic principles of the laser were described in "Infrared and Optical Masers," published in 1958 by the American physicists Arthur L. Schalow and Charles H. Townes (Schalow and Townes, 1958). The first MASER (microwave amplification through the stimulated emission of radiation, as the laser was called then) instrument was developed in 1959, and in the following year the first operational laser using ruby as an active medium was devised by American physicist Theodore Maiman (Maiman, 1960) at the Hughes Research Laboratories. Polanyi (1961) wrote about the possibility of using molecular vibrations for laser action in 1961, and Patel (1964) described the laser action on the vibrational-rotational

A. Rosenblatt, H. G. de Campos Guidi, *Human Papillomavirus*,
DOI: 10.1007/978-3-540-70974-9-10, © Springer-Verlag Berlin Heidelberg 2009

10

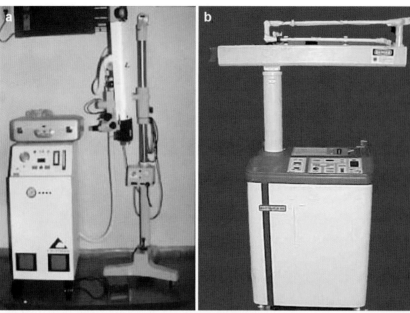

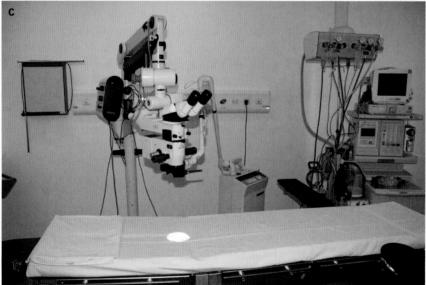

Fig. 10.1. (**a**) Cavitron (CO_2 laser) used in 1980 (**b**) CO_2 laser used in 1990 (**c**) CO_2 laser and microscope used in 2008

transitions of CO_2 in an electrical discharge in 1964. High power and efficiency have been attained with the addition of nitrogen (N_2) by Patel (1965) and helium (He) by Moeller and Rigden (1965).

10.3　CO_2 Laser Components

Laser medium: CO_2 gas

Optical cavity (also called resonator): The optical cavity is where the laser medium is enclosed and the amplification process takes place.

Pump (power supply): In the pump the atoms are excited, creating a population inversion (i.e., all the atoms are directly and continuously excited from the ground state to the excited state).

Delivery system: Typically, delivery is through an articulating arm containing mirrored joints (Fig. 10.2) to efficiently transmit the laser light through an output device, such as a handpiece (Fig. 10.3), colposcope (Fig. 10.4), or operating microscope (Fig. 10.5a, b). However, waveguide or fiberoptic cables may be used by some devices.

When using the laser connected to the operating microscope or colposcope, a joystick micromanipulator is

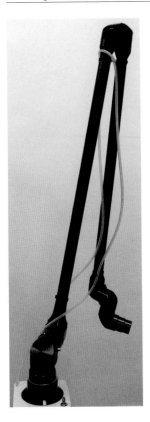

Fig. 10.2. Laser articulating arm

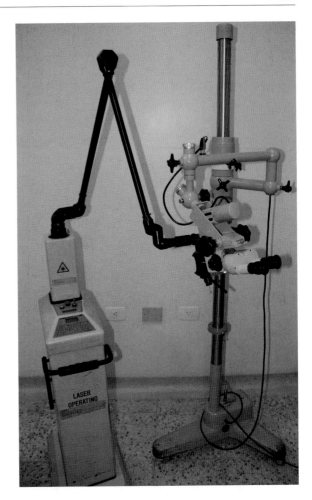

Fig. 10.4. CO$_2$ laser connected to colposcope

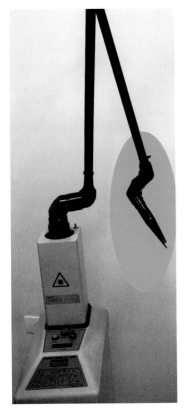

Fig. 10.3. Laser handpiece

operated to change the laser beam position (Fig. 10.6a, b). Each movement of the joystick is translated into the inclination of a movable mirror (Fig. 10.7). The surgeon then shifts the point irradiated with the laser beam by moving the joystick back and forth or right and left while observing the operative field through a microscope.

10.4 CO$_2$ Laser Beam

The laser beam in focus mode can be used like a scalpel to cut the tissue. Laser light is absorbed by blood, thus deep penetration of the laser beam with subsequent tissue damage is avoided.

Expert Advice

A dry operative field is required for effective CO$_2$ laser action.

10

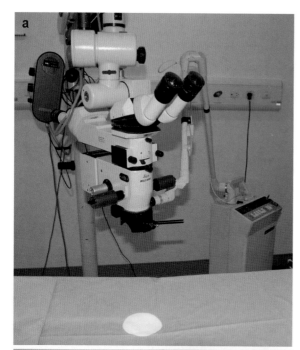

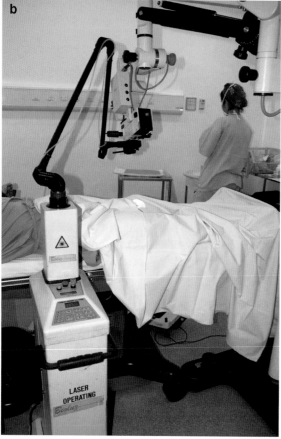

Fig. 10.5. (**a**) CO_2 laser connected to surgical microscope (**b**) Laser and operating microscope

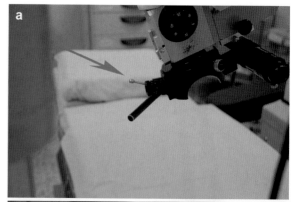

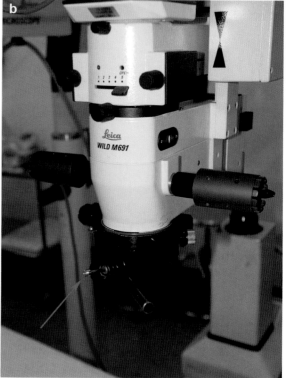

Fig. 10.6. (**a**) Joystick assembled into colposcope (*arrow*). (**b**) Joystick assembled into microscope (*arrow*)

Bleeding vessels can be coagulated by applying the laser beam in defocused mode or by directing the beam to the periphery of the lesion, causing the tissue (and the vessel within) to retract.

10.4.1 Laser Safety

Appropriate laser training is required to avoid risks to patients and operating room personnel, including the laser operator.

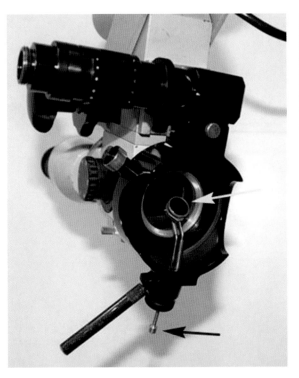

Fig. 10.7. Joystick (*black arrow*) and movable mirror (*white arrow*)

10.4.1.1   Eye Protection

Direct or reflected light from CO_2 lasers may damage the cornea, therefore special optically coated glasses and goggles should be used by the patient and operating room personnel. Adequate signage identifying laser usage should be displayed on the operating room doors, and these should be kept closed while the CO_2 laser is being used.

10.4.1.2   Laser Plume

Ferenczy and coworkers (1990) were the first to detect clinically active HPV particles within the plume of smoke that emanated from laser equipment, and Hallmo and Naess (1991) reported the occurrence of HPV-related laryngeal papillomatosis contracted by a laser surgeon. Therefore, the inadvertent inhalation of viral particles while performing laser surgery for HPV places the surgeon and other members of the operating team and room staff at risk of developing respiratory tract papillomatosis (Fig. 10.8). A laser-specific plume/smoke evacuator adapted with a filter (Fig. 10.9a, b) should be used and positioned close to the operative

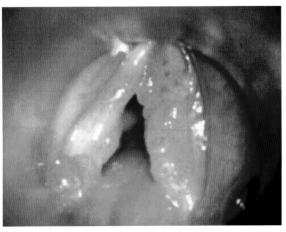

Fig. 10.8. Bilateral vocal cord papillomas (Source: Photograph courtesy of Reinaldo J. Gusmão, MD, PhD, São Paulo, Brazil)

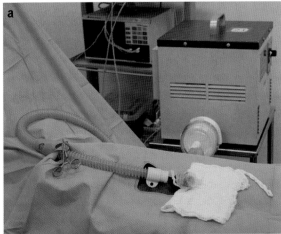

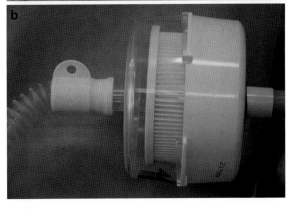

Fig. 10.9. (a) Laser plume/smoke evacuator with hose positioned close to the operative site. (b) Laser filter

site. In addition, maintaining appropriate room ventilation and wearing special mask protection should reduce inhalation risks.

10.5 CO_2 Laser Indications

- Extensive and exophytic lesions
- Multifocal recurring lesions
- Lesions unresponsive to other medical and/or surgical therapies
- Urethral lesions (see Chap. 4)
- Penile intraepithelial neoplasia (PIN) lesions (see Chap. 5)
- Perianal lesions associated with genital lesions

10.6 Personal Laser Technique

The CO_2 laser should preferably be connected to the operating microscope or colposcope (Fig. 10.10), because enhanced magnification is important in order to detect microscopic lesions. Lesions are then quickly and precisely vaporized under microscopic guidance using the laser joystick micromanipulator (Fig. 10.11).

However, the laser handpiece can also be used to treat extensive and multiple lesions (Fig. 10.12). The greater mobility of the device allows for the swift excision of exophytic lesions close to the base, which are then completely vaporized.

10.6.1 Preoperative Care

The topical anesthetic cream EMLA (eutectic mixture of lidocaine and prilocaine) is liberally applied to the genital area involved, with or without occlusion 30–60 min before the procedure (Fig. 10.13). For localized

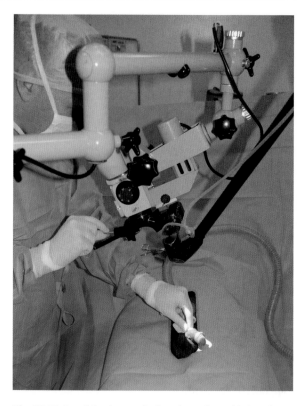

Fig. 10.11. Joystick micromanipulator is used to guide laser beam

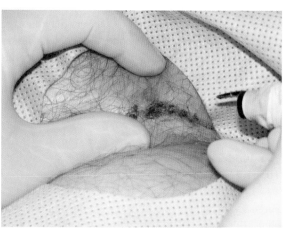

Fig. 10.12. Lesion is vaporized using the laser handpiece

lesions, local infiltration with lidocaine HCl 2% without epinephrine (Fig. 10.14) is used, and for extensive penile lesions a nerve block is preferred.

Acetic acid (5%) is applied to the genital area to identify and map areas to be treated (Fig. 10.15a, b) (see also How to Perform the Acetowhite Test in Chap. 3).

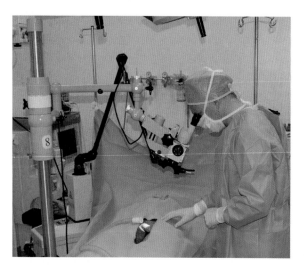

Fig. 10.10. Colposcope with connected laser is used to visualize and treat lesions

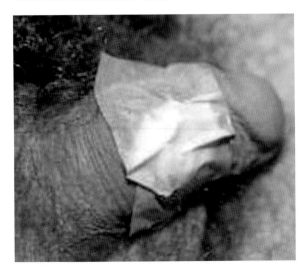

Fig. 10.13. EMLA is applied to involved area

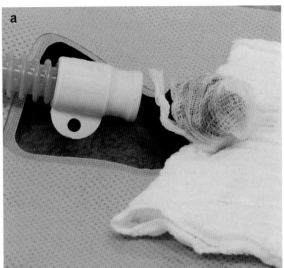

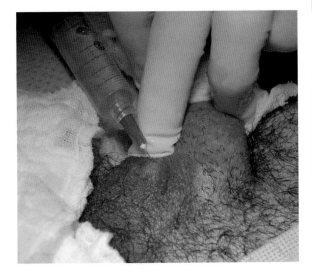

Fig. 10.14. Local infiltration of scrotal and penile lesions with lidocaine HCl 2% *without* epinephrine

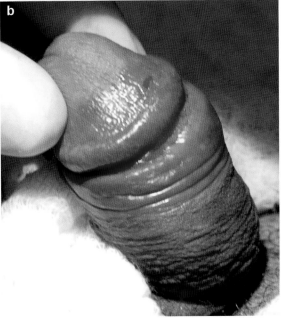

Fig. 10.15. (**a**) Acetowhite test performed to map areas to be treated (**b**) Acetowhite areas and diffuse hyperemic mucosa

A smoke evacuation system is always used and placed close to the vaporized area.

10.6.2 Settings

Power ranges between 4 W/cm^2 (urethra) and 5 W/cm^2 (external genitalia) in continuous (Fig. 10.16) or pulsed-wave mode for tissue vaporization, and between 5 and 10 W/cm^2 for excision of large exophytic lesions, are used.

Expert Advice

It is recommended to begin the laser procedure with the lowest possible power output, particularly for lesions located within the urethra, and power adjustments can be made accordingly during the laser session. This will reduce intraoperative complications and postoperative patient discomfort.

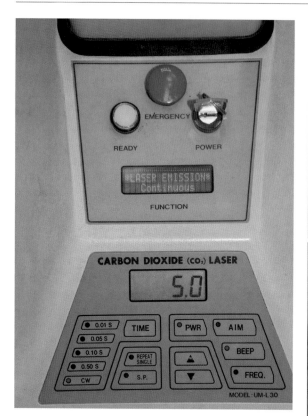

Fig. 10.16. Laser power 5 W/cm² in continuous mode

10.6.3   Procedure

Tissue vaporization is best accomplished when laser beam exposure times are shorter than 1 ms. Therefore, the laser beam should be moved in small and continuous movements until the area of interest is completely vaporized (Fig. 10.17a–c). The laser vaporization depth should not exceed 1 mm to prevent scarring and bleeding (particularly in the urethra). A 3-mm border of normal-appearing epithelium around the involved area is also vaporized to destroy any undetectable lesion (Fig. 10.18a, b). Bleeding is usually controlled with the defocused laser beam.

10.6.3.1   CO₂ Laser Vaporization of Penile Lesions

See Fig. 10.17a–c.

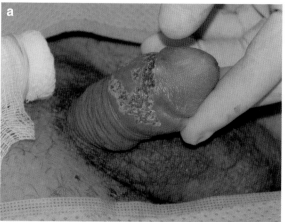

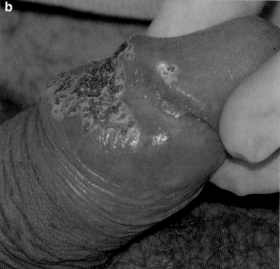

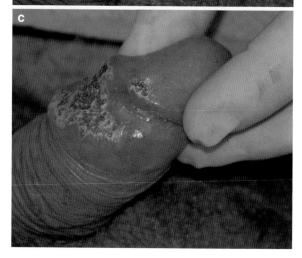

Fig. 10.17. (**a**) Laser directed to glans lesion. (**b**) Laser beam is moved in small and continuous movements. (**c**) Glans lesion is vaporized

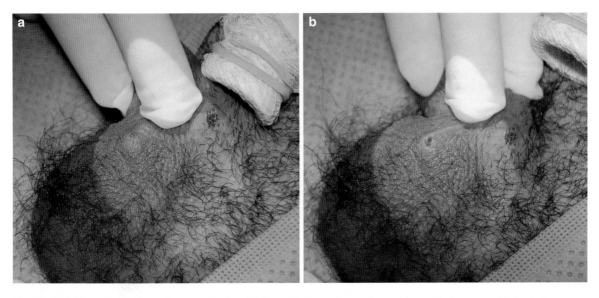

Fig. 10.18. (**a**) Laser beam directed to scrotal lesion. (**b**) Scrotal lesion and normal-appearing epithelium around lesion being vaporized (see laser plume)

10.6.3.2 CO$_2$ Laser Vaporization of Scrotal Lesions

See Fig. 10.18a, b.

10.6.3.3 CO$_2$ Laser Lesion Excision

The laser beam can also be used as a scalpel to cut the tissue and completely excise the affected area (Fig. 10.19a–d). The specimen obtained can be sent for histological analysis (Fig. 10.20).

10.6.3.4 CO$_2$ Laser Vaporization of Urethral Lesions

The urethral meatus is opened and the lesion is visualized (Fig. 10.21). It is very important to identify the lesion boundaries before vaporization begins, particularly at the deepest level, to avoid mucosal edema and loss of lesion margin definition. As soon as the lesion base is identified, the laser beam is applied to the wart's most exposed part to completely vaporize it down to its base (Fig. 10.22a, b). The laser is also applied to the areas adjacent to the urethral condyloma (Fig. 10.23). The unfocused beam is then quickly "flashed" over the remaining epithelium of

the fossa navicularis and urethral meatus, with the aim of destroying any clinically unapparent lesion contained within the area (Fig. 10.24). HPV-associated external lesions are treated during the same laser session (Fig. 10.25a, b).

> **Expert Advice**
>
> EMLA applied to the urethral meatus can produce mucosal edema (Figs. 10.22–10.24). This harmless side effect may cause undue difficulties during laser treatment, particularly in patients with deeper located lesions and/or narrow meatus. In these patients, the use of lidocaine gel may be a better topical anesthetic alternative.

10.6.4 Postoperative Care

Lidocaine gel is applied to all treated areas, which are then lightly covered with gauze mesh.

A topical collagenase-based ointment (sometimes associated with topical antibiotic after extensive vaporization) is applied on the first postoperative day and repeated thereafter two times a day with an open

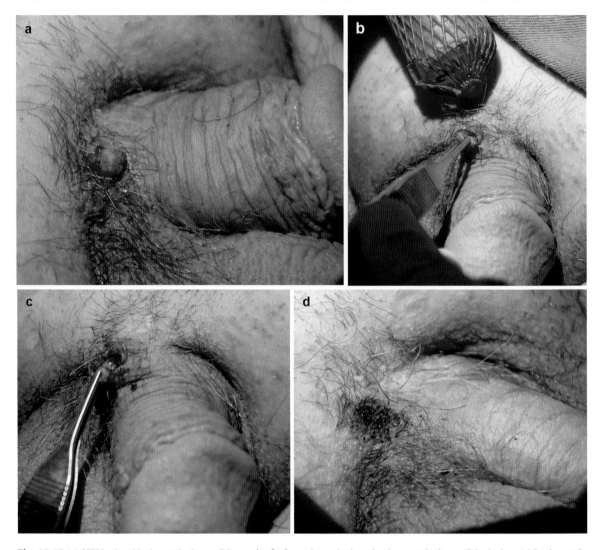

Fig. 10.19 (**a**) HPV-related lesion at the base of the penis. (**b**) Laser beam incises the tissue at the base of the lesion. (**c**) Lesion at the base of the penis being removed. (**d**) Final result

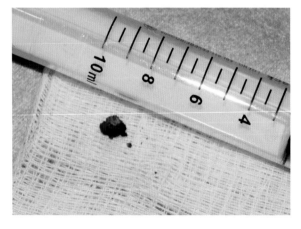

Fig. 10.20. Specimen obtained can be sent for histological and viral analysis

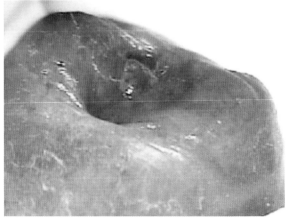

Fig. 10.21. Small urethral lesion

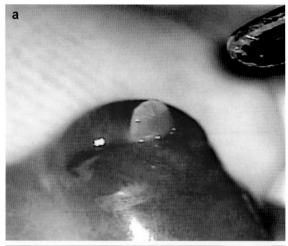

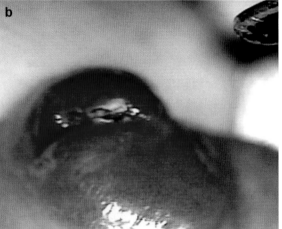

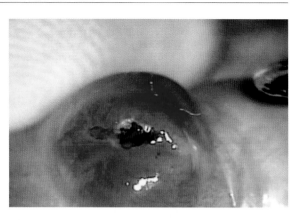

Fig. 10.23. Urethral mucosa adjacent to the lesion is also vaporized

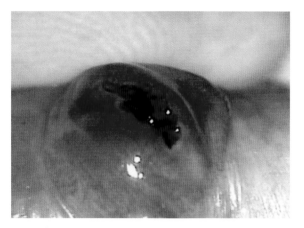

Fig. 10.22. (**a**) Laser beam directed to the lesion. (**b**) Urethral lesion is vaporized down to its base

Fig. 10.24. The unfocused beam is quickly flashed over the mucosa

dressing. Healing is usually completed in 2–3 weeks (Fig. 10.26–10.27) and sexual intercourse is deferred until complete healing occurs.

10.6.5 Complications

Postoperative swelling and ecchymosis usually subside in 2–5 days. Erythema and pruritus are usually due to contact dermatitis, and the cicatrizant cream should be removed or changed. Oral antifungal medications are occasionally required when erythema and pruritus associated with white discharge and odor persist.

Infection is an unusual event after genital laser treatment and topical and/or oral antibiotics are seldom recommended.

Pigmentary changes and scarring usually appear in areas where deep penetration of the laser beam has occurred.

10

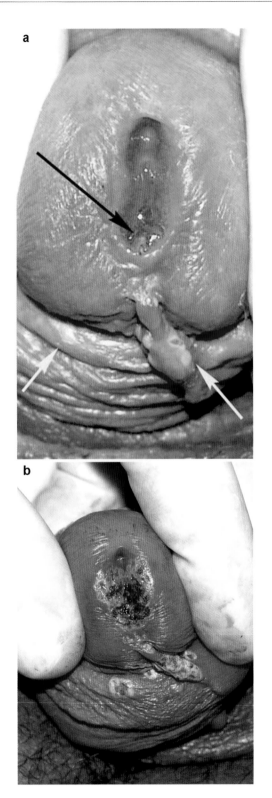

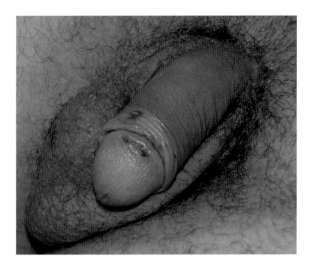

Fig. 10.26. Glans penis and preputial area on postoperative day 12

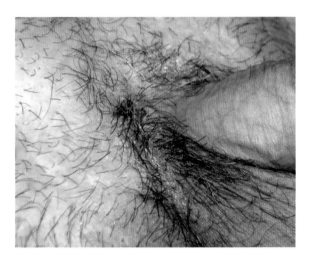

Fig. 10.27. Base of the penis on postoperative day 12

Fig. 10.25. (**a**) Broad-based urethral lesion (*black arrow*) and external lesions (*white arrows*). (**b**) Laser-treated areas

References

Einstein A (1917) Zur Quantentheorie der Strahlung (on the quantum mechanics of radiation). Physikalische Zeitschrift 18: 121–128

Ferenczy A, Bergeron C, Richart RM (1990) Carbon dioxide laser energy disperses human papillomavirus deoxyribonucleic acid onto treatment fields. Am J Obstet Gynecol 163: 1271–1274

Hallmo P, Naess O (1991) Laryngeal papillomatosis with human papillomavirus DNA contracted by a laser surgeon. Eur Arch Otorhinolaryngol 248: 425–427

Maiman T (1960) Stimulated optical radiation in ruby masers. Nature 187: 493–494

Moeller G, Rigden J (1965) High-power laser action in CO2-He mixtures. Appl Phys Lett 7: 274–276

Patel C (1964) Continuous-wave laser action on vibrational rotational transitions of CO2. Phys Rev 136: 1187–1193

Patel C (1965) High power N_2-CO_2 laser. Appl Phys Lett 7: 15–17

Polanyi J (1961) Proposal for an infrared Maser dependent on vibrational excitation. J Chem Phys 34: 347

Schalow A, Townes C (1958) Infrared and optical masers. Phys Rev 112: 1940–1949

Human Papillomavirus Vaccines

11

Alberto Rosenblatt and Homero Gustavo de Campos Guidi

Contents

A. Rosenblatt (✉)
Albert Einstein Jewish Hospital, Sao Paulo, Brasil
e-mail: albrose1@gmail.com

11.1   Introduction

Human papillomavirus (HPV) infection and HPV-associated anogenital diseases, such as warts, cancers precursors, as well as anogenital invasive cancers, are significant health care problems (Fig. 11.1). Current estimates of the worldwide prevalence of HPV indicate that approximately 10% of women in the general population will harbor cervical HPV infection at a given time (de Sanjose et al., 2007).

Furthermore, estimates of human cancer incidence linked to infectious agents suggest that HPV infections in female individuals presently contribute to more than 51% of cancer cases, whereas infection in male individuals accounts for slightly more than 4% of HPV-associated neoplasias (Hausen, 2008).

Cervical cancer causes considerable morbidity and mortality in the young female population and constitutes a significant economic burden to developing countries. According to 2002 data from the International Agency for Research on Cancer (Parkin et al., 2005), approximately half a million women worldwide develop cervical cancer every year (Fig. 11.1), and over two-thirds of these cases are associated with HPV infection of either oncogenic type 16 (51.0%) or HPV type 18 (16.2%). Consequently, successful strategies that can protect against HPV infection are expected to decrease the rates of HPV-related diseases.

Sexual abstinence is the most effective preventive measure against HPV infection and other sexually transmitted diseases (STDs). Although Winer et al. (2006) reported that the regular use of condoms may

A. Rosenblatt, H. G. de Campos Guidi, *Human Papillomavirus*,
DOI: 10.1007/978-3-540-70974-9-11, © Springer-Verlag Berlin Heidelberg 2009

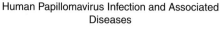

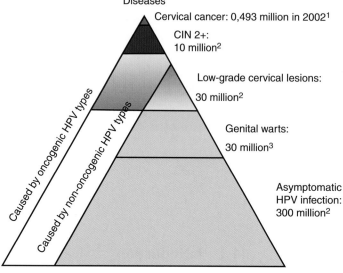

1.Parkin DM, Bray F, Ferlay J, Pisani P. *CA Cancer J Clin* 2005;55:74–108.
2.World Health Organization. Geneva, Switzerland: World Health Organization; 1999:1–22. 3. World Health Organization. WHO Office of Information. *WHO Features* 1990;152:1–6.

Fig. 11.1. HPV infection and associated diseases.(Source: Merck Sharp & Dohme. Reproduced with permission)

reduce the risk of genital HPV infection, transmission to the unprotected perigenital skin can still occur.

The interest in HPV immunology and vaccine development is not new. However, the practical obstacles involving the growth of papillomavirus in the laboratory and the oncogenic HPV proteins have been a hindrance to the generation of live attenuated HPV vaccines.

The recent licensure of two prophylactic vaccines against sexually transmitted HPV, developed with safe and effective recombinant DNA technology, has demonstrated that persistent HPV infection and more than 90% of precancerous lesions associated with types 16 or 18 among HPV-naive women can be effectively prevented.

This chapter begins with a brief introduction to the biology and life cycle of HPV, followed by a review of current information regarding the newly licensed prophylactic vaccines, as well as future developments in prophylactic and therapeutic strategies aimed at HPV-related diseases.

11.2   HPV: An Overview

HPV belongs predominately to the genus alphapapillomavirus, which can be further subdivided into species and then strains (de Villiers et al., 2004).

There are more than 30 strains of HPV that can infect the mucosa and genital tract, and between 13 and 18 HPV strains have been associated with an increased carcinogenic risk (Munoz et al., 2003; Trottier and Franco, 2006).

According to the epidemiologic classification of high-risk HPV types, 12 belong to the HPV species 7 (HPV 18, 39, 45, 59, 68) and HPV species 9 (HPV 16, 31, 33, 35, 52, 58, 67) (Munoz et al., 2003). However, strains that belong to the same species may differ biologically, and Viscidi et al. (2004, 2005) recently demonstrated that natural infection with high-risk HPV 16, 18, and 31 is not associated with immune protection from reinfection with homologous HPV strains or with genetically related types.

Evidence-based studies show that HPV infection with oncogenic types and viral persistence are highly associated with cervical cancer and to a lesser extent with vulvar, anal, and penile cancer.

A recent meta-analysis released by the Pan American Health Organization (2008) showed that the prevalence of HPV 16 and HPV 18 among a cohort of Latin–American women with invasive cervical cancer is 49.3% and 10%, respectively.

HPV vaccines can offer protection against high-risk HPV types responsible for approximately 70% of cervical cancers. However, due to several reasons (such as economic, religious, logistic), HPV vaccine introduction is a slow process. Therefore, for the present female population and particularly for those living in low-income countries, screening remains the primary option for cervical cancer prevention (Bosch et al., 2008).

> HPV vaccination is not a replacement for an effective screening program for cervical cancer, but rather a complement to it.

11.3 A Short Introduction to Papillomavirus Biology

Papillomaviruses are nonenveloped DNA viruses (i.e., the viral capsid (outer shell) lacks a lipid membrane). The HPV genome is a double-stranded circular DNA molecule that contains around 8,000 base pairs (bp), and the virus genome is divided into three portions (Munger and Howley, 2002; Munger et al., 2004):

1. A region of approximately 4,000 bp that encodes nonstructural early expressed (E) proteins primarily involved in viral DNA transcription and replication (E1, E2) and cell transformation (E5, E6, and E7)
2. A region containing around 3,000 bp that encodes the major late capsid protein (L1) and a minor capsid protein (L2)
3. A noncoding region (around 1,000 bp) that regulates viral DNA replication and gene expression

> There is no E3 protein and the E4 protein is encoded early but expressed late in infection, suggesting that it may facilitate virus escape from infected keratinocytes.

11.3.1 HPV Life Cycle (see graphic representation of HPV life cycle in Fig. 11.2)

HPV replication is restricted to the differentiated layers of the epidermis or mucosa (McMurray et al., 2001; Munger et al., 2004). Viral penetration occurs through microabrasions in the epithelium and HPV receptors have been identified on the surface of basal cells (Evander et al., 1997). According to de Witte et al. (2007), heparan sulfate proteoglycan syndecan-3 appears to be the initial cell surface attachment factor. It is currently believed that basal cell invasion occurs in a period of approximately 24 h, but viral gene expression is only initiated 2–3 days thereafter.

In the basal cells and their progeny, known as transit-amplifying cells, HPV DNA replication occurs with minimal gene expression (early genes E1 and E2).

The expression of early viral proteins E6 and E7 delay cell-cycle arrest and differentiation, and support the viral genome replication that occurs in the suprabasal epithelial layer cells (where some infected cells may persist for many years).

> High-risk HPV E6 and E7 oncoproteins lack intrinsic enzymatic activities, but interact with cellular proteins that are known cellular tumor suppressors, such as p53 and retinoblastoma tumor suppressor (pRB). Although p53 levels are unaffected by E6 proteins of low-risk HPV, oncogenic HPV E6 protein induces the degradation of p53 (Streeck, 2002).

In the differentiated keratinocyte, viral gene expression is upregulated and thousands of viral genomes are generated. High levels of late capsid viral proteins (L1 and L2) and proteins responsible for HPV DNA replication and encapsidation (E4) are expressed, with final virus assembly occurring in the superficial squames. Highly infectious virions are then shed into the environment.

> Stanley et al. (2007) showed that the time interval from infection to viral release is approximately 3 weeks, which coincides with the complete cycle of basal keratinocytes.

11.4 Significance of HPV Proteins in the Generation of Prophylactic and Therapeutic HPV Vaccines

The major late capsid protein (L1) of HPV spontaneously assembles into virus-like particles (VLPs) when synthesized by recombinant expression vector systems

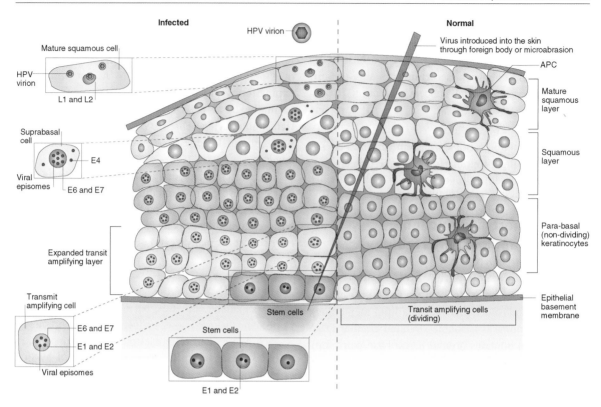

Fig. 11.2. HPV life cycle (see also text for further explanation). (Source: Frazer, 2004. Reproduced with permission from Macmillan)

(Zhou et al., 1991; Kirnbauer et al., 1992). Prophylactic vaccines use these noninfectious but immunogenic VLPs to generate neutralizing antibodies against HPV L1 protein (Wheeler, 2007).

According to studies performed by Hagensee et al. (1993), the minor viral capsid protein (L2) is not required for assembly, but it is integrated into VLPs when coexpressed together with L1. However, L2 protein is important for virus infectivity (Unckell et al., 1997) and it seems to play an essential role in viral morphogenesis (Day et al., 1998). Furthermore, according to some investigators the modification of current prophylactic HPV vaccines by insertion of cross-reactive L2-epitopes could be the basis for the production of broad-spectrum vaccines (Gambhira et al., 2007; Kondo et al., 2008).

Early expressed proteins (E6, E7), which are involved in uncontrolled proliferation and cellular transformation, have also been used as antigens for therapeutic vaccination against HPV-related anogenital diseases (Klencke et al., 2002; Sheets et al., 2003; Davidson et al., 2003; Baldwin et al., 2003; Hallez et al., 2004).

11.5   Natural History of HPV Antibodies

It is well known that HPV infection clearance often occurs in immunocompetent individuals (Schiffman and Kjaer, 2003), although the exact mechanisms involved remain uncertain. The regression, persistence, and progression of HPV-related lesions likely reflect the combined action of nonspecific innate immunity and antigen-specific adaptive immune components.

11.5.1   Humoral Responses

Since a bloodstream phase is not required in the life cycle of HPV, viral exposure to the systemic immune system is minimal. Consequently, host antibody levels following incident infection are very low and probably not sufficient to afford protection during the primary event. However, de Gruijl et al. (1997) found increased serum IgG antibody titers in patients with persistent HPV 16 infections and histologically confirmed high-grade lesions.

The main immunoglobulin present in the female genital tract is IgG, and these local neutralizing antibodies are the first line of defense against HPV infection. However, IgG antibodies are not produced locally, and transudation or exudation from serum to the cervical mucus must occur before antigen-specific immune components can exert their protective effects at the cervical mucosa (Parr and Parr, 1997; Nardelli-Haefliger et al., 2003; Kemp et al., 2008). In transudation, IgG is transferred from the intravascular compartment into the genital tract through ultrafiltration, while exudation involves the passage of fluid from damaged blood vessels (i.e., during intercourse) to the extravascular compartment (Fig. 11.3).

Most studies regarding antibody-mediated humoral immunity to naturally occurring HPV infection support the idea that minimal protection is exerted against HPV persistence or related diseases. The delay in response after infection suggests that HPV is able to efficiently evade the host immune system (see Chap. 9).

Ho et al. (2004) recently demonstrated that HPV 16-infected individuals elicited higher IgG and IgA antibodies titers than those infected with other HPV strains. IgG seropositivity appeared in 56.7% of cases within 8.3 months, and IgA appeared in 37% of subjects within 14 months after natural infection with HPV 16. Both IgG and IgA seroconversions lasted for approximately 36 months, and the same study showed that increased viral load and persistent HPV 16 infection may extend seropositivity duration.

Bontkes et al. (1999) found that systemic IgG responses were more frequently detected in patients with persistent HPV 16 infection. However, in a study evaluating antibody responses following incident HPV infection, Carter et al. (2000) reported that some subjects with persistent HPV 16 infection failed to seroconvert.

An epidemiologic analysis of mucosal immunoglobulin IgA and IgG responses to oncogenic HPV capsids has shown that IgA is associated with HPV infection, whereas IgG correlates with cervical squamous intraepithelial lesions (SIL) and invasive disease (Sasagawa et al., 2003).

Data evaluating the detection of HPV 16 antibody in HPV 16-associated cervical intraepithelial neoplasia (CIN) in Australian women reveal a more frequent seropositivity in women presenting HPV 16 DNA-positive lesions than in women with no HPV DNA. However, Tabrizi et al. (2006) reported that in this selected patient population HPV 16 serology was a poor predictor of the presence of HPV 16-associated CIN 3.

Mbulawa et al. (2008) recently demonstrated that serum and cervical HPV 16-neutralizing antibodies correlated with HPV 16 infection, and Bierl et al. (2005) suggested that cervical mucosal anti-HPV 16

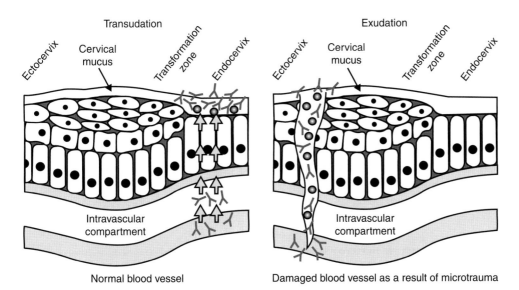

Fig. 11.3. Transudation and exudation of serum antibodies to the cervical mucus and cervical mucosa. (Source: Schwarz and Leo (2008). Reproduced with permission from Elsevier)

IgA and IgG antibodies may protect against HPV infection and cervical disease.

Therefore, it is likely that the primary mechanism of protection against persistent oncogenic HPV infection is the transudation of anti-HPV IgG antibodies from the serum to the cervical mucosa (Nardelli-Haefliger et al., 2003). However, the exact influence of seropositivity to oncogenic HPV 16, HPV 18, or HPV 31 after incident infection and protection to subsequent infections with homologous or genetically related HPV types must be further elucidated (Viscidi et al., 2004).

11.5.2 Cell Immune Responses

Cellular immunity plays a critical role in the eradication of HPV infection and related diseases, as well as in the protection against persistent viral infection and HPV-associated disease progression (Scott et al., 1999; Welters et al., 2003; Piketty and Kazatchkine, 2005; van Poelgeest et al., 2006).

T cells in the cervical epithelium belong mainly to the CD_8 suppressor/cytotoxic subgroup and to a lesser extent to the CD_4 helper/inductor subgroup. Stanley et al. (1994) demonstrated that HPV-related lesions that regress spontaneously usually exhibit a cellular infiltration composed essentially of CD_4 and macrophages.

In addition, other investigators have demonstrated that T helper 1 (Th1) responses are important in HPV control (Scott et al., 1999; de Jong et al., 2004).

Th 1 effector/memory cells secrete interferon-γ (IFN-γ), interleukin-2 (IL-2), and lymphotoxin, promoting a milieu in which important cytotoxic effectors (such as macrophages, natural killer cells, and cytotoxic CD8$^+$ T lymphocytes) are activated. This cell-mediated immune response is directed against intracellular pathogens (i.e., virus) and cancer cells.

Lee et al. (2004), in a recent study, found a reduction of Th1 cytokine production by activated CD4($^+$) T cells in female patients presenting with HPV-associated high-grade SIL, suggesting the deficient Th1 function may impair cytotoxic CD8($^+$) T cells responses.

The targets of the cell immune response include the early HPV oncoproteins E6 and E7 as well as HPV gene E2 (Stanley, 2006). However, CD4($^+$) T cell responses to HPV 16 oncoproteins are lacking or severely impaired in women presenting with CIN recurrence and invasive cervical cancer (de Jong et al., 2004; Sarkar et al., 2005).

These results demonstrate that HPV infection can interfere with local immune surveillance mechanisms and, according to Sheu et al. (2007), these interferences are probably related to cytokine immunomodulating actions and host genetic susceptibility (see also Chap. 9).

11.6   Prophylactic HPV Vaccination

The use of recombinant DNA technology to generate VLPs in 1991 (Zhou et al., 1991), and the subsequent improvements in VLPs assembly (Kirnbauer et al., 1992) (Fig. 11.4), contributed to the development of HPV vaccines. VLPs are noninfectious because the entire HPV genome is lacking, but they are readily recognized by the immune system and are able to elicit both humoral and cellular immune responses when injected into human hosts (Harro et al., 2001; Brown et al., 2001).

The mechanisms involved in vaccine protection against HPV infection have not been completely elucidated. However, several studies have demonstrated that high levels of HPV-specific neutralizing serum antibodies are essential for effective protection (Christensen et al., 1996; Suzich et al., 1995; Day et al., 2007).

HPV vaccines generate neutralizing antibodies against HPV capsid antigen L1 (Fig. 11.5a–c). Since viral neutralization is genotype-specific, HPV VLP vaccines need to be formulated with the most prevalent genital HPV types with the aim of inducing a broadly protective immunity against genital HPV disease.

There are two vaccines against HPV currently available (Table 11.1). Gardasil (Merck & Co., Whitehouse Station, NJ), the first vaccine to be licensed by the U.S. Food and Drug Administration (FDA, 2008), offers protection against high-risk HPV types 16 and 18, as well as low-risk HPV types 6 and 11. The oncogenic types 16 and 18 account for an estimated 70% of all cervical cancers worldwide, and the two low-risk types included in the vaccine are responsible for approximately 90% of genital warts.

Structural Model of Human Papillomavirus VLP

Fig. 11.4. Assembly of HPV virus-like particles (VLP). The rosette-like surface structures (*black arrow*) are pentamers, each consisting of five molecules of L1. (Source: Adapted from Kirnbauer et al., 1992; Syrjanen and Syrjanen, 2000; Reproduced with permission from Merck, Sharp & Dohme)

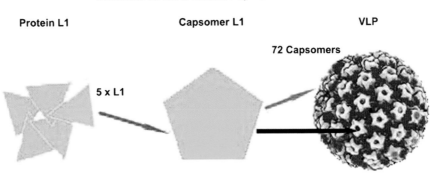

Cervarix (GlaxoSmithKline, Rixensart, Belgium), recently licensed in Europe, offers protection against oncogenic HPV types 16 and 18, and Paavonen et al. (2007) recently demonstrated that the bivalent vaccine may also prevent HPV infection with heterologous HPV strains 31/45/52 by cross-protection.

> The main target group for prophylactic vaccines is young girls before sexual onset, because the prevalence of HPV infection is dramatically increased thereafter (Brown et al., 2005).

Recent investigators have demonstrated that the bivalent and quadrivalent vaccine induce an enhanced and long-lasting immune response (Giannini et al., 2006; Olsson et al., 2007).

Furthermore, Giannini et al. (2006) showed that the adjuvant used in Cervarix (GSK AS04), a mixture of aluminum hydroxide and monophosphoryl lipid A, induced higher antibody responses than Merck's amorphous aluminum hydroxyphosphate sulfate adjuvant. However, no direct comparative studies have been performed to date between VLPs adjuvanted with AS04 and the aluminum salts of Gardasil.

Both Gardasil and Cervarix have been extensively tested in several randomized, double-blind, placebo-controlled phase-III clinical trials in North America, Latin America, Europe, and the Asia-Pacific region (Harper et al., 2004; Villa et al., 2005; Koutsky and Harper, 2006). Gardasil trials involved more than 30,000 women aged 16–26 who were seronegative and DNA-negative for the vaccine HPV types at the time of enrollment, and Cervarix phase-III trials are underway with more than 39,000 individuals planned to participate.

Results from the clinical trials published thus far have shown that prophylactic vaccines are safe and highly immunogenic (Future II Study Group, 2007; Villa, 2007; Paavonen et al., 2007; Rambout et al., 2007).

Gardasil showed sustained efficacy over 5 years (Villa et al., 2006) and it has reduced the combined

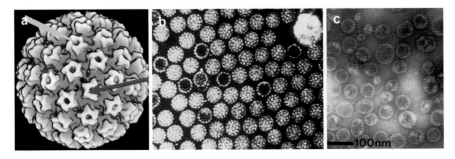

Fig. 11.5. (**a**) Model of papillomavirus capsid. The L1 pentamer is represented (gray *arrow*) and one molecule of L2 (not represented) fits into the central dimple of each pentamer (*yellow arrow*). (**b**) Papillomavirus particles with full (i.e., containing DNA) and empty particles represented. (**c**) HPV 16 L1 virus-like particles. (Source: Stanley et al., (2006). Reproduced with permission from Elsevier)

Table 11.1 Current HPV vaccines

	Quadrivalent vaccine	Bivalent vaccine
Trade name (manufacturer)	Gardasil® (Merck)	Cervarix® (GlaxoSmithKline)
VLPs of genotypes	6, 11, 16, 18	16, 18
Composition	20 μg HPV 6, 40 μg HPV 11, 40 μg HPV 16, 20 μg HPV 18	20 μg HPV 16, 20 μg HPV 18
Adjuvant	Proprietary aluminum hydroxyphosphate sulfate (225ug) (Merck aluminum adjuvant)	Proprietary aluminum hydroxide (500 μg) plus 50 μg 3-deacylated monophosphoryl lipid A (GSK AS04 adjuvant)
Dosage	Three 0.5-ml doses at 0, 2, 6 months	Three 0.5-ml doses at 0, 1, 6 months
Administration route	IM injections in the upper arm or thigh	IM injections in the upper arm
Recommended	11–12 year-old girls (FDA[3])	10–25-year-old female subjects
Licensed	FDA – girls/women between ages 9 and 26	European Commission – girls/women between the age of 10 and 25
Safety/immunogenicity bridging trials[a]	Girls and boys 9–15 years	Girls 10–14 years
		Boys 10–18 years
		Women 26–55 years
Cross-protection	HPV 31, 33, 35, 39, 45, 51, 52, 56, 58, and 59 (Brown et al., 2007)	HPV 45 (88%)
		HPV 31 (54.5%) (Harper et al., 2006)
		HPV 33 and 52 (Paavonen et al., 2007)
Cost[b]	(United States) U.S. $360 (three-dose regimen)	(United Kingdom) £240 (three-dose regimen)
Current duration of protection	5 years	6.4 years (Schwarz and Leo, 2008)

IM intramuscular
[a]Gardasil and Cervarix are not recommended for pregnant women (pregnancy category, B2 classification), although no greater risk of spontaneous pregnancy or fetal abnormality has been observed
[b]2008-based costs

incidence of HPV 6-, 11-, 16-, and 18-associated persistent infection or disease (CIN or adenocarcinoma in situ (AIS)) by 96% (Ault, 2007; Future II Study Group, 2007). The vaccine also prevented HPV 6-, 11-, 16-, or 18-related external genital lesions by 100% (Villa et al., 2006; Perez et al., 2008) (Table 11.2).

In addition, HPV prophylactic vaccination with quadrivalent vaccine resulted in 100% efficacy against HPV 16- and 18-related high-grade vulvar/vaginal neoplasias (VIN 2+/VaIN 2+) (Joura et al., 2007).

Giannini et al. (2006) demonstrated that the bivalent vaccine induced high frequencies of HPV L1 VLP-specific memory B cells, and Stanley et al. (2006)

showed that these cells are important for the long-term efficacy of vaccine-induced protection.

Phase-II and phase-III clinical trial results have shown that Cervarix-induced L1 VLP-specific antibody levels can be sustained for up to 6.4 years (Schwarz and Leo, 2008), with additional cross-protection against HPV 45, 31, and 52 (Gall and Teixeira, 2007; Paavonen et al., 2007). In addition, interim phase-III results showed vaccine efficacy in preventing 90.4% of CIN2+ lesions and 80% efficacy against persistent infections associated with HPV 16 and 18 (Paavonen et al., 2007).

The prophylactic HPV vaccines may also reduce the incidence of other HPV-related anogenital malignant diseases, such as anal and penile cancer (Hampl et al., 2006; Prowse et al., 2008). Current estimates of HPV-associated cancers in the United States showed that there were more than 3,000 HPV-associated anal cancers per year during the period 1998–2003 (Watson et al., 2008). In addition, Joseph et al. (2008) reported that the incidence rates of this disease increased 2.6% per year and women were more affected than men. Watson et al. (2008) also showed that penile cancer is relatively rare in the United States, with approximately 800 men affected each year, but the incidence of the disease can be as high as 17% of all male neoplasias in some low-resource countries. Moreover, in a recent study, Daling et al. (2005) reported a strong association between HPV DNA and penile cancer development, particularly with the high-risk HPV 16 strain.

Current HPV vaccines could also prevent HPV-associated benign and malignant neoplasms of the oral cavity and aerodigestive tracts. Low-risk HPV types 6 and 11 are almost always responsible for the development of juvenile laryngeal papillomas and recurrent respiratory papillomas (RRP) in adults. The former typically develops between birth and age 7 in children born to mothers with HPV-related genital lesions, while the adult-onset disease most likely occurs as a result of sexual transmission. Although both juvenile and adult RRP are rare (arising in perhaps 0.1–0.2% of exposed individuals), frequent surgeries are required to control the disease which imposes a significant burden on patients. Moreover, infected cells can also migrate down the airway causing tracheal, bronchial, and rarely pulmonary lesions.

Recently released data that evaluated HPV-associated cancers in the United States have shown that nearly 5,700 men and about 1,700 women develop cancers of the oral cavity and oropharynx per year (Watson et al., 2008). In addition, Ryerson et al. (2008) reported that the incidence rates for tonsil cancers and neoplasia of the tongue base increased 3% per year during the period 1998–2003, with a higher predilection for men. There is evidence to support a sexual transmission of HPV infection to the oral cavity (Frisch et al., 1999; Hemminki et al., 2000) and, in a systematic review of HPV types found in head and neck squamous cell carcinomas, Kreimer et al. (2005) reported that HPV 16 was associated with oropharyngeal carcinomas in more than 80% of cases.

Table 11.2 Key results from phase-III trials of HPV vaccines (Source: Bosch et al. (2008). Reproduced with permission from Macmillan)

Vaccine name	Gardasil®	Cervarix®
Time of follow-up	36 months (advanced)	15 months (interim)
HPV types included	6, 11, 16, 18	16, 18
Efficacy HPV16 or 18 CIN 2+	Yes	Yes
Efficacy HPV16 CIN 2+	Yes	Yes
Efficacy HPV18 CIN 2+	Yes	Not yet proven[a]
Efficacy HPV16 or 18 CIN 2	Yes	Yes
Efficacy HPV16 or 18 CIN 3	Yes	Not yet proven[a]
Therapeutic efficacy	None	None
Efficacy on VIN 2/3	Yes	Not yet reported
Efficacy on VaIN 2/3	Yes	Not yet reported
Efficacy on genital warts	Yes	Not in target
Safety at 6-year follow-up	Safe[b]	Safe[c]
Tolerability	Acceptable	Acceptable
Cross-protection (persistent HPV infection)	6 months	12 months
Cross-protection (lesions)	Reported	Not yet reported
Duration of protection[d]	5–6 years	6.4 years
Immunogenicity in preadolescents	Yes	Yes
Immunogenicity in older women	Yes	Yes
Immune memory at 6 years	Yes	Not yet reported

CIN cervical intraepithelial neoplasia; HPV human papillomavirus; VIN vulvar intraepithelial neoplasia; VaIN vaginal intraepithelial neoplasia
[a]Proven in combined analysis of phase-II/III trials
[b]In postlicencing evaluation (http://www.who.int/vaccine_safety/en/)
[c]In clinical trials
[d]Corresponds to duration of trials in 2007/2008

11.6.1 Gardasil®

11.6.1.1 Who Should Receive Gardasil?

Gardasil was approved by the U.S. Food and Drug Administration (FDA) and the European Medicines Agency (EMEA), and is currently licensed for use among female subjects aged 9–26 years.

The quadrivalent vaccine is currently recommended for 11–12-year-old girls, although HPV vaccination can begin at the age of 9. It is also recommended for 13–26-year-old girls/women who have not yet received or completed the three-dose vaccination regimen (Centers for Disease Control and Prevention-CDC).

In a recent analysis evaluating the epidemiological and economic impact of the quadrivalent HPV vaccine for preventing HPV-related diseases, Dasbach et al. (2008) reported that vaccination at 12 years of age combined with a 12- to 24-year-old catch-up strategy was cost-effective.

According to Luna and Saah (2007), the efficacy of Gardasil in HPV-naive women between the ages of 27 and 45 years is similar to that in younger women.

11.6.1.2 Indications

The quadrivalent vaccine is currently indicated for the prevention of incident and persistent HPV infections, external genital warts (condyloma acuminata), high-grade cervical dysplasia (precancerous cervical lesions), invasive cervical cancer, and high-grade vulvar and vaginal dysplastic lesions (precancerous vulvar and vaginal lesions) that are caused by HPV 6, 11, 16, or 18.

11.6.1.3 How to Administer

Gardasil is administered as three separate 0.5-ml intramuscular injections in the upper arm or thigh over a 6-month period. The initial dose is given anytime between the ages of 9 and 26 years; the second and third dose should be given 2 and 6 months, respectively, after the first injection.

11.6.1.4 Side Effects

- Injection site reactions such as pain (83.9%), swelling (25.4%), and erythema (24.6%)
- Low fever (13%)
- Nausea (6.7%)
- Nasopharyngitis (6.4%)
- Arthralgia, myalgia
- Asthenia, malaise
- Anaphylaxis (2.6 cases per 100,000 doses occurred in the Australian school-based program, according to Brotherton et al., 2008)

11.6.1.5 Cost

On the basis of 2008 prices, in the U.S. market, the cost of Gardasil per single dose is U.S. $120 (or U.S. $360 for a typical three-dose regimen), and in Europe the average price is 360 for the three doses of the vaccine.

11.6.2 Cervarix®

Cervarix was licensed in Australia and Europe, and is currently awaiting U.S. FDA approval.

11.6.2.1 Who Should Receive Cervarix?

The EMEA has licensed Cervarix for girls and women between the age of 10 and 25 years, and in Australia it is licensed for use among female individuals aged 10–45 years (Skinner et al., 2008).

Schwarz and Dubin (2007) recently demonstrated that the bivalent vaccine is safe and effective in women up to the age of 55 years.

11.6.2.2 Indications

The bivalent vaccine is currently indicated for the prevention of incident and persistent infections, high-grade cervical dysplasia (precancerous CIN 2 and 3) and invasive cervical cancer caused by HPV types 16 and 18.

Protection against persistent infections with HPV strains 45 and 31 (Harper et al., 2006; Paavonen et al., 2007) may broaden current indications.

11.6.2.3   How to Administer

Cervarix is administered as three separate 0.5-ml intramuscular injections in the upper arm over a 6-month period. The initial dose is given anytime between the ages of 10 and 25 years, and the second and third dose should be given 1 and 6 months, respectively, after the first injection.

11.6.2.4   Side Effects

- Headache
- Myalgia
- Mild soreness, hyperemia, and swelling around the injection site
- Fatigue
- Gastrointestinal symptoms
- Skin rash and itching
- Low fever (occasionally)

11.6.2.5   Cost

On the basis of 2008 prices, in the UK market, the cost of Cervarix per single dose is approximately £80 (or £240 for a typical three-dose regimen).

Both HPV vaccines can be administered simultaneously with other vaccines routinely given to individuals within this age-group, such as hepatitis B, quadrivalent meningococcal vaccine, and DTaP (Markowitz et al., 2007).

11.7   HPV Vaccination: Issues to Be Addressed

11.7.1   Duration of Protection

The duration of clinical trials that have evaluated the efficacy of current vaccines against HPV infection and SIL is approximately 6 years. Therefore, given the protracted natural history of HPV-related cervical cancer,

phase-IV studies using cervical carcinoma as endpoint are needed to demonstrate effective protection against the disease.

Population-based studies in Nordic countries are in progress to evaluate the efficacy of HPV vaccination with regard to carcinoma in situ (Lehtinen et al., 2006a) and invasive cervical cancer (Lehtinen et al., 2006b), and definitive results are expected by the years 2015–2020.

Villa et al. (2006) reported that a booster (fourth) dose of Gardasil at 5 years leads to a rapid increase in antibody levels, consistent with the presence of immune memory.

11.7.2   HPV Prophylactic Vaccine Cross-Protection

Current prophylactic vaccines only protect against HPV types targeted by the quadrivalent and bivalent vaccine (HPV 6, 11, 16, 18 and HPV 16, 18, respectively). Individuals can still be infected by other low- and high-risk types and secondary (screening) cancer prevention should continue even in vaccinated women.

There are conflicting results regarding cross-protection from naturally occurring HPV infection (Viscidi et al., 2004); however, recent studies have shown that HPV vaccination is likely to induce neutralizing antibodies across HPV species (Slupetzky et al., 2007; Gambhira et al., 2006).

Preliminary data reported by Brown (2007) showed that Gardasil provided cross-protection against ten HPV types (i.e., 31, 33, 35, 39, 45, 51, 52, 56, 58, and 59) associated with CIN2+ or adenocarcinoma in situ.

Cross-protection has also been demonstrated against persistent infections with HPV 45, 31, 33, and 52 following Cervarix vaccination, with vaccine efficacy against these types ranging from 31.6 to 59.9% at 6 months (Paavonen et al., 2007).

11.7.3   Vaccination of HPV-Infected Individuals

Hildesheim et al. (2007) recently showed that the administration of the prophylactic bivalent HPV vaccine to women already infected with HPV 16 and 18 failed to improve viral clearance. Therefore, bivalent HPV vaccine immunization has not been recommended in these subjects.

However, the Future II Study Group (2007) recommended HPV immunization with the quadrivalent vaccine for women already infected with 1–3 vaccine-related strains. The rationale is that the vaccine would still be effective against the remaining strain(s).

> Prevaccination HPV DNA testing is not necessary and is not recommended before vaccinating sexually active women.

11.7.4 HPV Vaccines in Developing Countries

The strategy of broad dissemination of HPV vaccines has the potential to reduce the burden of HPV-related diseases on individuals and subsequently decrease government-related health costs. The extent of the benefit of a specific population will be determined by the incidence rates of cervical cancer attributable to HPV 16 and 18, as well as the vaccine efficacy and coverage. Cervical cancer is a leading cause of cancer among young women as well as a leading cause of cancer-related deaths in poor countries. Recent data from the World Health Organization (WHO, 2006) reported that approximately 80% of the 250,000 cervical cancer deaths in 2005 occurred in poor-resource countries. Since this burden is predicted to increase in the coming years (Agosti and Goldie, 2007), the gains that can be obtained with even a partially effective HPV vaccine are likely to be substantial.

However, particularly in developing countries, the cost of the HPV vaccine and the cost-effectiveness of preventive vaccination relative to other established programs directed to the health care of female adolescents (the main vaccine target group) will greatly influence government policy recommendations for HPV immunization.

> VLP vaccines are relatively expensive, and it is predicted that vaccine cost will be one of the greatest barriers to the introduction of HPV immunization programs in developing countries (Saxenian and Hecht, 2006).

A recent economic report evaluating HPV vaccination in Latin American countries has shown that, based on current vaccine cost, cervical cancer screening was more cost-effective than vaccination as the main preventive measure against the disease (Pan American Health Organization, 2008).

In another recent analysis evaluating health and economic outcomes of HPV 16 and 18 vaccination for countries with a low GDP, Goldie, et al. (2008) reported that, to become cost-effective and affordable, each HPV vaccine dose should cost around U.S. $2.

Techakehakij and Feldman (2008) recently performed a systematic review of the literature regarding cost-effectiveness of HPV vaccination programs compared with Pap smear screening. Using guidelines of the World Health Organization to determine whether nation-wide application of the HPV vaccine would be cost-effective, they concluded that in only 46 high-income countries (i.e., with a per capita GDP higher than U.S. $8,505 in 2004) would an HPV vaccination program be cost-effective.

It is expected that HPV vaccines could receive subsidies from different public and private sectors, such as GAVI Alliance (Gavialliance), World Health Organization (WHO), UNICEF and others in a joint effort to bring HPV immunization to where it is most needed.

> It has been reported that both HPV vaccine manufacturers (Sanofi Pasteur MSD and Glaxo Smith Kline) have already submitted an application to seek WHO prequalification, an important step toward providing global access to vaccines (medical news today 2008b; The Henry J. Kaiser Family Foundation, 2007a).

11.7.5 Condoms vs. HPV Prophylactic Vaccines

Despite the high efficacy of current vaccines, vaccination does not offer 100% protection against HPV infection because HPV types not included in the formulation of Gardasil and Cervarix can also infect the anogenital region of both genders. Consistent condom use may offer some additional protection, although variable, against other low- and high-risk HPV types. In addition, condom use can protect against other common sexually transmitted infections.

11.8 Prophylactic HPV Vaccines in Men

Genital HPV infection is a sexually transmitted disease and it is predictable that male immunization may help prevent HPV transmission and subsequently reduce the burden of HPV infection and HPV-related diseases in women.

Studies show that HPV-infected men can transmit HPV infection to women, contributing to the development of cervical premalignant lesions and cervical cancer (Agarwal et al., 1993; Bosch et al., 1996).

According to Bosch et al. (1996), men with a history of multiple sexual partners are a known risk factor for cervical neoplasia, increasing by almost sevenfold the risk of the disease in the female partner (Castellsague et al., 2002).

Although HPV-infected men appear to have a lower antibody prevalence of HPV types 6, 11, 16, and 18 compared with women, recent studies evaluating immune responses using the HPV quadrivalent vaccine in male and female adolescents showed high antibody responses in both genders (Block et al., 2006; Reisinger et al., 2007). Seroprevalence in men peaks at an older age (around 30–39 years) when compared with women (20–29 years), and this biological difference might reflect a lower viral load, transient infections, or even decreased immunological responses in men compared with women (Partridge and Koutsky, 2006).

HPV-related lesions in men often present clinically as anogenital warts, and the development of these lesions has been associated with HPV types 6 and 11 (Greer et al., 1995). The quadrivalent vaccine proved effective in reducing HPV-related lesions in the vulva, suggesting that penile lesions could also be prevented because of epithelial similarities.

> A recent phase-III study that evaluated the efficacy of the quadrivalent vaccine in preventing HPV-related lesions in a large group of sexually active young men (3,400 heterosexuals and 600 men who have sex with men (MSM)), aged 16–26 and naïve to all four HPV vaccine types, showed that Gardasil was 89.4% effective in preventing external anogenital warts (Giuliano and Palefsky, 2008). Moreover, HPV-related persistent infections were reduced in 85.6% of the cases, with higher vaccine efficacy observed against persistent infection with HPV types 18 (96%) and 11 (93.4%) (Palefsky and Giuliano, 2008). HPV DNA detection was also decreased in almost 45% of the vaccinated individuals.
>
> Moreover, according to the investigators, the quadrivalent vaccine is safe to use in men with only minor injection site reactions reported (see also Sect. 3.11 in Chap. 3).

Anal HPV infection, anal intraepithelial neoplasia (AIN), and anal cancer are highly prevalent in MSM and in immunosuppressed patients, especially those with HIV (see also Chap. 7). Available data have shown that HPV infection with oncogenic type HPV 16 is closely involved in the development of AIN and anal squamous cell carcinoma (Varnai et al., 2006; Kagawa et al., 2006), but a recent study showed that the quadrivalent HPV vaccine was 100% effective in preventing AIN development in young male subjects (Giuliano and Palefsky, 2008).

Recent studies also reported a strong association between HPV DNA and penile cancer development, particularly with the high-risk HPV 16 strain (Daling et al., 2005; Pascual et al., 2007). However, in the study that evaluated the efficacy of the quadrivalent HPV vaccine in men, there were no penile intraepithelial neoplasia (PIN) cases in the vaccinated group, but three PIN cases were observed in the placebo group. Penile cancer was not reported in both groups (Giuliano and Palefsky, 2008).

Additional data from the ongoing Gardasil study in men will become available in the coming months and trials to evaluate Cervarix safety and immunogenicity in young males are also in progress (ClinicalTrials.gov).

11.8.1 Nongenital HPV Infections in Men

Current HPV vaccines could also prevent HPV-related oropharyngeal infection and disease in men.

Several studies suggest that oral HPV infection is sexually acquired (Schwartz et al., 1998; D'Souza et al., 2007) and HPV is considered an independent risk factor for oral cancer. Low-risk HPV types 6 and 11 are the viral genotypes most frequently associated with benign squamous cell lesions of the oral mucosa and the aerodigestive tract, while high-risk HPV 16 has been detected in up to 90% of HPV-related cases of head and neck squamous cell carcinomas (HNSCCs) (Gillison et al., 2000; Weinberger et al., 2006). Moreover, Syrjanen (2005) reported that tonsillar carcinoma was associated with the highest nongenital virus prevalence.

According to some investigators, there is a good level of evidence in these findings to argue in favor of the universal HPV vaccination of both boys and girls (Laurence, 2008). The quadrivalent HPV vaccine can be expected to significantly decrease HPV infection and related diseases of the head and neck region and respiratory tract.

11.8.2 Cost-Effectiveness of Male Vaccination

In a recent analysis using a dynamic model to evaluate cost-effectiveness of the quadrivalent HPV vaccine in the Mexican population, Insinga et al. (2007) showed that vaccination of 12-year-old girls and boys with a 12 to 24 year-old "catch-up" program was the most effective strategy to reduce HPV infection and related diseases in female subjects.

However, Kim et al. (2007), in another similar cost-effectiveness analysis showed little advantage of including boys in a preadolescent HPV vaccination program modeled in a low-resource setting.

A Nordic modeling study to evaluate the optimal vaccination strategies in the Swedish population has estimated the prevention of 5.8 million cumulative HPV 16 infections by the year 2055 with the vaccination of female subjects starting at age 12 in 2008 (Ryding et al., 2008). Moreover, the authors showed that vaccination of male subjects increased the protective effect by about 4%, yet the preventive effect per vaccination was reduced.

Currently, only UK, Mexico, Australia, New Zealand and South Korea have licensed HPV vaccination for both genders, where boys aged 9–15 years are able to receive the quadrivalent vaccine (May, 2007).

Although the European Union marketing authorization for Gardasil has not excluded its use in male subjects, at present only Austria opted to include boys aged 9–15 years into a government-based immunization program. The main goal of this policy is prevention of infection with HPV 6 or 11 and, as a result, reduction of the rate of genital warts in young male individuals.

11.9 Therapeutic HPV Vaccination and Future Vaccine Developments

Antibody-generating prophylactic vaccines are not effective against preexisting and persistent HPV infections (Future II Study Group, 2007; Hildesheim et al., 2007); however, HPV oncogenic proteins E6 and E7 are promising targets for therapeutic strategies aimed at these oncogenes, because they are the only proteins maintained and expressed in HPV-associated cancers (Bosch et al., 2002; Wentzensen et al., 2004). Therapeutic vaccines that elicit a cytolytic T-cell immune response to premalignant and malignant cells expressing HPV E6 and/or E7 have shown some degree of clinical efficacy against established HPV-associated malignancies (Lin et al., 2007; Hung et al., 2008; Huh and Roden, 2008).

Cellular immune responses directed against early expressed HPV 16 E7 protein have been associated with CIN 2 and CIN 3 regression and clearance of HPV infection (Kadish et al., 2002), suggesting the therapeutic potential of HPV E7-targeted vaccines in CIN patients (Hallez et al., 2004).

Viral vector vaccines can induce viral and recombinant protein expression, promoting strong cellular host responses. A phase-II trial using a modified vaccinia virus Ankara (MVA) expressing modified HPV 16 E6 and E7 proteins and coexpressed with T-cell cytokine IL-2 reported regression of CIN 2+ in 47.6% of vaccinated female subjects after 6 months (Transgene, 2006).

Although current HPV vaccines are comprised of L1 epitopes, Kondo et al. (2008) recently demonstrated that vaccine modification by insertion of cross-reactive L2 epitopes elicited antibodies that cross-neutralized against related HPV strains. This could potentially reduce the number of VLP types required for vaccine protection, suggesting it is a viable strategy for the generation of multivalent vaccines (Slupetzky et al., 2007; Xu et al., 2007).

In addition, new strategies aimed at improving HPV vaccine potency are being developed. The fusion of HPV 16 recombinant proteins E6 and E7 with heat shock protein (Hsp) 70 of *Mycobacterium tuberculosis* in an animal model study has elicited protection against challenge with transformed tumor cells (Qian et al., 2006). In another research study, Xu et al. (2008) showed that the fusion of effective adjuvant protein into chimeric VLPs induced increased titers of HPV 16-specific long-lasting neutralizing antibodies.

References

Agarwal SS, Sehgal A, Sardana S, Kumar A, Luthra UK (1993) Role of male behavior in cervical carcinogenesis among women with one lifetime sexual partner. Cancer 72: 1666–1669

Agosti JM, Goldie SJ (2007) Introducing HPV vaccine in developing countries – key challenges and issues. N Engl J Med 356: 1908–1910

Ault KA (2007) Effect of prophylactic human papillomavirus L1 virus-like-particle vaccine on risk of cervical intraepithelial neoplasia grade 2, grade 3, and adenocarcinoma in situ: A combined analysis of four randomised clinical trials. Lancet 369: 1861–1868

Baldwin PJ, van der Burg SH, Boswell CM, Offringa R, Hickling JK, Dobson J, Roberts JS, Latimer JA, Moseley RP, Coleman N, Stanley MA, Sterling JC (2003) Vaccinia-expressed human papillomavirus 16 and 18 e6 and e7 as a therapeutic vaccination for vulval and vaginal intraepithelial neoplasia. Clin Cancer Res 9: 5205–5213

Bierl C, Karem K, Poon AC, Swan D, Tortolero-Luna G, Follen M, Widerolf L, Unger ER, Reeves WC (2005) Correlates of cervical mucosal antibodies to human papillomavirus 16: Results from a case control study. Gynecol Oncol 99: S262–S268

Block SL, Nolan T, Sattler C, Barr E, Giacoletti KE, Marchant CD, Castellsague X, Rusche SA, Lukac S, Bryan JT, Cavanaugh PF, Jr., Reisinger KS (2006) Comparison of the immunogenicity and reactogenicity of a prophylactic quadrivalent human papillomavirus (types 6, 11, 16, and 18) L1 virus-like particle vaccine in male and female adolescents and young adult women. Pediatrics 118: 2135–2145

Bontkes HJ, de Gruijl TD, Walboomers JM, Schiller JT, Dillner J, Helmerhorst TJ, Verheijen RH, Scheper RJ, Meijer CJ (1999) Immune responses against human papillomavirus (HPV) type 16 virus-like particles in a cohort study of women with cervical intraepithelial neoplasia II. Systemic but not local IgA responses correlate with clearance of HPV-16. J Gen Virol 80(Pt 2): 409–417

Bosch FX, Castellsague X, de Sanjose S (2008) HPV and cervical cancer: Screening or vaccination? Br J Cancer 98: 15–21

Bosch FX, Castellsague X, Munoz N, de Sanjose S, Ghaffari AM, Gonzalez LC, Gili M, Izarzugaza I, Viladiu P, Navarro C, Vergara A, Ascunce N, Guerrero E, Shah KV (1996) Male sexual behavior and human papillomavirus DNA: Key risk factors for cervical cancer in Spain. J Natl Cancer Inst 88: 1060–1067

Bosch FX, Lorincz A, Munoz N, Meijer CJ, Shah KV (2002) The causal relation between human papillomavirus and cervical cancer. J Clin Pathol 55: 244–265

Brotherton JM, Gold MS, Kemp AS, McIntyre PB, Burgess MA, Campbell-Lloyd S (2008) Anaphylaxis following quadrivalent human papillomavirus vaccination. CMAJ 179: 525–533

Brown D (2007) HPV type 6/11/16/18 vaccine: First analysis of cross-protection against persistent infection, cervical intraepithelial neoplasia (CIN), and adenocarcinoma in situ (AIS) caused by oncogenic HPV types in addition to 16/18 In: 47th Interscience Conference on Antimicrobial Agents and Chemotherapy, Chicago

Brown DR, Bryan JT, Schroeder JM, Robinson TS, Fife KH, Wheeler CM, Barr E, Smith PR, Chiacchierini L, DiCello A, Jansen KU (2001) Neutralization of human papillomavirus type 11 (HPV-11) by serum from women vaccinated with yeast-derived HPV-11 L1 virus-like particles: correlation with competitive radioimmunoassay titer. J Infect Dis 184: 1183–1186

Brown DR, Shew ML, Qadadri B, Neptune N, Vargas M, Tu W, Juliar BE, Breen TE, Fortenberry JD (2005) A longitudinal study of genital human papillomavirus infection in a cohort of closely followed adolescent women. J Infect Dis 191: 182–192

Carter JJ, Koutsky LA, Hughes JP, Lee SK, Kuypers J, Kiviat N, Galloway DA (2000) Comparison of human papillomavirus types 16, 18, and 6 capsid antibody responses following incident infection. J Infect Dis 181: 1911–1919

Castellsague X, Bosch FX, Munoz N, Meijer CJ, Shah KV, de Sanjose S, Eluf-Neto J, Ngelangel CA, Chichareon S, Smith JS, Herrero R, Moreno V, Franceschi S (2002) Male circumcision, penile human papillomavirus infection, and cervical cancer in female partners. N Engl J Med 346: 1105–1112

CDC HPV Vaccine Information for Clinicians. Centers for Disease Control and Prevention, Atlanta

Christensen ND, Reed CA, Cladel NM, Han R, Kreider JW (1996) Immunization with virus like particles induces long-term protection of rabbits against challenge with cottontail rabbit papillomavirus. J Virol 70: 960–965

ClinicalTrials.gov In. U.S. National Institutes of Health

Daling JR, Madeleine MM, Johnson LG, Schwartz SM, Shera KA, Wurscher MA, Carter JJ, Porter PL, Galloway DA, McDougall JK, Krieger JN (2005) Penile cancer: Importance of circumcision, human papillomavirus and smoking in in situ and invasive disease. Int J Cancer 116: 606–616

Dasbach EJ, Insinga RP, Elbasha EH (2008) The epidemiological and economic impact of a quadrivalent human papillomavirus vaccine (6/11/16/18) in the UK. BJOG 115: 947–956

Davidson EJ, Boswell CM, Sehr P, Pawlita M, Tomlinson AE, McVey RJ, Dobson J, Roberts JS, Hickling J, Kitchener HC, Stern PL (2003) Immunological and clinical responses in women with vulval intraepithelial neoplasia vaccinated with a vaccinia virus encoding human papillomavirus 16/18 oncoproteins. Cancer Res 63: 6032–6041

Day PM, Roden RB, Lowy DR, Schiller JT (1998) The papillomavirus minor capsid protein, L2, induces localization of the major capsid protein, L1, and the viral transcription/replication protein, E2, to PML oncogenic domains. J Virol 72: 142–150

Day PM, Thompson CD, Buck CB, Pang YY, Lowy DR, Schiller JT (2007) Neutralization of human papillomavirus with monoclonal antibodies reveals different mechanisms of inhibition. J Virol 81: 8784–8792

de Gruijl TD, Bontkes HJ, Walboomers JM, Schiller JT, Stukart MJ, Groot BS, Chabaud MM, Remmink AJ, Verheijen RH, Helmerhorst TJ, Meijer CJ, Scheper RJ (1997) Immunoglobulin G responses against human papillomavirus type 16 virus-like particles in a prospective nonintervention cohort study of women with cervical intraepithelial neoplasia. J Natl Cancer Inst 89: 630–638

de Jong A, van Poelgeest MI, van der Hulst JM, Drijfhout JW, Fleuren GJ, Melief CJ, Kenter G, Offringa R, van der Burg SH (2004) Human papillomavirus type 16-positive cervical cancer is associated with impaired CD4 + T-cell immunity against early antigens E2 and E6. Cancer Res 64: 5449–5455

de Sanjose S, Diaz M, Castellsague X, Castellsague X, Clifford G, Bruni L, Munoz N, Bosch FX (2007) Worldwide prevalence and genotype distribution of cervical human papillomavirus DNA in women with normal cytology: A meta-analysis. Lancet Infect Dis 7: 453 – 459

de Villiers EM, Fauquet C, Broker TR, Bernard HU, zur Hausen H (2004) Classification of papillomaviruses. Virology 324: 17–27

de Witte L, Zoughlami Y, Aengeneyndt B, David G, van Kooyk Y, Gissmann L, Geijtenbeek TB (2007) Binding of human papilloma virus L1 virus-like particles to dendritic cells is mediated through heparan sulfates and induces immune activation. Immunobiology 212: 679–691

D'Souza G, Kreimer AR, Viscidi R, Pawlita M, Fakhry C, Koch WM, Westra WH, Gillison ML (2007) Case-control study of human papillomavirus and oropharyngeal cancer. N Engl J Med 356: 1944–1956

Evander M, Frazer IH, Payne E, Qi YM, Hengst K, McMillan NA (1997) Identification of the alpha6 integrin as a candidate receptor for papillomaviruses. J Virol 71: 2449–2456

FDA, (2008) Gardasil – Product Approval Information. U.S. Food and Drug Administration, Rockville

Frazer IH (2004) Prevention of cervical cancer through papillomavirus vaccination. Nat Rev Immunol 4: 46–54

Frisch M, Fenger C, van den Brule AJ, Sorensen P, Meijer CJ, Walboomers JM, Adami HO, Melbye M, Glimelius B (1999) Variants of squamous cell carcinoma of the anal canal and perianal skin and their relation to human papillomaviruses. Cancer Res 59: 753–757

Future II Study Group (2007b) Quadrivalent vaccine against human papillomavirus to prevent high-grade cervical lesions. N Engl J Med 356: 1915–1927

Gall S, Teixeira J (2007) Substantial impact on precancerous lesions and HPV infections through 5.5 years in women vaccinated with the HPV-16/18 L1 VLPAS04 candidate vaccine. In: Proceedings of the AACR Annual Meeting Los Angeles

Gambhira R, Gravitt PE, Bossis I, Stern PL, Viscidi RP, Roden RB (2006) Vaccination of healthy volunteers with human papillomavirus type 16 L2E7E6 fusion protein induces serum antibody that neutralizes across papillomavirus species. Cancer Res 66: 11120–11124

Gambhira R, Karanam B, Jagu S, Roberts JN, Buck CB, Bossis I, Alphs H, Culp T, Christensen ND, Roden RB (2007) A protective and broadly cross-neutralizing epitope of human papillomavirus. L2J Virol 81: 13927–13931

Gavialliance In. GAVI Alliance

Giannini SL, Hanon E, Moris P, Van Mechelen M, Morel S, Dessy F, Fourneau MA, Colau B, Suzich J, Losonksy G, Martin MT, Dubin G, Wettendorff MA (2006) Enhanced humoral and memory B cellular immunity using HPV16/18 L1 VLP vaccine formulated with the MPL/aluminium salt combination (AS04) compared to aluminium salt only. Vaccine 24: 5937–5949

Gillison ML, Koch WM, Capone RB, Spafford M, Westra WH, Wu L, Zahurak ML, Daniel RW, Viglione M, Symer DE, Shah KV, Sidransky D (2000) Evidence for a causal association between human papillomavirus and a subset of head and neck cancers. J Natl Cancer Inst 92: 709–720

Giuliano A, Palefsky J (2008) The efficacy of quadrivalent HPV (types 6/11/16/18) vaccine in reducing the incidence of HPV infection and HPV-related genital disease in young men In: European Research Organization on Genital Infection and Neoplasia – EUROGIN Nice, France

Goldie SJ, O'Shea M, Campos NG, Diaz M, Sweet S, Kim SY (2008) Health and economic outcomes of HPV 16,18 vaccination in 72 GAVI-eligible countries. Vaccine 26: 4080–4093

Greer CE, Wheeler CM, Ladner MB, Beutner K, Coyne MY, Liang H, Langenberg A, Yen TS, Ralston R (1995) Human papillomavirus (HPV) type distribution and serological response to HPV type 6 virus-like particles in patients with genital warts. J Clin Microbiol 33: 2058–2063

Hagensee ME, Yaegashi N, Galloway DA (1993) Self-assembly of human papillomavirus type 1 capsids by expression of the L1 protein alone or by coexpression of the L1 and L2 capsid proteins. J Virol 67: 315–322

Hallez S, Simon P, Maudoux F, Doyen J, Noel JC, Beliard A, Capelle X, Buxant F, Fayt I, Lagrost AC, Hubert P, Gerday C, Burny A, Boniver J, Foidart JM, Delvenne P, Jacobs N (2004) Phase I/II trial of immunogenicity of a human papillomavirus (HPV) type 16 E7 protein-based vaccine in women with oncogenic HPV-positive cervical intraepithelial neoplasia. Cancer Immunol Immunother 53: 642–650

Hampl M, Sarajuuri H, Wentzensen N, Bender HG, Kueppers V (2006) Effect of human papillomavirus vaccines on vulvar, vaginal, and anal intraepithelial lesions and vulvar cancer. Obstet Gynecol 108: 1361–1368

Harper DM, Franco EL, Wheeler C, Ferris DG, Jenkins D, Schuind A, Zahaf T, Innis B, Naud P, De Carvalho NS, Roteli-Martins CM, Teixeira J, Blatter MM, Korn AP, Quint W, Dubin G (2004) Efficacy of a bivalent L1 virus-like particle vaccine in prevention of infection with human papillomavirus types 16 and 18 in young women: A randomised controlled trial. Lancet 364: 1757–1765

Harper DM, Franco EL, Wheeler CM, Moscicki AB, Romanowski B, Roteli-Martins CM, Jenkins D, Schuind A, Costa Clemens SA, Dubin G (2006) Sustained efficacy up to 4.5 years of a bivalent L1 virus-like particle vaccine against human papillomavirus types 16 and 18: Follow-up from a randomised control trial. Lancet 367: 1247–1255

Harro CD, Pang YY, Roden RB, Hildesheim A, Wang Z, Reynolds MJ, Mast TC, Robinson R, Murphy BR, Karron RA, Dillner J, Schiller JT, Lowy DR (2001) Safety and immunogenicity trial in adult volunteers of a human papillomavirus 16 L1 virus-like particle vaccine. J Natl Cancer Inst 93: 284–292

Hausen HZ (2008) Papillomaviruses to vaccination and beyond. Biochemistry (Mosc) 73: 498–503

Hemminki K, Dong C, Frisch M (2000) Tonsillar and other upper aerodigestive tract cancers among cervical cancer patients and their husbands. Eur J Cancer Prev 9: 433–437

Hildesheim A, Herrero R, Wacholder S, Rodriguez AC, Solomon D, Bratti MC, Schiller JT, Gonzalez P, Dubin G, Porras C, Jimenez SE, Lowy DR (2007) Effect of human papillomavirus 16/18 L1 viruslike particle vaccine among young women with preexisting infection: A randomized trial. JAMA 298: 743–753

Ho GY, Studentsov YY, Bierman R, Burk RD (2004) Natural history of human papillomavirus type 16 virus-like particle antibodies in young women. Cancer Epidemiol Biomarkers Prev 13: 110–116

Huh WK, Roden RB (2008) The future of vaccines for cervical cancer. Gynecol Oncol 109: S48–S56

Hung CF, Ma B, Monie A, Tsen SW, Wu TC (2008) Therapeutic human papillomavirus vaccines: Current clinical trials and future directions. Expert Opin Biol Ther 8: 421–439

Insinga RP, Dasbach EJ, Elbasha EH, Puig A, Reynales-Shigematsu LM (2007) Cost-effectiveness of quadrivalent human papillomavirus (HPV) vaccination in Mexico: A transmission dynamic model-based evaluation. Vaccine 26: 128–139

Joseph DA, Miller JW, Wu X, Chen VW, Morris CR, Goodman MT, Villalon-Gomez JM, Williams MA, Cress RD (2008) Understanding the burden of human papillomavirus-associated anal cancers in the US. Cancer 113: 2892–2900

Joura EA, Leodolter S, Hernandez-Avila M, Wheeler CM, Perez G, Koutsky LA, Garland SM, Harper DM, Tang GW, Ferris DG, Steben M, Jones RW, Bryan J, Taddeo FJ, Bautista OM, Esser MT, Sings HL, Nelson M, Boslego JW, Sattler C, Barr E, Paavonen J (2007) Efficacy of a quadrivalent prophylactic human papillomavirus (types 6, 11, 16, and 18) L1 virus-like-particle vaccine against high-grade vulval and vaginal lesions: A combined analysis of three randomised clinical trials. Lancet 369: 1693–1702

Kadish AS, Timmins P, Wang Y, Ho GY, Burk RD, Ketz J, He W, Romney SL, Johnson A, Angeletti R, Abadi M (2002) Regression of cervical intraepithelial neoplasia and loss of human papillomavirus (HPV) infection is associated with cell-mediated immune responses to an HPV type 16 E7 peptide. Cancer Epidemiol Biomarkers Prev 11: 483–488

Kagawa R, Yamaguchi T, Furuta R (2006) Histological features of human papilloma virus 16 and its association with the development and progression of anal squamous cell carcinoma. Surg Today 36: 885–891

Kemp TJ, Hildesheim A, Falk RT, Schiller JT, Lowy DR, Rodriguez AC, Pinto LA (2008) Evaluation of two types of sponges used to collect cervical secretions and assessment of antibody extraction protocols for recovery of neutralizing anti-human papillomavirus type 16 antibodies. Clin Vaccine Immunol 15: 60–64

Kim JJ, Andres-Beck B, Goldie SJ (2007) The value of including boys in an HPV vaccination programme: A cost-effectiveness analysis in a low-resource setting. Br J Cancer 97: 1322–1328

Kirnbauer R, Booy F, Cheng N, Lowy DR, Schiller JT (1992) Papillomavirus L1 major capsid protein self-assembles into virus-like particles that are highly immunogenic. Proc Natl Acad Sci U S A 89: 12180–12184

Klencke B, Matijevic M, Urban RG, Lathey JL, Hedley ML, Berry M, Thatcher J, Weinberg V, Wilson J, Darragh T, Jay N, Da Costa M, Palefsky JM (2002) Encapsulated plasmid DNA treatment for human papillomavirus 16-associated anal dysplasia: A Phase I study of. ZYC101Clin Cancer Res 8: 1028–1037

Kondo K, Ochi H, Matsumoto T, Yoshikawa H, Kanda T (2008) Modification of human papillomavirus-like particle vaccine by insertion of the cross-reactive L2-epitopes. J Med Virol 80: 841–846

Koutsky LA, Harper DM (2006) Chap. 13: Current findings from prophylactic HPV vaccine trials. Vaccine 24(Suppl 3): S3/114–S3/121

Kreimer AR, Clifford GM, Boyle P, Franceschi S (2005) Human papillomavirus types in head and neck squamous cell carcinomas worldwide: a systematic review. Cancer Epidemiol Biomarkers Prev 14: 467–475

Laurence J (2008) HPV-linked oral cancer: another argument for universal HPV vaccination of boys and girls. AIDS Read 18: 345–346

Lee BN, Follen M, Shen DY, Malpica A, Adler-Storthz K, Shearer WT, Reuben JM (2004) Depressed type 1 cytokine synthesis by superantigen-activated CD4 + T cells of women with human papillomavirus-related high-grade squamous intraepithelial lesions. Clin Diagn Lab Immunol 11: 239–244

Lehtinen M, Apter D, Dubin G, Kosunen E, Isaksson R, Korpivaara EL, Kyha-Osterlund L, Lunnas T, Luostarinen T, Niemi L, Palmroth J, Petaja T, Rekonen S, Salmivesi S, Siitari-Mattila M, Svartsjo S, Tuomivaara L, Vilkki M, Pukkala E, Paavonen J (2006a) Enrolment of 22,000 adolescent women to cancer registry follow-up for long-term human papillomavirus vaccine efficacy: guarding against guessing. Int J STD AIDS 17: 517–521

Lehtinen M, Idanpaan-Heikkila I, Lunnas T, Palmroth J, Barr E, Cacciatore R, Isaksson R, Kekki M, Koskela P, Kosunen E, Kuortti M, Lahti L, Liljamo T, Luostarinen T, Apter D, Pukkala E, Paavonen J (2006b) Population-based enrolment of adolescents in a long-term follow-up trial of human papillomavirus vaccine efficacy. Int J STD AIDS 17: 237–246

Lin YY, Alphs H, Hung CF, Roden RB, Wu TC (2007) Vaccines against human papillomavirus. Front Biosci 12: 246–264

Luna J, Saah A (2007) Safety, efficacy, and immunogenicity of quadrivalent HPV vaccine (Gardasil) in women aged 24–45.In: 24th International Papillomavirus Congress, Beijing

Markowitz LE, Dunne EF, Saraiya M, Lawson HW, Chesson H, Unger ER (2007) Quadrivalent human papillomavirus vaccine: Recommendations of the Advisory Committee on

Immunization Practices (ACIP). MMWR Recomm Rep 56: 1–24

May J (2007) HPV vaccination – a paradigm shift in public health. Aust Fam Physician 36: 106–111

Mbulawa ZZ, Williamson AL, Stewart D, Passmore JA, Denny L, Allan B, Marais DJ (2008) Association of serum and mucosal neutralizing antibodies to human papillomavirus type 16 (HPV-16) with HPV-16 infection and cervical disease. J Gen Virol 89: 910–914

McMurray HR, Nguyen D, Westbrook TF, McAnce DJ (2001) Biology of human papillomaviruses. Int J Exp Pathol 82: 15–33

MediLexicon International Ltd (2008) Gardasil® applies for WHO certification to reinforce global access to the vaccine – Approval would qualify Gardasil® for procurement by United. medicalnewstoday.

Munger K, Baldwin A, Edwards KM, Hayakawa H, Nguyen CL, Owens M, Grace M, Huh K (2004) Mechanisms of human papillomavirus-induced oncogenesis. J Virol 78: 11451–11460

Munger K, Howley PM (2002) Human papillomavirus immortalization and transformation functions. Virus Res 89: 213–228

Munoz N, Bosch FX, de Sanjose S, Herrero R, Castellsague X, Shah KV, Snijders PJ, Meijer CJ (2003) Epidemiologic classification of human papillomavirus types associated with cervical cancer. N Engl J Med 348: 518–527

Nardelli-Haefliger D, Wirthner D, Schiller JT, Lowy DR, Hildesheim A, Ponci F, De Grandi P (2003) Specific antibody levels at the cervix during the menstrual cycle of women vaccinated with human papillomavirus 16 virus-like particles. J Natl Cancer Inst 95: 1128–1137

Olsson SE, Villa LL, Costa RL, Petta CA, Andrade RP, Malm C, Iversen OE, Hoye J, Steinwall M, Riis-Johannessen G, Andersson-Ellstrom A, Elfgren K, von Krogh G, Lehtinen M, Paavonen J, Tamms GM, Giacoletti K, Lupinacci L, Esser MT, Vuocolo SC, Saah AJ, Barr E (2007) Induction of immune memory following administration of a prophylactic quadrivalent human papillomavirus (HPV) types 6/11/16/18 L1 virus-like particle (VLP) vaccine. Vaccine 25: 4931–4939

Paavonen J, Jenkins D, Bosch FX, Naud P, Salmeron J, Wheeler CM, Chow SN, Apter DL, Kitchener HC, Castellsague X, de Carvalho NS, Skinner SR, Harper DM, Hedrick JA, Jaisamrarn U, Limson GA, Dionne M, Quint W, Spiessens B, Peeters P, Struyf F, Wieting SL, Lehtinen MO, Dubin G (2007) Efficacy of a prophylactic adjuvanted bivalent L1 virus-like-particle vaccine against infection with human papillomavirus types 16 and 18 in young women: An interim analysis of a phase III double-blind, randomised controlled trial. Lancet 369: 2161–2170

Palefsky J, Giuliano A (2008) Efficacy of the quadrivalent HPV vaccine against HPV 6/11/16/18-related genital infection in young men In: European Research Organization on Genital Infection and Neoplasia – EUROGIN, Nice, France

Pan American Health Organization (2008) Burden of Human Papillomavirus (HPV) Infection and HPV-Related Disease in Latin America and the Caribbean, and Health and Economic Outcomes of HPV Vaccination in Selected Countries in LatinAmerica, Executive Summary. Pan American Health Organization, Washington

Parkin DM, Bray F, Ferlay J, Pisani P (2005) Global cancer statistics, 2002. CA Cancer J Clin 55: 74–108

Parr EL, Parr MB (1997) Immunoglobulin G is the main protective antibody in mouse vaginal secretions after vaginal immunization with attenuated herpes simplex virus type 2. J Virol 71: 8109–8115

Partridge JM, Koutsky LA (2006) Genital human papillomavirus infection in men. Lancet Infect Dis 6: 21–31

Pascual A, Pariente M, Godinez JM, Sanchez-Prieto R, Atienzar M, Segura M, Poblet E (2007) High prevalence of human papillomavirus 16 in penile carcinoma. Histol Histopathol 22: 177–183

Perez G, Lazcano-Ponce E, Hernandez-Avila M, Garcia PJ, Munoz N, Villa LL, Bryan J, Taddeo FJ, Lu S, Esser MT, Vuocolo S, Sattler C, Barr E (2008) Safety, immunogenicity, and efficacy of quadrivalent human papillomavirus (types 6, 11, 16, 18) L1 virus-like-particle vaccine in Latin American women. Int J Cancer 122: 1311–1318

Piketty C, Kazatchkine MD (2005) Human papillomavirus-related cervical and anal disease in HIV-infected individuals in the era of highly active antiretroviral therapy. Curr HIV/AIDS Rep 2: 140–145

Prowse DM, Ktori EN, Chandrasekaran D, Prapa A, Baithun S (2008) Human papillomavirus-associated increase in p16INK4A expression in penile lichen sclerosus and squamous cell carcinoma. Br J Dermatol 158: 261–265

Qian X, Lu Y, Liu Q, Chen K, Zhao Q, Song J (2006) Prophylactic, therapeutic and anti-metastatic effects of an HPV-16mE6Delta/mE7/TBhsp70Delta fusion protein vaccine in an animal model. Immunol Lett 102: 191–201

Rambout L, Hopkins L, Hutton B, Fergusson D (2007) Prophylactic vaccination against human papillomavirus infection and disease in women: A systematic review of randomized controlled trials. CMAJ 177: 469–479

Reisinger KS, Block SL, Lazcano-Ponce E, Samakoses R, Esser MT, Erick J, Puchalski D, Giacoletti KE, Sings HL, Lukac S, Alvarez FB, Barr E (2007) Safety and persistent immunogenicity of a quadrivalent human papillomavirus types 6, 11, 16, 18 L1 virus-like particle vaccine in preadolescents and adolescents: A randomized controlled trial. Pediatr Infect Dis J 26: 201–209

Ryding J, French KM, Naucler P, Barnabas RV, Garnett GP, Dillner J (2008) Seroepidemiology as basis for design of a human papillomavirus vaccination program. Vaccine 26: 5263–5268

Ryerson AB, Peters ES, Coughlin SS, Chen VW, Gillison ML, Reichman ME, Wu X, Chaturvedi AK, Kawaoka K (2008) Burden of potentially human papillomavirus-associated cancers of the oropharynx and oral cavity in the US, 1998–2003. Cancer 113: 2901–2909

Sarkar AK, Tortolero-Luna G, Follen M, Sastry KJ (2005) Inverse correlation of cellular immune responses specific to synthetic peptides from the E6 and E7 oncoproteins of HPV-16 with recurrence of cervical intraepithelial neoplasia in a cross-sectional study. Gynecol Oncol 99: S251–S261

Sasagawa T, Rose RC, Azar KK, Sakai A, Inoue M (2003) Mucosal immunoglobulin-A and -G responses to oncogenic human papilloma virus capsids. Int J Cancer 104: 328–335

Saxenian H, Hecht R (2006) HPV vaccines: Costs and financing. In: Stop Cervical Cancer: Accelerating Global Access to HPV vaccines, London

Schiffman M, Kjaer SK (2003) Chapter 2: Natural history of anogenital human papillomavirus infection and neoplasia. J Natl Cancer Inst Monogr (31): 14–19

Schwartz SM, Daling JR, Doody DR, Wipf GC, Carter JJ, Madeleine MM, Mao EJ, Fitzgibbons ED, Huang S, Beckmann AM, McDougall JK, Galloway DA (1998) Oral cancer risk in relation to sexual history and evidence of human papillomavirus infection. J Natl Cancer Inst 90: 1626–1636

Schwarz TF, Dubin G (2007) Human papillomavirus (HPV) 16/18 L1 AS04 virus-like particle (VLP) cervical cancer vaccine is immunogenic and well-tolerated 18 months after vaccination in women up to age 55 years. J Clin Oncol 25: abstract 3007

Schwarz TF, Leo O (2008) Immune response to human papillomavirus after prophylactic vaccination with AS04-adjuvanted HPV-16/18 vaccine: Improving upon nature. Gynecol Oncol 110: S1–S10

Scott M, Stites DP, Moscicki AB (1999) Th1 cytokine patterns in cervical human papillomavirus infection. Clin Diagn Lab Immunol 6: 751–755

Sheets EE, Urban RG, Crum CP, Hedley ML, Politch JA, Gold MA, Muderspach LI, Cole GA, Crowley-Nowick PA (2003) Immunotherapy of human cervical high-grade cervical intraepithelial neoplasia with microparticle-delivered human papillomavirus 16 E7 plasmid DNA. Am J Obstet Gynecol 188: 916–926

Sheu BC, Chang WC, Lin HH, Chow SN, Huang SC (2007) Immune concept of human papillomaviruses and related antigens in local cancer milieu of human cervical neoplasia. J Obstet Gynaecol Res 33: 103–113

Skinner SR, Garland SM, Stanley MA, Pitts M, Quinn MA (2008) Human papillomavirus vaccination for the prevention of cervical neoplasia: Is it appropriate to vaccinate women older than 26? Med J Aust 188: 238–242

Slupetzky K, Gambhira R, Culp TD, Shafti-Keramat S, Schellenbacher C, Christensen ND, Roden RB, Kirnbauer R (2007) A papillomavirus-like particle (VLP) vaccine displaying HPV16 L2 epitopes induces cross-neutralizing antibodies to. HPV11 Vaccine 25: 2001–2010

Stanley M (2006) Immune responses to human papillomavirus. Vaccine 24(Suppl 1): S16–S22

Stanley M, Coleman N, Chambers M (1994) The host response to lesions induced by human papillomavirus. Ciba Found Symp 187: 21–32; discussion 32–44

Stanley M, Lowy DR, Frazer I (2006) Chapter 12: Prophylactic HPV vaccines: Underlying mechanisms. Vaccine 24(Suppl 3): S3/106–S3/113

Stanley MA, Pett MR, Coleman N (2007) HPV: From infection to cancer. Biochem Soc Trans 35: 1456–1460

Streeck RE (2002) A short introduction to papillomavirus biology. Intervirology 45: 287–289

Suzich JA, Ghim SJ, Palmer-Hill FJ, White WI, Tamura JK, Bell JA, Newsome JA, Jenson AB, Schlegel R (1995) Systemic immunization with papillomavirus L1 protein completely prevents the development of viral mucosal papillomas. Proc Natl Acad Sci U S A 92: 11553–11557

Syrjanen KJ, Syrjanen SM (2000) Papillomavirus infections in human pathology. Wiley & Sons, Chichester, pp 11–51.

Syrjanen S (2005) Human papillomavirus (HPV) in head and neck cancer. J Clin Virol 32(Suppl 1): S59–S66

Tabrizi SN, Frazer IH, Garland SM (2006) Serologic response to human papillomavirus 16 among Australian women with high-grade cervical intraepithelial neoplasia. Int J Gynecol Cancer 16: 1032–1035

Techakehakij W, Feldman RD (2008) Cost-effectiveness of HPV vaccination compared with Pap smear screening on a national scale: A literature review. Vaccine 26(49): 6258–6265

The Henry J. Kaiser Family Foundation (2007a) Public Health & Education | GSK Applies for WHO Prequalification of HPV Vaccine Cervarix. kaisernetwork.org.

Transgene (2006) Sustained response at month 12 for transgene's TG 4001 in HPV-induced precancerous lesions of the cervix and next clinical development steps. http://www. transgene.fr/us/pdf/communique_presse/communiques_divers_2006/PR-US_TG4001-HPV_13-11-2006.pdf

Trottier H, Franco EL (2006) The epidemiology of genital human papillomavirus infection. Vaccine 24(Suppl 1): S1–S15

Unckell F, Streeck RE, Sapp M (1997) Generation and neutralization of pseudovirions of human papillomavirus type 33. J Virol 71: 2934–2939

van Poelgeest MI, Nijhuis ER, Kwappenberg KM, Hamming IE, Wouter Drijfhout J, Fleuren GJ, van der Zee AG, Melief CJ, Kenter GG, Nijman HW, Offringa R, van der Burg SH (2006) Distinct regulation and impact of type 1 T-cell immunity against HPV16 L1, E2 and E6 antigens during HPV16-induced cervical infection and neoplasia. Int J Cancer 118: 675–683

Varnai AD, Bollmann M, Griefingholt H, Speich N, Schmitt C, Bollmann R, Decker D (2006) HPV in anal squamous cell carcinoma and anal intraepithelial neoplasia (AIN). Impact of HPV analysis of anal lesions on diagnosis and prognosis. Int J Colorectal Dis 21: 135–142

Villa LL (2007) Overview of the clinical development and results of a quadrivalent HPV (types 6, 11, 16, 18) vaccine. Int J Infect Dis 11(Suppl 2): S17–S25

Villa LL, Costa RL, Petta CA, Andrade RP, Ault KA, Giuliano AR, Wheeler CM, Koutsky LA, Malm C, Lehtinen M, Skjeldestad FE, Olsson SE, Steinwall M, Brown DR, Kurman RJ, Ronnett BM, Stoler MH, Ferenczy A, Harper DM, Tamms GM, Yu J, Lupinacci L, Railkar R, Taddeo FJ, Jansen KU, Esser MT, Sings HL, Saah AJ, Barr E (2005) Prophylactic quadrivalent human papillomavirus (types 6, 11, 16, and 18) L1 virus-like particle vaccine in young women: A randomised double-blind placebo-controlled multicentre phase II efficacy trial. Lancet Oncol 6: 271–278

Villa LL, Costa RL, Petta CA, Andrade RP, Paavonen J, Iversen OE, Olsson SE, Hoye J, Steinwall M, Riis-Johannessen G, Andersson-Ellstrom A, Elfgren K, Krogh G, Lehtinen M, Malm C, Tamms GM, Giacoletti K, Lupinacci L, Railkar R, Taddeo FJ, Bryan J, Esser MT, Sings HL, Saah AJ, Barr E (2006) High sustained efficacy of a prophylactic quadrivalent human papillomavirus types 6/11/16/18 L1 virus-like particle vaccine through 5 years of follow-up. Br J Cancer 95: 1459–1466

Viscidi RP, Schiffman M, Hildesheim A, Herrero R, Castle PE, Bratti MC, Rodriguez AC, Sherman ME, Wang S, Clayman B, Burk RD (2004) Seroreactivity to human papillomavirus (HPV) types 16, 18, or 31 and risk of subsequent HPV infection: Results from a population-based study in Costa Rica. Cancer Epidemiol Biomarkers Prev 13: 324–327

Viscidi RP, Snyder B, Cu-Uvin S, Hogan JW, Clayman B, Klein RS, Sobel J, Shah KV (2005) Human papillomavirus capsid antibody response to natural infection and risk of subsequent HPV infection in HIV-positive and HIV-negative women. Cancer Epidemiol Biomarkers Prev 14: 283–288

Watson M, Saraiya M, Ahmed F, Cardinez CJ, Reichman ME, Weir HK, Richards TB (2008) Using population-based cancer registry data to assess the burden of human papillomavirus-associated cancers in the United States: Overview of methods. Cancer 113: 2841–2854

Weinberger PM, Yu Z, Haffty BG, Kowalski D, Harigopal M, Brandsma J, Sasaki C, Joe J, Camp RL, Rimm DL, Psyrri A (2006) Molecular classification identifies a subset of human Papillomavirus – associated oropharyngeal cancers with favorable prognosis. J Clin Oncol 24: 736–747

Welters MJ, de Jong A, van den Eeden SJ, van der Hulst JM, Kwappenberg KM, Hassane S, Franken KL, Drijfhout JW, Fleuren GJ, Kenter G, Melief CJ, Offringa R, van der Burg SH (2003) Frequent display of human papillomavirus type 16 E6-specific memory T-helper cells in the healthy population as witness of previous viral encounter. Cancer Res 63: 636–641

Wentzensen N, Vinokurova S, von Knebel Doeberitz M (2004) Systematic review of genomic integration sites of human papillomavirus genomes in epithelial dysplasia and invasive cancer of the female lower genital tract. Cancer Res 64: 3878–3884

Wheeler CM (2007) Advances in primary and secondary interventions for cervical cancer: human papillomavirus prophylactic vaccines and testing. Nat Clin Pract Oncol 4: 224–235

WHO In. World Health Organization (WHO)

WHO (1990) Sexually transmitted infections increasing – 250 million new infections annually. WHO Feature 152: 1–6

WHO (1990) The current status of development of prophylactic vaccines against human papillomavirus infection. Report of a technical meeting, Geneva, 16–18 February 1999, pp 1–22

WHO (2006) Comprehensive cervical cancer control: a guide to essential practice. World Health Organization p284

Winer RL, Hughes JP, Feng Q, O'Reilly S, Kiviat NB, Holmes KK, Koutsky LA (2006) Condom use and the risk of genital human papillomavirus infection in young women. N Engl J Med 354: 2645–2654

Xu Y, Wang Q, Han Y, Song G, Xu X (2007) Type-specific and cross-reactive antibodies induced by human papillomavirus 31 L1/L2 virus-like particles. J Med Microbiol 56: 907–913

Xu Y, Zhang H, Xu X (2008) Enhancement of vaccine potency by fusing modified LTK63 into human papillomavirus type 16 chimeric virus-like particles. FEMS Immunol Med Microbiol 52: 99–109

Zhou J, Sun XY, Stenzel DJ, Frazer IH (1991) Expression of vaccinia recombinant HPV 16 L1 and L2 ORF proteins in epithelial cells is sufficient for assembly of HPV virion-like particles. Virology 185: 251–257

Index

Printing and Binding: Stürtz GmbH, Würzburg